Common Neurologic Disorders

Guest Editor

RANDOLPH W. EVANS, MD

MEDICAL CLINICS OF NORTH AMERICA

www.medical.theclinics.com

March 2009 • Volume 93 • Number 2

SAUNDERS an imprint of ELSEVIER, Inc.

W.B. SAUNDERS COMPANY
A Division of Elsevier Inc.

1600 John F. Kennedy Boulevard • Suite 1800 • Philadelphia, Pennsylvania 19103-2899

http://www.theclinics.com

MEDICAL CLINICS OF NORTH AMERICA Volume 93, Number 2
March 2009 ISSN 0025-7125, ISBN-13: 978-1-4377-0500-3, ISBN-10: 1-4377-0500-6

Editor: Rachel Glover
Developmental Editor: Donald Mumford

Medical Clinics of North America (ISSN 0025-7125) is published bimonthly by W.B. Saunders, 360 Park Avenue South, New York, NY 10010-1710. Business and editorial offices: 1600 John F. Kennedy Boulevard, Suite 1800, Philadelphia, PA 19103-2899. Accounting and circulation offices: 6277 Sea Harbor Drive, Orlando, FL 32887-4800. Periodicals postage paid at New York, NY, and additional mailing offices. Subscription prices are USD 187 per year for US individuals, USD 334 per year for US institutions, USD 96 per year for US students, USD 238 per year for Canadian individuals, USD 434 per year for Canadian institutions, USD 151 per year for Canadian students, USD 288 per year for international individuals, USD 434 per year for international institutions and USD 151 per year for international students. To receive student/resident rate, orders must be accompanied by name of affiliated institution, date of term, and the *signature* of program/residency coordinator on institution letterhead. Orders will be billed at individual rate until proof of status is received. Foreign air speed delivery is included in all *Clinics* subscription prices. All prices are subject to change without notice. POSTMASTER: Send address changes to *Medical Clinics of North America*, Elsevier Periodicals Customer Service, 11830 Westline Industrial Drive, St. Louis, MO 63146. Customer Service (orders, claims, online, change of address): Elsevier Periodicals Customer Service, 11830 Westline Industrial Drive, St. Louis, MO 63146. Tel: 1-800-654-2452 (U.S. and Canada); 314-453-7041 (outside U.S. and Canada). Fax: 314-453-5170. E-mail: journalscustomerservice-usa@elsevier.com (for print support); journalsonlinesupport-usa@elsevier.com (for online support).

Reprints. For copies of 100 or more of articles in this publication, please contact the Commercial Reprints Department, Elsevier Inc., 360 Park Avenue South, New York, NY 10010-1710. Tel.: 212-633-3812; Fax: 212-462-1935; E-mail: reprints@elsevier.com.

Medical Clinics of North America is also published in Spanish by McGraw-Hill Interamericana Editores S. A., P.O. Box 5-237, 06500 Mexico, D.F., Mexico.

Medical Clinics of North America is covered in *MEDLINE/PubMed (Index Medicus), Current Contents, ASCA, Excerpta Medica, Science Citation Index,* and *ISI/BIOMED.*

Printed in the United States of America.

GOAL STATEMENT
The goal of *Medical Clinics of North America* is to keep practicing physicians up to date with current clinical practice by providing timely articles reviewing the state of the art in patient care.

ACCREDITATION
The *Medical Clinics of North America* is planned and implemented in accordance with the Essential Areas and Policies of the Accreditation Council for Continuing Medical Education (ACCME) through the joint sponsorship of the University of Virginia School of Medicine and Elsevier. The University of Virginia School of Medicine is accredited by the ACCME to provide continuing medical education for physicians.

The University of Virginia School of Medicine designates this educational activity for a maximum of 90 *AMA PRA Category 1 Credits*™. Physicians should only claim credit commensurate with the extent of their participation in the activity.

The American Medical Association has determined that physicians not licensed in the US who participate in this CME activity are eligible for *AMA PRA Category 1 Credits*™.

Credit can be earned by reading the text material, taking the CME examination online at: http://www.theclinics.com/home/cme, and completing the evaluation. After taking the test, you will be required to review any and all incorrect answers. Following completion of the test and evaluation, your credit will be awarded and you may print your certificate.

FACULTY DISCLOSURE/CONFLICT OF INTEREST
The University of Virginia School of Medicine, as an ACCME accredited provider, endorses and strives to comply with the Accreditation Council for Continuing Medical Education (ACCME) Standards of Commercial Support, Commonwealth of Virginia statutes, University of Virginia policies and procedures, and associated federal and private regulations and guidelines on the need for disclosure and monitoring of proprietary and financial interests that may affect the scientific integrity and balance of content delivered in continuing medical education activities under our auspices.

The University of Virginia School of Medicine requires that all CME activities accredited through this institution be developed independently and be scientifically rigorous, balanced and objective in the presentation/discussion of its content, theories and practices.

All authors/editors participating in an accredited CME activity are expected to disclose to the readers relevant financial relationships with commercial entities occurring within the past 12 months (such as grants or research support, employee, consultant, stock holder, member of speakers bureau, etc.). The University of Virginia School of Medicine will employ appropriate mechanisms to resolve potential conflicts of interest to maintain the standards of fair and balanced education to the reader. Questions about specific strategies can be directed to the Office of Continuing Medical Education, University of Virginia School of Medicine, Charlottesville, Virginia.

The authors/editors listed below have identified no professional or financial affiliations for themselves or their spouse/partner:
Aimee Borazanci, MD; Louis R. Caplan, MD; Ardith M. Courtney, DO; Rachel Glover (Acquisitions Editor); Meghan K. Harris, MD; Fong Kwong Sonny Hon, FRCP; Elena Korniychuk, MD; Alireza Minagar, MD; Lori A. Panossian, MD; Robert M. Pascuzzi, MD; David C. Preston, MD; D. Eric Searls, MD; Barbara E. Shapiro, MD, PhD; Natalya Shneyder, MD; Katherine Treadaway, LCSW-ACP; Ronald J. Tusa, MD, PhD; Louis H. Weimer, MD; Andrew Wolf, MD (Test Author); and Pezhman Zadeh, MD.

The authors/editors listed below identified the following professional or financial affiliations for themselves or their spouse/partner:
Alon Y. Avidan, MD, MPH serves on the Speakers Bureau for Takeda Pharmaceuticals, Sepracor, Inc., Cephalon, and Pfizer.
Michael Devereaux, MD, FACP receives a salary from Digitrace.
Randolph W. Evans, MD (Guest Editor) is a consultant and serves on the Speakers Bureau for GlaxoSmithKline, Merck, Pfizer, UCB, and Lilly.
Elliot M. Frohman, MD, PhD is a consultant and serves on the Advisory Board for Biogen Idec and TEVA and serves on the Advisory Board for Bayer.
Roger E. Kelley, MD is an industry funded research/investigator for Sanofi-Aventis and Elan Pharmaceuticals.
Gina Remington, BSN, RN serves on the Advisory Board for TEVA Neuroscience, Biogen/Elan, and NMSS, and serves on the Speakers Bureau for TEVA Neuroscience.
Steven C. Schachter, MD is an Editor-in-Chief for the Epilepsy Therapy Project, is a chair for Johnson & Johnson, and serves as a consultant for Sepracor and Biogen Idec.

Disclosure of Discussion of Non-FDA Approved Uses for Pharmaceutical Products and/or Medical Devices:
The University of Virginia School of Medicine, as an ACCME provider, requires that all faculty presenters identify and disclose any off label uses for pharmaceutical and medical device products. The University of Virginia School of Medicine recommends that each physician fully review all the available data on new products or procedures prior to clinical use.

TO ENROLL
To enroll in the *Medical Clinics of North America* Continuing Medical Education program, call customer service at 1-800-654-2452 or visit us online at: http://www.theclinics.com/home/cme. The CME program is available to subscribers for an additional fee of USD 205.

THE CLINICS ARE NOW AVAILABLE ONLINE!

Access your subscription at:
www.theclinics.com

Contributors

GUEST EDITOR

RANDOLPH W. EVANS, MD
Clinical Professor of Neurology, Baylor College of Medicine, Houston, Texas

AUTHORS

ALON Y. AVIDAN, MD, MPH
UCLA Neurology Residency Program Director; UCLA Neurology Clinic Director; UCLA Sleep Disorders Center Associate Director, UCLA Medical Center, Los Angeles, California

AIMEE BORAZANCI, MD
Department of Neurology, Louisiana State University Health Sciences Center, Shreveport, Louisiana

LOUIS R. CAPLAN, MD
Department of Neurology, Beth Israel Deaconess Medical Center; Cerebrovascular Division, Department of Neurology, Harvard University, School of Medicine, Boston, Massachusetts

ARDITH M. COURTNEY, DO
Department of Neurology, University of Texas Southwestern Medical Center at Dallas, Dallas, Texas

MICHAEL DEVEREAUX, MD, FACP
Professor of Neurology, Neurological Institute, University Hospitals, Case Medical Center, Cleveland, Ohio

RANDOLPH W. EVANS, MD
Clinical Professor of Neurology, Baylor College of Medicine, Houston, Texas

ELLIOT FROHMAN, MD, PhD
Department of Neurology, University of Texas Southwestern Medical Center at Dallas; Department of Ophthalmology University of Texas Southwestern Medical Center at Dallas, Dallas, Texas

MEGHAN K. HARRIS, MD
Department of Neurology, Louisiana State University Health Sciences Center, Shreveport, Louisiana

FONG KWONG SONNY HON, FRCP
Department of Medicine, Pamela Youde Nethersole Eastern Hospital, Hong Kong, China

ROGER E. KELLEY, MD
Professor and Chairman, Department of Neurology, Louisiana State University Health Sciences Center, Shreveport, Louisiana

ELENA KORNIYCHUK, MD
Department of Neurology, Louisiana State University Health Sciences Center, Shreveport, Louisiana

ALIREZA MINAGAR, MD
Associate Professor of Neurology, Department of Neurology, Louisiana State University Health Sciences Center, Shreveport, Louisiana

LORI A. PANOSSIAN, MD
Resident, UCLA Department of Neurology, UCLA Medical Center, Los Angeles, California

ROBERT M. PASCUZZI, MD
Professor and Chair of Neurology, Department of Neurology, Indiana University School of Medicine; Clarian Health, Indianapolis, Indiana

DAVID C. PRESTON, MD
Professor of Neurology, Neurological Institute, University Hospitals Case Medical Center, Cleveland, Ohio

GINA REMINGTON, BSN, RN
Department of Neurology, University of Texas Southwestern Medical Center at Dallas, Dallas, Texas

STEVEN C. SCHACHTER, MD
Professor, Department of Neurology, Harvard Medical School; Director of Clinical Research, Department of Neurology, Beth Israel Deaconess Medical Center, Boston, Massachusetts

D. ERIC SEARLS, MD
Department of Neurology, Beth Israel Deaconess Medical Center; Cerebrovascular Division, Department of Neurology, Harvard University, School of Medicine, Boston, Massachusetts

BARBARA E. SHAPIRO, MD, PhD
Associate Professor of Neurology, Neurological Institute, University Hospitals Case Medical Center, Cleveland, Ohio

NATALYA SHNEYDER, MD
Department of Neurology, Louisiana State University Health Sciences Center, Shreveport, Louisiana

KATHERINE TREADAWAY, LCSW-ACP
Department of Neurology, University of Texas Southwestern Medical Center at Dallas, Dallas, Texas

RONALD J. TUSA, MD, PhD
Professor of Neurology, Department of Neurology and Otolaryngology; Director, Dizziness and Balance Center, Emory University, Center for Rehabilitation Medicine, Atlanta, Georgia

LOUIS H. WEIMER, MD
Associate Clinical Professor of Neurology; Director, EMG Laboratory; Director, Clinical Autonomic Laboratory, Columbia University Medical Center; The Neurological Institute of New York, New York, New York

PEZHMAN ZADEH, MD
The Neurological Institute of New York, New York, New York

Contents

Although there are at least a thousand different causes for peripheral neuropathy, the majority of patients can be properly diagnosed (and managed) based on framing the diagnostic possibilities within one of six typical scenarios. The case presentations in this article illustrate common and less common but essential presentations and the approach to evaluation and treatment. For these patients the key to success lies in the history and clinical examination findings.

The diagnosis and management of patients with epilepsy is often undertaken by pediatricians, internists, and geriatricians (primary care physicians [PCPs]). Although referral to a neurologist may be necessary if the diagnosis of epilepsy is unclear or if the patient does not respond to initial therapy with antiepileptic drugs, PCPs may subsequently follow-up with patients to implement the recommendations of the neurologist. To maximize the likelihood of treatment success, PCPs should supplement antiepileptic drug therapy with patient education and referrals for psychosocial and vocational support when needed. Special considerations are warranted for women of childbearing potential and elderly patients.

Effective management of patients who have cerebrovascular disease depends on accurate diagnosis. Many conditions cause clinical findings that closely mimic cerebrovascular disorders and are often ruled out through brain imaging or laboratory findings. Diagnosis of cerebrovascular disorders is based on the presence of risk factors for vascular disease, the tempo of onset, the presence of concurrent conditions, and the clinical course of development of neurologic symptoms and signs. This article shares a process by which clinicians can combine a patient's history, neurologic examination, and brain and vascular imaging to localize a lesion and diagnose cerebrovascular disease.

Abnormal involuntary movements are major features of a large group of neurologic disorders, some of which are neurodegenerative and pose a significant diagnostic and treatment challenge to treating physicians. This article presents a concise review of clinical features, pathogenesis, epidemiology, and management of seven of the most common movement disorders encountered in a primary care clinic routinely. The disorders discussed are Parkinson disease, essential tremor, restless legs syndrome, Huntington disease, drug-induced movement disorder, Wilson disease, and Tourette syndrome.

With people having the luxury of living longer there is an increasing epidemic of dementia throughout the world. It is important to distinguish true dementia from the not-unexpected loss of mental acuity as people age. This latter process has been termed "benign forgetfulness of senescence." We are all probably susceptible to memory loss if we live long enough. Progressive cognitive impairment to a clinically significant degree, with no obvious identifiable factor, such as a metabolic disturbance, drug intoxication, or medication effect, probably indicates a dementing illness, however.

Sleep disorders are common and may result in significant morbidity. Examples of the major sleep disturbances in primary care practice include insomnia; sleep-disordered breathing, such as obstructive sleep apnea; central nervous system hypersomnias, including narcolepsy; circadian rhythm sleep disturbances; parasomnias, such as REM sleep behavior disorder; and sleep-related movement disorders, including restless legs syndrome. Diagnosis is based on meticulous inventory of the clinical history and careful physical examination. In some cases referral to a sleep laboratory for further evaluation with polysomnography, a sleep study, is indicated.

Sudden falling with loss of consciousness from syncope and symptoms of orthostatic intolerance are common, dramatic clinical problems of diverse cause, but cerebral hypoperfusion is the ultimate mechanism in most. Cardiac, reflex, and orthostatic hypotension are important forms to consider. Syncope must be differentiated from seizures, psychiatric events, drop attacks, and other mimics. However, factors such as syncopal induced movements, ictal bradycardia, and insufficient clinical information can confound accurate diagnosis and hamper appropriate treatment. Progress in the diagnosis, treatment, and understanding of underlying mechanisms is continually advancing.

Multiple sclerosis is the most common disabling neurologic disease affecting young adults and adolescents in the United States. The first objective of this article is to familiarize nonspecialists with the cardinal features of multiple sclerosis and our current understanding of its etiology, epidemiology, and natural history. The second objective is to explain the approach to diagnosis. The third is to clarify current evidence-based treatment strategies and their roles in disease modification. The overall goal is to facilitate the timely evaluation and confirmation of diagnosis and enhance effective management through collaboration among primary physicians, neurologists, and other care providers who are confronted with these formidably challenging patients.

Michael Devereaux

General internists and family practitioners play an important role in the initial evaluation and treatment of acute low back pain and chronic low back pain. Given the usual time constraints placed on the primary care physician for evaluation of a patient with back pain, it is imperative that the generalist be acquainted and comfortable with the salient points in the history, the essentials of the examination, the appropriate use of diagnostic tests, and the effectiveness (or lack thereof) of available treatments.

Preface

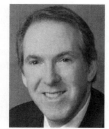

Randolph W. Evans, MD
Guest Editor

Consider the epidemiology of the following neurologic disorders...

Migraine: over 30 million persons have attacks per year in the United States
Vertigo: the third most common complaint among outpatients
Lifetime prevalence of "significant" neck pain: 40% to 70%
Lifetime prevalence of "significant" low back pain: 60% to 90%; fifth most common reason for physician visits
Carpal tunnel syndrome: 3% of the general population
Diabetic polyneuropathy: 30% of diabetics
Seizure: 10% risk of having at least one by age 80
Strokes: 780,000 yearly in the United States
Parkinson's disease:1 million people diagnosed in the United States
Essential tremor: prevalence of up to 5% of the population
Restless legs syndrome: 10% of adults
Alzheimer's disease: 4.5 million persons in the United States
Chronic insomnia: up to 15% of the population
Obstructive sleep apnea: 3% of those ages 30–60 years and 25% in those with mean age of 76 years
Syncope: 3% of visits to the emergency department
Multiple sclerosis: 350,000 persons in the United States

It is hardly surprising that internists frequently see patients with these common neurologic disorders. Some disorders, such as headaches, dizziness, and back pain, are distinctly unpopular among many internists (and neurologists). Other internists may be interested in neurological disorders but feel that their training was inadequate or find it difficult to keep current. However, many patients have to be managed without neurological consultations.

Whatever the level of your neurological expertise, this issue of *Medical Clinics of North America* reviews common neurological disorders including migraine, vertigo, neck and low back pain, entrapment neuropathies, peripheral neuropathies, seizure disorders, cerebrovascular disease, movement disorders, memory complaints and

Med Clin N Am 93 (2009) xi–xii
doi:10.1016/j.mcna.2009.01.001
0025-7125/09/$ – see front matter

dementia, sleep disorders, syncope, and multiple sclerosis. As a change from the usual format, the articles use a question and answer approach that I hope will facilitate review of the topics and stimulate your interest in neurology. Eight of the articles have been revised and updated from the well-received 2004 issue of *Primary Care: Clinics in Office Practice*: "Neurology for the Primary Care Physician," which I edited.

I thank our distinguished contributors for their outstanding articles. I also thank Rachel Glover, editor; Don Mumford, senior developmental editor; and the Elsevier production team for an excellent job. Finally, I am grateful for the support of my wife Marilyn and our children Elliott, Rochelle, and Jonathan.

Randolph W. Evans, MD
Baylor College of Medicine
1200 Binz Street, #1370
Houston, TX 77004

E-mail address:
rwevans@pol.net (R.W. Evans)

Migraine: A Question and Answer Review

Randolph W. Evans, MD

KEYWORDS

- Migraine • Clinical features • Diagnosis • Diagnostic testing
- Treatment

EPIDEMIOLOGY AND PATHOPHYSIOLOGY
Where does the Word Migraine Originate?

Migraine comes from a Greek word meaning "hemicrania" or "half the head," which, as discussed later, is only a partial description.

What is the Prevalence of Migraine in the United States?

The 1-year period prevalence is 11.7% (17.1% in women and 5.6% in men), some 29 million people.[1] An additional 4.5% have probable migraine, which fulfills all but one criterion for migraine with or without aura and responds to migraine medication.[2] The lifetime prevalence is 25% of women and 8% of men. Chronic migraine, which occurs on 15 or more days per month for at least 3 months, may occur in 1% to 2% of the population yearly.

Migraine prevalence is highest in those aged 30 to 39 years for both men (7.4%), and women (24.4%) and lowest in those aged 60 years or older at 1.6% in men and 5.0% in women (**Fig. 1**). The frequency of migraines per month is as follows: less than one, 23%; 1 to 4, 63%; 5 to 9, 9.6%, and 9 to 14, 4.2%.

Who are Some Famous Male Migraineurs?

Because migraine is much more common in women, including Joan of Arc and Elizabeth Taylor, men who have migraine may get ignored. Famous historical figures suspected of having migraine include Julius Caesar, Napoleon Bonaparte, Thomas Jefferson, Ulysses Grant, Friedrich Nietzsche, Sigmund Freud, Claude Monet, Alexander Graham Bell, and Lewis Carroll. Elvis Presley had migraine—the sunglasses were not just to look cool.

Probably the most witnessed migraine took place in Super Bowl XXXII in 1998. Running back Terrell Davis, who had a history of migraine, developed a migraine with visual aura after a ding on the helmet at the end of the first quarter. After

Dr. Evans is a consultant or on the speakers bureau (or both) of GlaxoSmithKline, Merck, Pfizer, and UCB.
Baylor College of Medicine, 1200 Binz #1370, Houston, TX 77004, USA
E-mail address: rwevans@pol.net

Med Clin N Am 93 (2009) 245–262
doi:10.1016/j.mcna.2008.09.003
0025-7125/08/$ – see front matter © 2009 Elsevier Inc. All rights reserved.

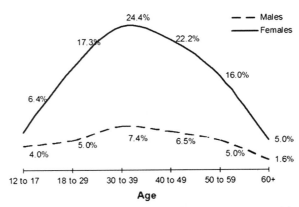

Fig. 1. One-year period prevalence of migraine by age and sex adjusted for demographics. (*Reproduced from* Lipton RB, Bigal ME, Diamond M, et al. Migraine prevalence, disease burden, and the need for preventive therapy. Neurology 2007;68:343; with permission.)

successfully using dihydroergotamine (DHE) nasal spray, he was able to return for the third quarter, scored the winning touchdown, set a Super Bowl rushing record, and was voted Most Valuable Player. Early treatment does make a difference.

It is not surprising that Freud was a migraineur because he was a psychiatrist and also a neurologist. More than 50% of neurologists and 75% of headache specialists have migraines, including this author.[3]

What is the Genetics of Migraine?

Migraine often runs in families with the risk for migraine increased in first-degree relatives by 1.5 to 4 fold. The risk is greatest for those who have migraine with aura, young age at onset, and a high attack severity and disease disability. Up to 61% of migraine is heritable.[4] There is an unclear mode of transmission, however, which is genetically heterogeneous.

What is the Cause of Migraine?

The cause of migraine is not known. Migraine is an often inherited episodic disorder with a disturbance in the perception of normal sensory input, such as pain, light, and sound signals.[5] Migraine may be a disorder of ion channels, as suggested by the rare example of familial hemiplegic migraine. Functional imaging studies have demonstrated migraine-related activation of the dorsolateral pons. Associated neurologic symptoms (the aura) are likely to be the human homolog of the experimental phenomenon known as cortical spreading depression (in the occipital cortex in visual aura).

What Disorders are Comorbid with Migraine?

Numerous disorders are comorbid with migraine, including the following: cardiovascular and cerebrovascular (hypertension/hypotension, Raynaud, mitral valve prolapse, angina/myocardial infarction, stroke), psychiatric; neurologic (epilepsy, essential tremor, benign positional vertigo, and restless legs syndrome), gastrointestinal (irritable bowel syndrome), and other (asthma, atopic allergies, endometriosis, and fibromyalgia).

Psychiatric disorders are among the most common migraine comorbidities.[6,7] Migraineurs are from 2.2 to 4.0 times more likely to have depression. Migraine is also comorbid with generalized anxiety disorder (odds ratio [OR] 3.5 to 5.3), panic disorder (OR 3.7), and bipolar disorder (OR 2.9 to 7.3).

Is Syncope More Common in Migraineurs?

In a population-based study among migraineurs with and without aura (n = 323) and control subjects (n = 153), migraineurs had a higher lifetime prevalence of syncope (46% versus 31%; P = .001), frequent syncope (five or more attacks) (13% versus 5%; P = .02), and orthostatic intolerance (32% versus 12%; P<.001) compared with controls of uncertain etiology.[8] There was no association between autonomic nerve system symptoms and the severity of migraine or type of migraine. Cardiovascular measurements and the prevalence of postural tachycardia syndrome and orthostatic hypotension did not differ significantly between migraineurs and controls. Migraineurs who have syncopal episodes require diagnostic testing as appropriate.

How Often do Sufferers Know That They Have Migraine?

Only 56% of migraineurs know that they have migraine. In a recent study, sinus headache (39%), tension-type headache (31%), and stress headache (29%) were common self-reported diagnoses among migraineurs (subjects could list more than one probable diagnosis).[9]

How often do Patients who Have Self- or Physician-Diagnosed Sinus Headaches Actually Have Migraines?

In a study of 2991 patients who had a history of self-described or physician-diagnosed sinus headache, 88% were diagnosed as fulfilling migraine (80% of patients) or migrainous criteria (8% of patients).[10]

CLINICAL FEATURES
What are the International Classification of Headache Disorders Second Edition (ICHD-2) Criteria for Migraine without Aura?

The duration of untreated or unsuccessfully treated episodes ranges from 4 to 72 hours. The headaches are associated with at least two of the following pain characteristics: unilateral location, pulsating quality, moderate or severe intensity, and aggravation by or causing avoidance of routine physical activity (eg, walking or climbing stairs). The pain is accompanied by at least one of the following symptoms: nausea or vomiting, sensitivity to light (photophobia), and sensitivity to sound (phonophobia). Also, the patient must have a history of at least five previous attacks that meet these criteria. If there are no indications that other primary causes may be responsible for the headaches, a diagnosis of migraine without aura can be reasonably established.[11] Migraine without aura accounts for about 70% to 80% of migraine attacks.

What are the General Features of Migraine?

Although the International Classification of Headache Disorders second edition (ICHD-2) criteria have been useful for research purposes, most clinicians recognize migraine through familiarity with the general features. Migraine pain is unilateral in 60% of cases and bilateral in 40%. About 15% of migraineurs report so-called "side-locked" headaches, with migraine always occurring on the same side. The pain is often more intense in the frontotemporal and ocular regions before spreading to the parietal and occipital areas. Any region of the head or face may be affected, including the parietal region, the upper or lower jaw or teeth, the malar eminence, and the upper anterior neck. Throbbing pain is present in 85% of episodes of migraine, although up to 50% of patients describe non-throbbing pain during some attacks. Up to 75% of migraineurs report, along with the head pain, unilateral or bilateral tightness, stiffness, or throbbing pain in the posterior neck. The neck pain can occur during the migraine prodrome, the attack itself, or the postdrome.

Migraines last 4 to 72 hours if left untreated or if unsuccessfully treated. Migraine persisting for more than 72 hours is termed status migrainosus. Without treatment, 80% of patients have moderate to severe pain and 20% have mild pain. The pain, which is usually increased by physical activity or movement, is associated with nausea in about 80% of episodes, vomiting in about 30%, photophobia in about 90%, and phonophobia in about 80%.[12]

When patients deny a history of light and noise sensitivity, the questions should be asked, "During a headache, would you prefer to be in bright sunlight or in a dark room?" and "During a headache, would you prefer to be in a room with loud music or in a quiet room?" About 20% additional patients become aware of associated light and noise sensitivity by use of the follow-up questions.[13]

Forty-five percent of migraineurs have at least one autonomic symptom (ie, lacrimation, eye redness, ptosis, eyelid edema, nasal congestion, or rhinorrhea) during an attack. These symptoms are caused by parasympathetic activation of the sphenopalatine ganglion, which innervates the tear ducts and sinuses, and these symptoms can lead to confusion of migraine with sinus headaches. Of patients who have autonomic symptoms, 45% have both nasal and ocular symptoms, 21% have nasal symptoms only, and 34% have ocular symptoms only.[14]

How many Patients are Impaired During Migraine Attacks?

A large study found that 54% have severe impairment or require bed rest, 39% have some impairment, and 7% report no impairment.[1] In the prior 3 months, 25% missed at least 1 day of school or work, 28% had work or school productivity reduced by at least 50%, 34% had household productivity reduced by at least 50%, 47% did no household work, and 29% missed family or social activities.

How do you Distinguish Migraine from Other Primary Headaches?

Table 1 compares the features of migraine, tension-type, and cluster headaches.

Why are Migraines Commonly Misdiagnosed as Sinus and Stress Headaches?

Migraine can be confused with sinus headache because the pain can be referred to the face or forehead, associated with nasal or ocular symptoms, such as nasal congestion, eye redness, or lacrimation, and can be triggered by changes in the weather. Migraine can be misdiagnosed as stress or tension headaches because 75% of headaches may be referred to the neck and 50% can be triggered by stress. Again, the history of other associated symptoms makes the diagnosis.

What are Migraine Prodromal Symptoms?

Prodromal or premonitory symptoms, which may be present in up to 80% of cases and precede the migraine attack by hours or up to 1 or 2 days, include changes in mental state, such as depression, hyperactivity, euphoria, talkativeness, irritability, drowsiness, or restlessness. Neurologic symptoms may include photophobia, difficulty concentrating, phonophobia, dysphasia, hyperosmia, and yawning. General symptoms may include stiff neck, food cravings, feeling cold, anorexia, sluggishness, diarrhea or constipation, thirst, and fluid retention. Migraineurs have an average of seven prodromal symptoms per attack, including the following most common: anxiety, irritability,

Table 1
Features of some primary headaches

Feature	Migraine	Episodic Tension-Type	Episodic Cluster
Epidemiology	18% of women, 6% of men 4% of children before puberty	90% of adults 35% of children aged 3–11 y	0.4% for men 0.08% for women
Female/male	3/1 after puberty, 1/1 before	5/4	1/5
Family history	80% of first-degree relatives	Frequent	Rare
Typical age at onset (y)	92% before age 40, 2% after age 50	20–40	20–40
Visual aura	In 20%	No	Occasional
Location	Unilateral, 60%; bilateral, 40%	Bilateral > unilateral	Unilateral Especially orbital, periorbital, frontotemporal
Quality	Pulsatile or throbbing in 85%	Pressure, aching, tight, squeezing	Boring, burning, or stabbing
Severity	Mild to severe	Mild to moderate	Severe
Onset to peak pain	Minutes to hours	Hours	Minutes
Duration	4–72 h May be <1 h in children	Hours to days	15–180 min
Frequency	Rare to frequent	Rare to frequent	1–8 per d during clusters
Periodicity	Menstrual migraine	No	Yes Average bouts 4–8 weeks Average 1 or 2 bouts yearly
Associated features	Nausea in 90%, vomiting in 30%, light and noise sensitivity in 80%	Occasional nausea	Ipsilateral conjunctival injection, tearing, and nasal congestion or drainage Ptosis and miosis in 30%
Triggers	Present in 85% Present in 85%	Stress, lack of sleep	Alcohol, nitrates
Behavior during headache	Still, quiet, tries to sleep	No change	Often paces
Awakens from sleep	Can occur	Rare	Frequently

Data from Evans RW. Diagnosis of headaches. In Evans RW, Mathew NT, editors. Handbook of headache. 2nd edition. Philadelphia: Lippincott Williams & Wilkins; 2005. p. 14–5.

yawning, unhappiness, concentration difficulties, somnolence, light and noise sensitivity, flatulence, and constipation.[15]

What are Migraine Triggers?

Migraines are often triggered by environmental or other factors; 85% of migraineurs report triggers. Patients typically have multiple triggers, with a mean of three. Up to 53% of migraineurs report that a change of weather is a trigger.[16] Other environmental triggers are heat, high humidity, and high altitude. There are numerous additional triggers, including stress (reported by up to 80% of patients), letdown after stress, vacations, and crying. Missing a meal (57%), lack of sleep, oversleeping, and fatigue are also commonly reported as triggers. Sensory triggers include bright lights, glare, flickering lights, loud noise, and strong smells, such as perfume or cigarette smoke. Up to 50% of patients report alcohol as a trigger; this can be all forms of alcohol or only one type, such as red wine or beer. Up to 45% report food triggers, such as chocolate, dairy products (particularly cheese), citrus fruit, fried foods, and nitrates and nitrites in cured meats or fish (eg, frankfurters, bacon, and smoked salmon). Other triggers include minor head trauma, exertion, and nitroglycerin.

There are triggers unique to women. Half of women who have migraine report menses as a trigger, and 14% have migraines associated only with their menses. During pregnancy, the frequency of migraines decreases (especially during the second and third trimesters) in 60%, remains the same in 20%, and increases in 20%. Migraines may occur for the first time when women start using oral contraceptives (OCs). Low-estrogen OCs usually have no effect on migraine or may even improve it, although frequency can increase. Of patients who have new-onset migraine or increased frequency of migraine associated with OCs, 30% to 40% may improve when OCs are discontinued, although improvement may not occur for up to 1 year. Two thirds of women who have prior migraine improve with physiologic menopause. Surgical menopause results in worsening of migraine in two thirds of cases.

What is Central Sensitization?

As the headache progresses, central sensitization can cause cutaneous allodynia (pain provoked by stimulation of the skin that would ordinarily not produce pain; this is seen especially in the head and face, but it can also be generalized), and triptans are unlikely to be an effective treatment.[17]

What is a Migraine Aura?

The migraine aura has a total duration of usually less than 1 hour and frequently less than 30 minutes.[18] An aura lasting more than 1 hour but less than 1 week is termed migraine with prolonged aura, or complicated migraine. The most common aura is a visual one, which is present in 99% of cases and has two types: positive visual phenomena, with hallucinations; and negative visual phenomena or scotomas, with either an incomplete or complete loss of vision in a portion or all of the visual field. Most visual auras have a hemianoptic distribution. Photopsias consist of small spots, dots, stars, unformed flashes or streaks of light, or simple geometric forms and patterns that typically flicker or sparkle.

A scintillating scotoma, also called a fortification (because of its resemblance to a medieval fortified town as viewed from above) spectrum or teichopsia (seeing fortifications), is present in about 10% of cases. The scotoma, which is frequently semicircular or horseshoe shaped, usually begins in the center of the visual field and then slowly extends laterally. The scotomatous arc or band is a shimmering or glittering, bright, zigzag border. Most visual auras consist of flickering, colored or uncolored, unilateral or bilateral zig-zag lines or patterns, semicircular or arcuate patterns, wavy lines, or irregular patterns. Rare visual auras include metamorphopsia (objects appear to change in size and shape), macropsia, micropsia, telescopic vision (objects appear larger than normal), teleopsia (objects appear to be far away), mosaic vision, Alice in Wonderland syndrome (distorted body image), and multiple images. Headaches, when unilateral, usually occur on the side contralateral to the visual symptoms but can occasionally be ipsilateral.

What Other Type of Auras can Occur?

A sensory aura, which is present in about 30% of episodes of migraine with aura, consists of numbness, tingling, or a pins-and-needles sensation. The aura, which is usually unilateral, commonly affects the hand and then the face, or it may affect either one alone. Paresthesia of one side of the tongue is typical. Less often, the leg and trunk may be involved. A true motor aura is rare, but sensory ataxia or a heavy feeling is often misinterpreted as weakness.

Speech and language disturbances may occur in up to 20% of cases. Patients often report a speech disturbance when the spreading paresthesias reach the face or tongue. Slurred speech may be present. With involvement of the dominant hemisphere, paraphasic errors and other types of impaired language production and comprehension may occur. Rarely, other aura symptoms may be described, including déjà vu and olfactory and gustatory hallucinations.

Although visual symptoms frequently occur by themselves, combinations of aura symptoms can occur. Sensory, speech, and motor symptoms are usually associated with visual symptoms or with one or more other symptoms. When two or more aura symptoms are present, they almost always occur in succession rather than simultaneously.

Migraine aura can occur without headache (acephalgic migraine), often in patients who typically have migraine with or without aura. A visual aura is the most common in these cases. Another type of acephalgic migraine is episodic vertigo without a headache, auditory disturbances, or other neurologic symptoms, lasting minutes to days. Rarely, migraineurs may have persistent visual aura. This aura usually consists of simple, unformed hallucinations in the entire visual field of both eyes, including innumerable dots, television static, clouds, heat waves, flashing or flickering lights, lines of ants, a rainlike or snowlike pattern, squiggles, bubbles, and grainy vision. Occasionally, palinopsia (the persistence of visual images), micropsia, or formed hallucinations occur.

What are Late-Life Migraine Accompaniments?

Late-life migraine accompaniments are transient visual, sensory, motor, or behavioral neurologic manifestations of the migraine aura.[19] More than 1% of the population has a first episode of migraine aura after the age of 50 years. Headache is associated with only 50% of cases and may be mild. These accompaniments occur more often in men than in women. From most to least common, migraine accompaniments consist of visual symptoms (transient blindness, homonymous hemianopsia, and blurring of vision), paresthesias (numbness, tingling, pins-and-needles sensation, or a heavy feeling of an extremity), brain stem and cerebellar dysfunction (ataxia, clumsiness, hearing loss, tinnitus, vertigo, and syncope), and disturbances of speech (dysarthria or dysphasia).

Other causes of transient cerebral ischemia should be considered, especially when the patient is seen after the first episode or if the case has unusual aspects. The usual diagnostic evaluation for transient ischemic attacks (TIAs) or seizures is performed.

Features that help distinguish migraine accompaniments from TIAs include a gradual build-up of sensory symptoms, a march of sensory paresthesias, serial progression from one accompaniment to another, longer duration (90% of TIAs last for less than 15 minutes), and multiple stereotypical episodes. If the episodes are frequent, the usual preventive medications may be considered.

What is Basilar-Type Migraine?

Basilar-type migraine is a rare disorder that most often occurs in children and rarely presents in patients older than 50 years. According to ICHD-2 criteria, attacks are marked by two or more of the following fully reversible aura symptoms originating from the brain stem or both occipital lobes, but no motor weakness: dysarthria, vertigo, tinnitus, hypacusia, diplopia, visual symptoms simultaneously in both temporal and nasal field of both eyes, ataxia, decreased level of consciousness, and simultaneously bilateral paresthesias. There is also at least one of the following: at least one aura symptom develops gradually over 5 minutes or more or different aura symptoms occur in succession over 5 minutes or more; each aura symptom lasts between 5 and 60 minutes. Patients who have basilar-type migraine may also have other types of migraine. Visual symptoms—which usually take the form of blurred vision, shimmering colored lights accompanied by blank spots in the visual field, scintillating scotoma, and graying of vision—may start in one visual field and then spread to become bilateral. Diplopia occurs in up to 16% of cases. Vertigo may be present, either alone or accompanied by various combinations of tinnitus, dysarthria, gait ataxia, and paresthesias (usually bilateral, but sometimes affecting alternate sides in successive episodes). Impairment of consciousness is common and may include obtundation, amnesia, syncope, and, rarely, prolonged coma. A severe throbbing headache, typically with a bilateral occipital location, is present in 96% of cases. Nausea and vomiting typically occur, with light and noise sensitivity in up to 50% of cases.

DIAGNOSTIC TESTING
Is Neuroimaging Warranted in Migraineurs?

A report of the Quality Standards Subcommittee of the American Academy of Neurology makes the following recommendation: "Neuroimaging is not usually warranted in patients with migraine and a normal neurologic examination."[20] Numerous CT and MRI studies have been done in migraineurs, all finding a small percentage of significant abnormalities, with the most recent large study finding abnormalities in only 0.4%.[21]

What are Some Reasons to Consider Neuroimaging in Migraineurs?

Indications to consider neuroimaging include the following: unusual, prolonged, or persistent aura; increasing frequency, severity, or change in clinical features; first or worst migraine; basilar; confusional; hemiplegic; late-life migraine accompaniments; aura without headache; possibly headaches always on the same side; posttraumatic; and when patient or family and friends request. In the case of patient or their family or friend's request for imaging, often medically unnecessary imaging can be avoided with a brief discussion of their concerns (eg, brain tumor or aneurysm as the cause of the migraines) and why their headaches are typical of migraine, which is diagnosed clinically, whereas scanning has a minimal yield of incidental findings. If they are concerned about intracranial saccular aneurysm, I explain that the chance of an adult having an incidental aneurysm is about 2% but that an incidental aneurysm would not be responsible for migraines.

There are many reasons that physicians recommend diagnostic testing, including neuroimaging: aiming for diagnostic certainty, faulty cognitive reasoning, the medical decision rule that holds that it is better to impute disease than to risk overlooking it, busy practice conditions in which tests are ordered as shortcuts, patient and family expectations, financial incentives, and medicolegal issues. In the era of managed care, equally compelling reasons for not ordering diagnostic studies include physician fears of deselection and at-risk capitation. Lack of funds and underinsurance continue to be barriers for appropriate diagnostic testing for many patients.

Is it Preferable to Obtain a CT or MRI for the Evaluation of Headache?

CT detects most abnormalities that may cause headaches, which are also visualized on MRI.[22] CT is generally preferred over MRI for the evaluation of acute subarachnoid hemorrhage, acute head trauma, and bony abnormalities. There are several disorders that may be missed on routine CT of the head, including vascular disease, neoplastic disease, cervicomedullary lesions, infections, and low cerebrospinal fluid (CSF) pressure syndrome.

MRI is more sensitive than CT in the detection of posterior fossa and cervicomedullary lesions, ischemia, white matter abnormalities, cerebral venous thrombosis, subdural and epidural hematomas, neoplasms (especially in the posterior fossa), meningeal disease (such as carcinomatosis, diffuse dural enhancement in low CSF pressure syndrome, and sarcoid), and cerebritis and brain abscess. Pituitary pathology is more likely to be detected on a routine MRI of the brain than a routine CT. In addition, CT exposes the patient to ionizing radiation, which raises the long-term risk for cancer.[23] MRI is thus generally preferred over CT for the evaluation of headaches.

The yield of MRI may vary depending on the field strength of the magnet, the use of paramagnetic contrast, the selection of acquisition sequences, and the use of magnetic resonance angiography and venography. MRI has contraindications, however, such as the presence of some aneurysm clips or a pacemaker. In addition, about 8% of patients are claustrophobic and about 2% are unable tolerate the study.

What are White Matter Abnormalities and How often are they Detected in Migraineurs?

A patient wanted to be reassured that her 10-year history of typical migraines were not due to a brain tumor. She had a MRI scan and the report came back discussing a few scattered deep white matter abnormalities (WMA); you should consider microvascular ischemic disease or perhaps demyelinating disease (especially if you have an overzealous radiologist). Migraine should be listed in the differential.

WMA are foci of hyperintensity on both proton density and T2-weighted images in the deep and periventricular white matter caused by either interstitial edema or perivascular demyelination.[22] WMA are easily detected on MRI but are not seen on CT scan. The percentages of WMA for all types of migraine range from 12% to 46%, whereas the incidence of WMA in controls ranges from 2% to 14%. Although the cause of WMA in migraine is not certain, various hypotheses have been advanced, including increased platelet aggregability with microemboli, abnormal cerebrovascular regulation, and repeated attacks of hypoperfusion during the aura.

ACUTE TREATMENT
Are Over-the-Counter Medications Effective?

Over-the-counter medications are effective, especially for mild to moderate migraine pain when taken at the onset of headache. All migraine medications are more effective if taken when the headache is mild. Aspirin, acetaminophen, and caffeine combination medications; aspirin; acetaminophen; and nonsteroidal anti-inflammatory medications can reduce the headache to mild or none 2 hours after dosing in up to 59% of patients. Use of these medications (naproxen sodium may be an exception) more than 2 to 3 days per week for several months may result in rebound headaches (the precise duration has not been determined). Isometheptene combination prescription medications may be similarly effective for some patients.

What about Butalbital Combinations and Opiates?

There is no evidence for efficacy from randomized controlled trials for the use of butalbital combinations. In addition, butalbital combinations are frequently associated with medication overuse or rebound headaches and can be habituating. In one study, use of butalbital as infrequently as 5 days per month was linked to transformation into chronic daily headache and medication overuse headache.[24] Patients on butalbital require careful monitoring with use preferably limited to no more than two to three treatment days per week or less.

Opiate combinations may be effective as rescue medication if a triptan did not work or for those who are triptan nonresponders or who have triptan contraindications. Opiates are also associated with a risk for dependency and medication overuse headaches. Preferably, patients' use should be limited to no more than 2 days per week.

What are Triptans and How Effective are They?

Triptan medications are selective 5-hydroxytryptamine (5-HT1B/1D) receptor agonists that share a basic indole ring structure with different side chains. Triptans have three potential mechanisms of action: cranial vasoconstriction, peripheral neuronal inhibition, and inhibition of transmission through second-order neurons of the trigeminocervical complex. These mechanisms inhibit the effects of activated nociceptive trigeminal afferents and control acute migraine attacks.

Over the past 16 years, seven triptans have become available: sumatriptan, zolmitriptan, naratriptan, rizatriptan, almotriptan, frovatriptan, and eletriptan (**Table 2**).[25] Sumatriptan is also recently available in a combination with naproxen sodium, a bilayer tablet of 85 mg of rapid-release sumatriptan on the top and 500 mg of naproxen sodium on the bottom. If oral triptans are taken when the pain is moderate to severe in intensity, the 2-hour response rate (no pain or mild pain) is about 45% for naratriptan and frovatriptan and about 65% to 70% for the others. If taken when the headache is mild, the 2-hour pain-free responses are much higher for all of the triptans and may be greater than 70% depending on the drug. About 25% of patients do not respond to any of the triptans, however.[26]

The oral triptans may not be equally effective for different patients. If a patient has an unsatisfactory or inconsistent response, unpleasant side effects, or tachyphylaxis with one triptan, a different triptan may prove effective and tolerable. Patients who have prominent vomiting or nausea or who desire the quickest relief may benefit from subcutaneous sumatriptan (at 2 hours, 79% of patients show a response and 60% are pain-free) or intranasal sumatriptan or zolmitriptan. A non-triptan option is DHE nasal spray, which can be about as effective as any oral or nasal triptan and may also be effective in some patients who do not respond to any triptan.

Patients may experience recurrence, which is defined as the return of headache (usually of moderate or severe intensity) within 24 hours after an initial response to acute treatment, at which time patients may need to take a second dose of medication. When taken for moderate to severe pain, sumatriptan/naproxen sodium, naratriptan, frovatriptan, almotriptan, and eletriptan have the lowest recurrence rates of about

Table 2
Available triptan preparations

Drug	Formulation	Strengths (mg)
Almotriptan	Tablets	12.5
Eletriptan	Tablets	40
Frovatriptan	Tablets	2.5
Naratriptan	Tablets	1, 2.5
Rizatriptan	Tablets	5, 10
	Orally disintegrating preparation[a]	5, 10
Sumatriptan	Subcutaneous injection	4, 6
	Tablets	25, 50, 100
	Nasal spray	5, 20
Sumatriptan/naproxen sodium	Tablets	85/100
Zolmitriptan	Tablets	2.5, 5
	Orally disintegrating preparation[a]	2.5, 5
	Nasal spray	5

[a] Dissolves on the tongue; can be taken without water (efficacy similar to that of tablet form).

14% to 25%. The recurrence rates for the other triptans are about 30% to 40%. The time to recurrence is generally about 12 hours.[23]

What are the Contraindications for the use of Triptans?

Triptans are contraindicated in those who have ischemic heart disease, Prinzmetal angina, cerebrovascular disease, peripheral vascular syndromes, or uncontrolled hypertension and for use within 24 hours of ergotamine or dihydroergotamine.

Triptans can stimulate 5-HT1B receptors on coronary arteries and result in constriction, which may become clinically significant in patients who have coronary artery stenosis or vasospastic disease. The common triptan side effects—tightness, heaviness, pressure, or pain in the chest, neck, or throat—are not associated with electrocardiogram changes and are not caused by coronary vasoconstriction.

Should you be Concerned About Serotonin Syndrome When Prescribing Triptans and Antidepressants?

The serotonin syndrome is an adverse drug reaction that results from therapeutic single or combination medication use or overdose of medication that increase serotonin levels and stimulates central and peripheral postsynaptic serotonin receptors. Medications associated with the serotonin syndrome include selective serotonin reuptake inhibitors (SSRIs), selective serotonin/norepinephrine reuptake inhibitors (SNRIs), monoamine oxidase inhibitors, tricyclic antidepressants, opiate analgesics, over-the-counter cough medicines, antibiotics, weight-reduction agents, antiemetics, drugs of abuse, and herbal products. The syndrome has also been associated with the withdrawal of medications. Sixty percent of patients who have serotonin syndrome present within 6 hours of medication initiation, overdose, or change in dosage, and 74% present within 24 hours.

The serotonin syndrome presents with one or a combination of mental status changes (with a range including anxiety, agitation, confusion, delirium and hallucinations, drowsiness, and coma), autonomic hyperactivity in about 50% of affected individuals (including hyperthermia, diaphoresis, sinus tachycardia, hypertension or hypotension, flushing of the skin, diarrhea, and vomiting), and neuromuscular dysfunction (including myoclonus, hyperreflexia, muscle rigidity, tremor, and severe shivering).[27] The presentation may range from diarrhea and tremor in a mild case to life-threatening complications, such as seizures, coma, rhabdomyolysis, and disseminated intravascular coagulation. The diagnosis is one of exclusion based on the history of medication use, the physical examination, and ruling out other neurologic disorders, such as meningoencephalitis, delirium tremens, heat stroke, neuroleptic malignant syndrome, malignant hyperthermia, and anticholinergic poisoning.

In 2006, the Food and Drug Administration (FDA) issued an alert, "Potentially Life-Threatening Serotonin Syndrome with Combined Use of SSRIs or SNRIs and Triptan Medications"[28] stating, "The FDA has reviewed 27 reports of serotonin syndrome reported in association with concomitant SSRI or SNRI and triptan use. Two reports described life-threatening events, and 13 reports stated that the patients required hospitalization. Some of the cases occurred in patients who had previously used concomitant SSRIs or SNRIs and triptans without experiencing serotonin syndrome." The warning concluded, "The FDA recommends that patients treated concomitantly with a triptan and an SSRI/SNRI be informed of the possibility of serotonin syndrome (which may be more likely to occur when starting or increasing the dose of an SSRI, SNRI, or triptan) and be carefully followed."[28]

Through a Freedom of Information Act request, The FDA provided me with their complete reports of 29 possible serotonin syndrome cases (2 more than described in the alert), which I analyzed as previously reported.[29] Eight of the cases have been published; the rest were submitted to the FDA through the MedWatch reporting system. Of the 29 cases, 7 meet the Sternbach toxicity criteria but not the Hunter criteria. No cases meet both the Sternbach and Hunter criteria or the Hunter criteria but not the Sternbach. Even among those meeting criteria, however, there are questions as to whether other disorders were excluded in 6 cases.

During 2003 to 2004 alone, an annualized mean of 694,276 patients were simultaneously prescribed or continued use of a triptan along with an SSRI or SNRI. Millions of patients have been exposed to the triptan combinations worldwide and, according to my analysis, only 7 cases meet the Sternbach criteria, and none meet the more sensitive and specific Hunter criteria for serotonin syndrome.[30] Does this justify routinely advising our patients of this possibility as the FDA advisory recommends and perhaps unnecessarily alarming them? Some migraineurs on an SSRI or SNRI might be so alarmed that they would not want to take a triptan that could be effective, or those already taking a triptan may not want to take an indicated SSRI or SNRI. It is certainly possible that additional definite cases may be reported with greater physician awareness of these potential drug interactions and serotonin syndrome, although I am not aware of any definite cases in the 2 years since the release of the alert.

How do you Treat an Intractable Acute Migraine or Migraine Status (Persisting for more than 72 hours) in the Urgent Care Clinic or Emergency Department?

About 2% of patients in emergency rooms have migraines of the following types: first or worst attacks, those who have not taken or not responded to drugs, frequent attendees, those who have acute exacerbation of chronic migraine, and those who have migraine with neurologic symptoms and signs (with aura). These patients may receive a less-than warm welcome when they present with "just a headache." The migraines may be difficult to treat because the pain persists or recurs within 24 hours of discharge from the emergency department regardless of treatment in more than half of patients.

Intravenous fluids and electrolyte replacement may be necessary for the patient who has intractable vomiting from migraines. Evidence-based guidelines recommend the first-line use of DHE (0.5–1 mg intravenous [IV], intramuscular [IM], or subcutaneous [SC]), SC sumatriptan 4 to 6 mg (DHE and triptans should not be used within 24 hours of each other), dopamine antagonists (metoclopramide 10 mg IV, prochlorperazine 10 mg IV, and chlorpromazine 0.1 mg/kg), and ketorolac 30 mg IV or 30 to 60 mg IM, which have response rates of up to 70%.[31] Narcotic analgesics, recommended as rescue drugs, are still widely used, even though their administration may result in significantly longer stays in the emergency department compared with nonnarcotic treatments.[32] Narcotics, such as parenteral meperidine may be as effective as ketorolac but less effective than DHE and cause more sedation and dizziness.[33]

Intravenous valproate sodium (500 mg diluted in 50 mL of saline, administered intravenously over 5 to 10 minutes) and droperidol (2.5 mg IV or IM) may also be effective. Intravenous corticosteroids, such as a single dose of 10 to 24 mg of dexamethasone, are not effective for termination of the acute attack but may prevent recurrence of the headache with a number needed to treat of nine.[34]

There are the usual contraindications to the use of triptans and DHE and risk for administration with some of the drugs if the patient is pregnant. There is a small risk for prolonged QT intervals and torsade de pointes with the use of neuroleptics, such as prochlorperazine and droperidol.

PREVENTIVE TREATMENT
What are the Indications for Preventive Medications?

Indications for preventive treatment are as follows: the headaches significantly interfere with the patient's daily routine despite acute treatment; acute medications are contraindicated, ineffective, or overused, or have intolerable side effects; frequent migraines (two or more attacks a week); uncommon migraine types (hemiplegic, basilar, prolonged aura, or migrainous infarction); the cost of acute medications is significantly greater than the cost of preventive medication; and patient preference (ie, the patient is willing to risk the possibility of side effects from the preventive medication to reduce the frequency of headaches).[35]

What are the General Principles for use of Preventives?

The clinician should start with a low dose of medication and increase it slowly, depending on the response and whether side effects occur.

Each medication should be given a trial of 2 to 3 months at adequate doses.

Overused medications that may be causing rebound headache and may decrease the efficacy of preventive treatment should be discontinued or tapered (depending on the drug).

The patient should keep a headache diary to monitor his or her headaches.

The clinician should educate the patient about the rationale for treatment and possible side effects and should address the patient's expectations for treatment. Many patients want a complete cure, and although this is certainly understandable, it is usually not possible.

Consider coexistent or comorbid conditions. Some medications may be effective for both migraine and another disorder. Other disorders, along with the migraine medications that may be effective for them, include epilepsy (divalproex sodium, topiramate, and gabapentin), hypertension (beta-blockers), depression (tricyclic antidepressants), bipolar disorder (divalproex sodium), insomnia (tricyclic antidepressants), essential tremor (beta-blockers and topiramate), and overweight or obesity (topiramate). On the other hand, coexistent diseases, such as depression or asthma, may be relative contraindications to the use of beta-blockers. In a woman who is pregnant or may become pregnant, the potential for teratogenicity should be considered. Patients who have mild responses to one preventive agent may benefit from the addition of a second agent. Finally, when some drugs, such as tricyclic antidepressants and beta-blockers, are discontinued, they may need to be tapered off.

What Preventive Medications may be Effective?

Based on class I evidence, the beta-blocker propranolol, the tricyclic antidepressant amitriptyline, and the antiseizure medications divalproex sodium and topiramate are the most effective preventive medications, reducing the frequency of migraines by more than 50% in about 50% of patients.[36] In general, preventive medications are more effective when patients are placed on a titration schedule with a minimum target dose. Some titration schedules and minimum target doses are as follows: propranolol (either regular or long acting) 40 mg/d increased by 40 mg/wk to 120 to 160 mg; amitriptyline 10 to 25 mg at bedtime increased by 10 to 25 mg per week to 50 to 75 mg; divalproex sodium (either regular or extended release) 500 mg/d for 1 week and then 1000 mg daily; and topiramate 25 mg for the first week, increased by 25 mg/wk in divided doses to 50 mg twice daily.[37]

Other beta-blockers may also be effective (see **Table 3**). Regarding the tricyclic antidepressants, the quality of evidence for nortriptyline is not as good as that for amitriptyline, but the clinical impression is one of similar efficacy with less sedation. Venlafaxine may be as effective as amitriptyline with fewer side effects.[38] SSRIs are probably not effective for migraine prevention. Verapamil and gabapentin are only modestly effective for migraine prevention.

There are natural products that may be beneficial for migraine prevention, including the herb feverfew (*Tanacetum parthenium*; 50–82 mg daily); extract from the butterbur plant, *Petasites hybridus* (75 mg twice a day); riboflavin (200 mg twice a day); coenzyme Q10 (100 mg three times daily); and oral magnesium supplements. Botulinum toxin injections may also be of benefit in some patients who have chronic migraine but the evidence does not support the use in episodic migraine (less than 15 days per month). The relative benefit of these treatments may become clearer with additional studies, but for now, some migraineurs may prefer them because they have few if any side effects.

For many migraineurs, the avoidance of triggers may be useful. Examples include adequate sleep at set hours, routine exercise, regular meals, avoiding triggering foods and beverages, and wearing sunglasses in bright sunlight or glare. Some patients may benefit from biofeedback, relaxation training, and psychotherapy.

When Should an Effective Preventive Medication be Discontinued?

Only one randomized, placebo-controlled trial has been performed to investigate migraine frequency after preventive treatment has been discontinued. Patients were treated with topiramate for 6 months and then randomly assigned to continue this dose or switch to placebo for 6 months with 254 patients on topiramate and 258 on placebo.[39] Discontinuation "...was associated with persistent benefits compared with values before treatment, although numbers of migraine days were higher and quality of life was lower in patients who discontinued topiramate use than in those who continued treatment. Patients should therefore be treated for 6 months, with the option to continue treatment to 12 months in some patients, particularly those whose migraine frequency decreased substantially with topiramate."[39]

Table 3
Preventive medications for migraine

Drug Class	Agent	Dosage	Typical Side Effects
Beta-blockers	Propranolol	40–120 mg bid	Hypotension, tiredness, exacerbation of asthma
	Propranolol long acting	60–160 mg/d	
	Metoprolol	50–100 mg/d	
	Nadolol	40–160 mg/d	
	Atenolol	50–100 mg/d	
	Timolol	10–20 mg bid	
Antidepressants	Amitriptyline	25–150 mg hs	Drowsiness, dry mouth, weight gain, constipation
	Nortriptyline	25–150 mg hs	
	Venlafaxine XR	37.5 mg for 1 wk then 75 mg/d for 1 wk then 150 mg/d as tolerated	Nausea, vomiting, insomnia, drowsiness
	Divalproex sodium	500–1000 mg in divided doses or once daily with extended-release formulation	Nausea, tremor, drowsiness, weight gain, alopecia, hematologic and liver abnormalities, fetal abnormalities
Anticonvulsants	Topiramate	50–200 mg/d in divided doses	Weight loss, paresthesias, cognitive disturbances, kidney stones
	Gabapentin	300–800 mg tid	Dizziness, fatigue, drowsiness

Are you Unhappy with Current Acute and Preventive Medication Options?

Physicians and migraineurs would like to see more effective and more tolerable medications. There is some research going on at pharmaceutical companies but more needs to be done when the large number of migraineurs is considered. Physicians and migraine advocacy groups should lobby for increased government funding for migraine research, which is only about $13 million in the United States and €6 million in Europe annually.[40] Also consider joining the American Headache Society (www.ahsnet.org), which has been lobbying Congress.

WOMEN'S TREATMENT ISSUES
How do you Treat Menstrual Migraine?

Menstrual migraine is treated with the same acute medications as other migraines. Interval or short-term preventive treatment of menstrual migraine, starting 2 or 3 days before menses and continuing during the menses, may be helpful for some women who have regular menses and migraines that are poorly responsive to symptomatic medications.[41] Potentially effective medications include the following: nonsteroidal anti-inflammatory drugs, such as naproxen sodium 550 mg twice daily; ergotamine 1 mg once or twice a day; or DHE 1 mg subcutaneously or intramuscularly; naratriptan 1 mg orally twice daily for 6 days started 2 days before predicted menses; frovatriptan 2.5 mg twice daily (with double loading dose on day 1) for 6 days starting 2 days before predicted menstrual migraine; transdermal estradiol, 100 µg applied 3 days before the expected start of menses and replaced after 3 days or a 6-day patch; continuous combined oral contraceptive use, with a lower estrogen dose given during the menses; and extended-duration oral contraceptive use.

Are Combined Estrogen Oral Contraceptives Safe for Migraineurs?

Although there is controversy whether low-estrogen OCs increase the risk for stroke, most women who have migraine without aura can safely take low-estrogen OCs if they have no other contraindications or risk factors. When taking low-estrogen OCs, women less than 35 years old who have migraine with aura, such as visual symptoms lasting less than 1 hour, have a risk for ischemic stroke of about 30/100,000 annually, which is twice the risk of those who have migraine without aura.[42] A task force of the International Headache Society to assess the use of OCs in women who have migraine concluded that "there is a potentially increased risk of ischemic stroke in women with migraine who are using combined estrogen oral contraceptives (COCs) and have additional risk factors which cannot easily be controlled, including migraine with aura. One must individually assess and evaluate these risks. Combined oral contraceptive use may be contraindicated"[43] Women who have aura symptoms, such as hemiparesis or aphasia, or prolonged focal neurologic symptoms and signs lasting more than 1 hour, should avoid starting low-estrogen OCs and should stop the medication if they are already taking it. Progestin-only OCs and the many other contraceptive options can be considered, as appropriate. Cigarette smoking should be strongly discouraged because female migraineurs who smoke one or more packs of cigarettes per day raise their risk for ischemic stroke by a factor of about 10.

What is the Effect of Estrogen Replacement Therapy?

Estrogen replacement therapy has a variable effect on migraine: 77.5% show no change or improved and 22.5% worsen. If migraines increase when a patient starts estrogen replacement, the following strategies may be beneficial:

Reduce the estrogen dose.
Change the estrogen type to one less likely to promote migraine. From most to least likely to promote migraine, these are, in order, conjugated estrogens, pure estradiol, synthetic estrogen, and pure estrogen.
Convert from interrupted to continuous dosing, in the case of estrogen withdrawal migraine.
Convert from oral to parenteral administration (eg, a transdermal patch).
Add androgens.[44]

REFERENCES

1. Lipton RB, Bigal ME, Diamond M, et al. Migraine prevalence, disease burden, and the need for preventive therapy. Neurology 2007;68:343–9.
2. Silberstein S, Loder E, Diamond S, et al. Probable migraine in the United States: results of the American Migraine Prevalence and Prevention (AMPP) study. Cephalalgia 2007;27:220–34.
3. Evans RW, Lipton RB, Silberstein SD. The prevalence of migraine in neurologists. Neurology 2003;61:1271–2.
4. Ferrari MD. Migraine genetics: a fascinating journey towards improved migraine therapy. Headache 2008;48:697–700.
5. Goadsby PJ. Emerging therapies for migraine. Nat Clin Pract Neurol 2007;3: 610–9.

6. Hamelsky SW, Lipton RB. Psychiatric comorbidity of migraine. Headache 2006; 46:1327–33.

7. Evans RW, Rosen N. Migraine, psychiatric comorbidities, and treatment. Headache 2008;48:952–8.

8. Thijs RD, Kruit MC, van Buchem MA, et al. Syncope in migraine: the population-based CAMERA study. Neurology 2006;66:1034–7.

9. Diamond S, Bigal ME, Silberstein S, et al. Patterns of diagnosis and acute and preventive treatment for migraine in the United States: results from the American Migraine Prevalence and Prevention study. Headache 2007;47:355–63.

10. Schreiber CP, Hutchinson S, Webster CJ, et al. Prevalence of migraine in patients with a history of self-reported or physician-diagnosed "sinus" headache. Arch Intern Med 2004;164:1769–72.

11. Headache Classification Subcommittee of the International Headache Society. The international classification of headache disorders 2nd edition. Cephalalgia 2004;24(Suppl 1):1–232.

12. Lipton RB, Scher AI, Kolodner K, et al. Migraine in the United States. Neurology 2002;58:885.

13. Evans RW, Seifert T, Kailasam J, et al. The use of questions to determine the presence of photophobia and phonophobia during migraine. Headache 2008;48: 395–7.

14. Barbanti P, Fabbrini G, Pesare M, et al. Neurovascular symptoms during migraine attacks. Cephalalgia 2001;21:295.

15. Quintela E, Castillo J, Muñoz P, et al. Premonitory and resolution symptoms in migraine: a prospective study in 100 unselected patients. Cephalalgia 2006;26: 1051–60.

16. Kelman L. The triggers or precipitants of the acute migraine attack. Cephalalgia 2007;27:394–402.

17. Bigal ME, Ashina S, Burstein R, et al. Prevalence and characteristics of allodynia in headache sufferers: a population study. Neurology 2008;70:1525–33.

18. Cutrer FM, Huerter K. Migraine aura. Neurologist 2007;13:118–25.

19. Purdy RA. Late-life migrainous accompaniments. In: Gilman S, editor. MedLink neurology. San Diego: MedLink Corporation. Available at: www.medlink.com. Accessed October 20, 2008.

20. Silberstein SD. Practice parameter: evidence-based guidelines for migraine headache (an evidence-based review): report of the Quality Standards Subcommittee of the American Academy of Neurology. Neurology 2000;55: 754–62.

21. Sempere AP, Porta-Etessam J, Medrano V, et al. Neuroimaging in the evaluation of patients with non-acute headache. Cephalalgia 2005;25:30–5.

22. Evans RW, Rozen TD, Mechtler L. Neuroimaging and other diagnostic testing in headache. In: Silberstein SD, Lipton RB, Dodick DW, editors. Wolff's headache and other head pain. 8th ed. New York: Oxford; 2008. p. 63–93.

23. Brenner DJ, Hall EJ. Computed tomography—an increasing source of radiation exposure. N Engl J Med 2007;357:2277–84.

24. Bigal ME, Serrano D, Buse D, et al. Acute migraine medications and evolution from episodic to chronic migraine: a longitudinal population-based study. Headache 2008;48:1157–68.

25. Silberstein SD. Migraine. Lancet 2004;363:381–91.

26. Diener HC, Limmroth V. Specific acute migraine treatment: ergotamine and triptans. In: Lipton R, Bigal M, editors. Migraine and other headache disorders: tools and rules for diagnosis and treatment. Ontario: BC Decker; 2006. p. 289–310.

27. Boyer EW, Shannon M. The serotonin syndrome. N Engl J Med 2005;35:1112–20.
28. Available at: http://www.fda.gov/cder/drug/InfoSheets/HCP/triptansHCP.htm. Accessed on August 3, 2008.
29. Evans RW. The FDA alert on serotonin syndrome with combined use of SSRIs or SNRIs and triptans: an analysis of the 29 case reports. Medscape Gen Med. 2007;9:48. Available at: http://www.medscape.com/viewarticle/561741. Accessed October 20, 2008.
30. Sclar DA, Robison LM, Skaer TL, et al. Concomitant triptan and SNRI use: a risk for serotonin syndrome. Headache 2008;48:126–9.
31. Ducharme J. Canadian Association of Emergency Physicians guidelines for the acute management of migraine headache. J Emerg Med 1999;17:137–44.
32. Tornabene SV, Deutsch R, Davis DP, et al. Evaluating the use and timing of opioids for the treatment of migraine headaches in the emergency department. J Emerg Med 2008 [Epub ahead of print].
33. Friedman BW, Kapoor A, Friedman MS, et al. The Relative efficacy of meperidine for the treatment of acute migraine: a meta-analysis of randomized controlled trials. Ann Emerg Med. 2008 Jul 14 [Epub ahead of print].
34. Evans RW. Treating migraine in the emergency department. BMJ 2008;336:1320.
35. Silberstein SD, Rosenberg J. Multispecialty consensus on diagnosis and treatment of headache. Neurology 2000;54:1553.
36. Silberstein SD. Preventive migraine treatment. Neurol Clin 2009, in press.
37. Evans RW, Bigal ME, Grosberg B, et al. Target doses and titration schedules for migraine preventive medications. Headache 2006;46:160–4.
38. Bulut S, Berilgen MS, Baran A, et al. Venlafaxine versus amitriptyline in the prophylactic treatment of migraine: randomized, double-blind, crossover study. Clin Neurol Neurosurg. 2004;107(1):44–8.
39. Diener HC, Agosti R, Allais G, et al. Cessation versus continuation of 6-month migraine preventive therapy with topiramate (PROMPT): a randomised, double-blind, placebo-controlled trial. Lancet Neurol 2007;6:1054–62.
40. Shapiro RE, Goadsby PJ. The long drought: the dearth of public funding for headache research. Cephalalgia 2007;27:991–4.
41. MacGregor EA. Menstrual migraine. Curr Opin Neurol 2008;21:309–15.
42. Evans RW, Becker WJ. Migraine and oral contraceptives. Headache 2006;46:328–31.
43. International Headache Society Task Force. Recommendations on the use of oral contraceptives in women with migraine. Cephalalgia 2000;20:155–6.
44. Ashkenazi A, Silberstein SD. Hormone-related headache: pathophysiology and treatment. CNS Drugs 2006;20:125–41.

Dizziness

Ronald J. Tusa, MD, PhD

KEYWORDS

- Dizziness • Vertigo • Vestibular • Imbalance
- Falls • Rehabilitation

DEFINITION, EPIDEMIOLOGY
What is the Definition of Dizziness?

Dizziness is an imprecise term used to describe various symptoms, each of which has a different pathophysiologic mechanism and significance (**Table 1**). If the patient cannot describe the symptoms, ask the patient if the problem primarily causes problems in the head or problems with balance. If the patient has spells, have the patient describe in detail the initial spell and the last severe spell.

How Common is Dizziness in the United States?

Dizziness is the third most common complaint among outpatients.[1] Only chest pain and fatigue are more common. In 80% of these cases, the dizziness is severe enough to require medical intervention. Dizziness affects more than 50% of the elderly population and is the most common reason for visiting a physician after the age of 75 years.[2]

CAUSE
What are the Causes of Dizziness?

The causes of dizziness in patients seen at our Dizziness and Balance Center since 2000 are shown in **Fig. 1**.

BEDSIDE ASSESSMENT
What are the Key Elements of the History?

The tempo, symptoms, and circumstances of the complaint are three key items in the history (**Table 2**).

Tempo
Determine if the patient has an acute attack of dizziness (3 days or fewer), chronic dizziness (more than 3 days), or spells of dizziness. Most disorders of acute dizziness lead to chronic dizziness. If the patient suffers from spells, try to determine the average duration of the spells in seconds, minutes, or hours.

Department of Neurology and Otolaryngology, Dizziness and Balance Center, Emory University, Center for Rehabilitation Medicine, 1441 Clifton Road, NE, Atlanta, GA 30322, USA
E-mail address: rtusa@emory.edu

Med Clin N Am 93 (2009) 263–271
doi:10.1016/j.mcna.2008.09.005
0025-7125/08/$ – see front matter. Published by Elsevier Inc.

medical.theclinics.com

Table 1
Symptoms of dizziness

Symptoms	Mechanism
Dysequilibrium: imbalance or unsteadiness while standing or walking	Loss of vestibulospinal, proprioceptive, visual, or motor function; joint pain or instability; psychologic factors
Lightheadedness or presyncope	Decreased blood flow to the brain
Sense of rocking or swaying as if on a ship (mal de debarquement)	Vestibular system adapts to continuous, passive motion and must readapt once environment is stable. Anxiety.
Motion sickness	Visual-vestibular mismatch
Nausea and vomiting	Stimulation of medulla
Oscillopsia: illusion of visual motion	Spontaneous: acquired nystagmus. Head-induced: severe, bilateral loss of the vestibulo-ocular reflex
Floating, swimming, rocking, and spinning inside of head (psychologically induced).	Anxiety, depression, and somatoform disorders
Vertical diplopia	Skew eye deviation
Vertigo: rotation, linear movement, or tilt	Imbalance of tonic neural activity to vestibular cerebral cortex

Symptoms

What is meant by "dizziness" should be determined. If the patient cannot describe the symptoms then ask the patient if the problem primarily causes problems in the head or problems with balance. If the patient has spells, have them describe in detail the initial spell and the last severe spell.

Circumstance

Determine the circumstances in which dizziness occurs. Dizziness may be provoked by only certain movements, such as standing up after lying down for at least 10 minutes in

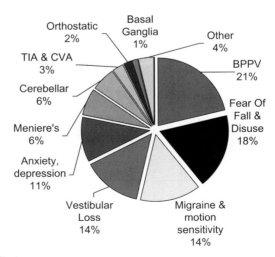

Fig. 1. Causes of dizziness.

Table 2
Key items in the history of the dizzy patient

Disorder	Tempo	Symptoms	Circumstances
Vestibular neuritis	Acute dizziness	Vertigo, dysequilibrium, nausea/vomiting, oscillopsia	Spontaneous, exacerbated by head movements
Labyrinthitis	Acute dizziness	Vertigo, dysequilibrium, nausea/vomiting, oscillopsia, hearing loss and tinnitus	Spontaneous, exacerbated by head movements
Wallenberg infarct	Acute dizziness	Vertigo, dysequilibrium, nausea/vomiting, tilt, lateropulsion, ataxia, crossed sensory loss, oscillopsia	Spontaneous, exacerbated by head movements
Bilateral vestibular deficit or >3 d from a unilateral vestibular defect	Chronic dizziness	Dizzy, dysequilibrium, occasionally oscillopsia.	Induced by head movements, walking. Exacerbated when walking in the dark or on uneven surfaces.
Mal de debarquement	Chronic dizziness	Rocking or swaying as if on a boat	Spontaneous while lying or sitting. Rarely occurs while in motion
Oscillopsia	Chronic dizziness	Subjective illusion of visual motion	Spontaneous with eyes open
Anxiety/depression	Chronic dizziness	Lightheaded, floating or rocking	Induced by eye movements with head still
Benign paroxysmal positional vertigo	Spells: seconds	Vertigo, lightheaded, nausea	Positional: lying down, sitting up or turning over in bed, bending forward
Orthostatic hypotension	Spells: seconds	Lightheaded	Positional: standing up
Transient ischemic attacks	Spells: minutes	Vertigo, lightheaded, dysequilibrium	Spontaneous
Migraine	Spells: minutes	Vertigo, dizziness, motion sickness	Usually movement-induced
Panic attack	Spells: minutes	Dizzy, nausea, diaphoresis, fear, palpitations, paresthesias	Spontaneous or situational
Motion sickness	Spells: hours	Nausea, diaphoresis, dizzy,	Movement-induced, usually visual-vestibular mismatch
Ménière disease	Spells: hours	Vertigo, dysequilibrium, ear fullness from hearing loss and tinnitus	Spontaneous, exacerbated by head movements

orthostatic hypotension, or may occur after vertical or oblique head movements, such as lying down, turning over in bed, or sitting up in benign paroxysmal positional vertigo (BPPV). If the individual tells you that simply moving the eyes with the head stationary causes dizziness and there is no eye movement disorder (eg, ocular misalignment or an internuclear ophthalmoparesis), then dizziness is likely to be the result of anxiety. When dizziness occurs without provocation (spontaneous) and is vestibular in origin, it frequently is exacerbated by head movements.

How Does the History Help Determine Management?

One of the most useful questions to ask to determine appropriate management is "How does dizziness affect your life?" A peripheral vestibular loss from vestibular neuritis on one side may yield different responses in different individuals. Patients may state that they are not affected at all by the dizziness, but they want to be reassured that nothing is seriously wrong. These patients may not require extensive evaluations and management. Other patients may state they have no unsteadiness while walking, but they can no longer play golf or tennis because of their imbalance. These patients may require limited balance rehabilitation. Other patients state they are completely devastated by their dizziness and they do not leave the house, drive, or participate in any social activities. These patients require extensive counseling and physical therapy, and may require medication.

What Portion of the Bedside Examination Should be Done in Every Dizzy Patient?

Box 1 lists the portions of the examination that should be performed on all patients who have dizziness to facilitate diagnosis. Visual fixation reduces or suppresses horizontal and vertical nystagmus generated by peripheral vestibular defects. The head thrust test is shown in **Fig. 2**. **Fig. 3** shows the Hallpike-Dix test.

What are the Characteristics of Nystagmus in Individuals Who Have Acute, Unilateral Peripheral Vestibular Loss?

The characteristics of nystagmus in individuals who have acute unilateral peripheral vestibular loss (eg, vestibular neuritis) are shown in **Fig. 4**.

MANAGEMENT
What are Vestibular Suppressant Medications and When Should They be Used?

Various vestibular suppressant medications can be used for symptomatic treatment of acute vertigo and nausea (**Table 3**). These should be used for 1 week or less, when the symptoms of spontaneous vertigo and nausea are most intense. I give promethazine (25–50 mg intramuscularly [IM]) in the office at the onset of severe vertigo, and then send the patient home for 3 days of bed rest with promethazine suppositories to be taken as needed. This medication causes sedation and reduces nausea. Ondansetron may also be appropriate for patients who have severe vertigo and nausea, but currently this is only approved for chemotherapy-induced nausea.[3]

Box 1
Routine physical examination

Check for spontaneous nystagmus in the light when the patient is fixating a target and also with fixation blocked.

Check the vestibulo-ocular reflex by doing a head thrust test.

Do the Hallpike-Dix test to check for benign paroxysmal positional vertigo and central positional vertigo.

Check smooth pursuit and saccadic eye movements.

Check standing balance (Romberg and sharpened Romberg); check gait.

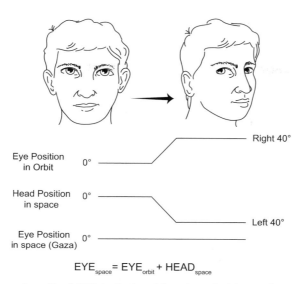

Eye Position in Orbit   0°   Right 40°

Head Position in space   0°

Eye Position in space (Gaza)   0°   Left 40°

$$EYE_{space} = EYE_{orbit} + HEAD_{space}$$

Fig. 2. Vestibulo-ocular reflex (VOR) during head thrust test. In this test, the examiner holds the head firmly between the hands. Tell the patient to fixate your nose. Then quickly thrust the head 10° to 20° to either side and determine if the patient is still fixating on your nose immediately after the head thrust. If the patient has to make a corrective saccade to refixate your nose after the head thrust, the VOR is impaired (*Adapted from* Leigh RJ, Zee DS. The neurology of eye movements. New York: Oxford University Press; 1999. p. 646; with permission.)

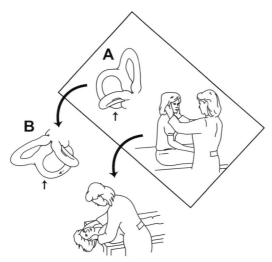

Fig. 3. Hallpike-Dix test for BPPV. (*A*) In this test, the patient sits on the examination table and the head is turned 45° horizontally. (*B*) The head and trunk are quickly brought straight back en bloc so that the head is hanging over the edge of the examination table by 20°. Nystagmus is looked for and the patient is asked if they have vertigo. Although not shown in the figure, the patient is then brought up slowly to a sitting position with the head still turned 45° and nystagmus is looked for again. This test is repeated with the head turned 45° in the other direction. This figure also shows movement of debris in the right posterior semicircular canal (*black arrows*) during the test. In this example, the patient would have nystagmus and vertigo when the test is performed on the right side, but not when the test is performed on the left side. (*From* Tusa RJ. Vertigo. Neurol Clin 2001;19:39; with permission.)

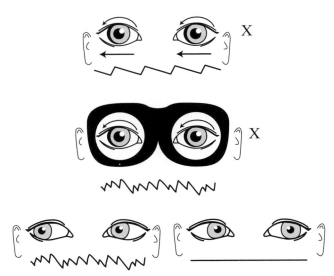

Fig. 4. Peripheral vestibular nystagmus. This figure depicts disruption of the left superior division of the 8th nerve from vestibular neuritis. Top figures show vigorous right beating and right torsional nystagmus when subject views straight ahead through Frenzel glasses, and mild nystagmus when patient does not have the glasses on. Arrows indicate the direction of the quick phases of nystagmus. Frenzel glasses block the patient's ability to visually fixate. Nystagmus is labeled according to the direction of the quick phases. Eye movement trace is shown below the face. Bottom figures illustrate the effect of horizontal eye position on nystagmus. The intensity of nystagmus increases when the patient looks in the direction of the quick phases (*Adapted from* Brandt T. Vertigo: its multisensory syndrome. London: Springer-Verlag; 1991. p. 329; with permission.)

Table 3
Vestibular suppressant drugs

Drug	Major Action	Indication	Dosage
Alprazolam	GABA agonists	Acute UVL	0.25 mg prn
Meclizine	Antihistamine, anticholinergic	Acute UVL	25–50 mg q6h × 3 d max
Ondansetron	Serotonin agonist	Severe nausea from central vertigo	4 mg q8h for 3 d
Scopolamine	Anticholinergic	Motion sickness	1 patch for 3 d
Promethazine	Phenothiazine (antidopa)	Acute UVL	25 mg po, IM, supp q 6h
Prochlorperazine	Phenothiazine (antidopa)	Acute UVL	25 mg po, IM, or supp q12h

Abbreviations: supp, suppository; UVL, unilateral vestibular loss.

What Therapeutic Medications are Available and When Should They be Used?

There are various medications that may be therapeutic for different causes of dizziness (**Table 4**). For example, prednisone and acyclovir during the first 10 days of the attack may shorten the course of the illness in patients who have Ramsay Hunt syndrome.[4] Prednisone alone may be useful in patients who have vestibular neuritis.[5-7] Midodrine and fludrocortisone are useful in treating orthostatic hypotension.[8]

What Medications can Cause Dizziness or be Harmful to the Dizzy Patient?

Several medications may cause subjective symptoms of dizziness, especially in those patients older than 65 years of age.[9-11] **Table 5** lists the more common medications along with their primary effects. Certain drugs cause dysequilibrium and lightheadedness. These include anticonvulsants, antidepressants, antihypertensives, anti-inflammatory agents, hypnotics, muscle relaxants, tranquilizers, and chronic use of vestibular suppressants. Sensitization may occur to meclizine and scopolamine after a few days of continuous use, and withdrawal symptoms will occur when the medication is discontinued. This may be misinterpreted as recurrence of the disorder itself, so that physicians should be cautious about restarting these medications.

Certain drugs may cause vestibular ototoxicity and spare hearing, yet lead to dysequilibrium. These include certain aminoglycosides (streptomycin, gentamicin, tobramycin), furosemide and ethacrynic acid. The other aminoglycosides affect hearing primarily. Treatment of bilateral vestibular defects should include avoidance of all ototoxins that may cause further permanent peripheral vestibular damage (gentamicin, streptomycin, tobramycin, ethacrynic acid, furosemide, quinine, cisplatinum) and avoidance of drugs that may transiently impair balance (sedative, antianxiety, antiepileptics, and antidepressants). Vestibular rehabilitation may be helpful for these patients.

Table 4
Therapeutic medications for dizziness

Drug	Major Action	Indications	Dosage
Acetazolamide	Diuretic	Ménière disease	250 mg bid to tid
Acyclovir	Antiviral	Ramsay Hunt syndrome	400 mg 5×/d × 10 d
Fludrocortisone	Mineral corticoid	Orthostatic hypotension	0.1–0.6 mg/d
Midodrine	Alpha1 adrenergic stimulant	Orthostatic hypotension	10 mg tid
Paroxetine	Selective serotonin reuptake inhibitor (antidepressant)	Anxiety	10–20 mg q AM
Prednisone	Anti-inflammation	Acute vestibular neuritis and Ramsay Hunt syndrome	60 mg qd, then taper over 10 d
Propranolol	Beta-blocker	Migraine	At least 80 mg qd split up in several doses
Valproic Acid	GABA agonist	Migraine	250–500 mg po bid

Table 5
Drugs that can induce dizziness or be harmful to the dizzy patients

Drug	Drugs that can Cause Dizziness	Drugs that Interfere with Vestibular Compensation	Ototoxic (Vestibular) Drugs
Antiarrhythmics			
Amiodarone, quinine			X (synergistic)
Anticonvulsants			
Barbiturates	X		
Carbamazepine, phenytoin, ethosuximide	X		
Antidepressants			
Amitriptyline, imipramine	X		
Antihypertensives			
Diuretics			
Hydrochlorothiazide	X		
Furosemide, ethacrynic acid			X (synergistic)
Alpha1-blockers			
Prazosin, Terazosin	X		
Beta-blockers			
Atenolol, propranolol	X		
Calcium antagonists			
Nifedipine, verapamil	X		
Anti-inflammatory drugs			
Ibuprofen, indomethacin	X		
Acetylsalicylic acid			X (reversible)
Antibiotics			
Streptomycin, gentamicin			X
Tobramycin			X
Chemotherapeutics			
Cisplatinum			X
Hypnotics			
Flurazepam, triazolam	X		
Muscle relaxants			
Cyclobenzaprine,	X		
Orphenadrine	X		
Methocarbamol			
Tranquilizers			
Chlordiazepoxide Meprobamate	X		
Vestibular suppressants			
Chlordiazepoxide, diazepam	X	X	
Meclizine, scopolamine,	X	X	

REFERENCES

1. Kroenke K, Mangelsdorff D. Common symptoms in ambulatory care: incidence, evaluation, therapy and outcome. Am J Med 1989;86:262–6.
2. National Health and Nutrition Examination Survey. Balance Procedures Manual, 2001. Available at: http://www.cdc.gov/nchs/data/nhanes/ba.pdf. Accessed January 19, 2009.
3. Rice GPA, Ebers GC. Ondansetron for intractable vertigo complicating acute brainstem disorders. Lancet 1995;345:1182–3.
4. Murakami S, Hato N, Horiuchi J, et al. Treatment of Ramsay Hunt syndrome with acyclovir-prednisone: significance of early diagnosis and treatment. Ann Neurol 1997;41:353–7.
5. Ariyasu L, Byl FM, Sprague MS, et al. The beneficial effect of methylprednisolone in acute vestibular vertigo. Arch Otolarygol Head Neck Surg 1990;116:700–3.
6. Ohbayashi S, Oda M, Yamamoto M, et al. Recovery of vestibular function after vestibular neuronitis. (Stockh). Acta Otolaryngol Suppl 1993;503:31–4.
7. Strupp M, Zingler VC, Arbusow V, et al. Methylprednisolone, valacyclovir, or the combination for vestibular neuritis. N Engl J Med 2004;351(4):354–61.
8. Jankovic J, Gilden JL, Hiner BC, et al. Neurogenic orthostatic hypotension: a double-blind, placebo-controlled study with midodrine. Am J Med 1993;95:38–48.
9. Ballantyne J, Ajodhia J. Iatrogenic dizziness. In: Dix MR, Hood JD, editors. Vertigo. Chichester (NY): John Wiley and Sons; 1984. p. 217–47.
10. Wennmo K, Wennmo C. Drug-related dizziness. (Stockh). Acta Otolaryngol Suppl 1988;455:11–3.
11. Klockhoff I, Lindblom U, Stahle J. Diuretic treatment of Ménière disease. long-term results with chlorthalidone. Arch Otolaryngol 1974;100:262–5.

Neck Pain

Michael Devereaux, MD, FACP

KEYWORDS

- Neck pain • Cervicalgia • Acute neck pain
- Chronic neck pain • Cervical spondylosis
- Cervical radiculopathy • Cervical myelopathy

Neck pain due to cervical spine and related disorders, although not as common as low back pain, is nonetheless a common and often debilitating problem and an important reason for seeking medical attention. Although patients with neck pain secondary to trauma may be seen initially in an emergency department or in some cases by a specialist, such as an orthopedic surgeon, neck pain more often is spontaneous in onset without correlation with a specific activity or neck trauma.[1] Patients with neck pain frequently see their primary care physician first, which is most appropriate given that many of these patients can be treated effectively without extensive diagnostic testing or referral to a specialist. It is important that the generalist have a good working knowledge of how to evaluate patients with neck pain and the differential diagnosis of disorders of the neck. It is also important to remember that patients presenting with neck and shoulder pain, particularly when it extends into the upper extremities, may have disorders of the brachial plexus rather than a cervical radiculopathy.

WHAT IS THE PREVALENCE OF NECK PAIN?

The lifetime prevalence of neck pain is less than that of low back pain. At the same time, there are fewer epidemiologic studies on neck pain available for review.[1,2] Studies suggest that perhaps two thirds of individuals experience neck pain at least once during their lifetime.[3,4] Visits to a primary care physician for the treatment of neck pain, particularly in the geriatric population, is not uncommon.[1,5] The prevalence of neck pain increases with age and is more common in women than men.[6]

WHAT ARE THE RISK FACTORS FOR NECK PAIN?

Risk factors are better established for low back pain than neck pain, but many risk factors probably are common to both (see the article on low back pain elsewhere in this issue). As noted in the discussion on whiplash to follow, gender and rear-end automobile accidents are risk factors. Older age also is a risk factor.[7,8]

Neurological Institute, University Hospitals, Case Medical Center, 11100 Euclid Avenue, Cleveland, OH 44106, USA
E-mail address: michael.devereaux@uhhospitals.org

Med Clin N Am 93 (2009) 273–284
doi:10.1016/j.mcna.2008.11.001
0025-7125/08/$ – see front matter © 2009 Elsevier Inc. All rights reserved.

WHAT ANATOMIC ESSENTIALS DOES A PRIMARY CARE PHYSICIAN NEED TO KNOW TO DIAGNOSE AND TREAT THE CAUSES OF NECK PAIN?

The spinal column must be rigid enough to support the trunk and the extremities, strong enough to protect the spinal cord and cauda equina and to anchor the erector spinae and other muscles, and yet sufficiently flexible to allow for movement of the head and trunk in multiple directions. The anatomic organization of the spinal column and related structures allows for all of this, but at a price because the combined properties of rigidity and mobility can lead to many problems. The spine is most flexible in the neck, permitting multiple head movements over a wide arc.

Much of the basic organization of the spine is reviewed in the article on low back pain and is not repeated here. Instead, basic differences between the cervical and lumbar spine are emphasized. The two vertebrae in the spinal column, which vary from all the rest, are the atlas and axis. The atlas is composed of a ring of bone without a body, and the axis has the odontoid process around which the atlas rotates. The vertebral arteries pass through the transverse foramina of the first six vertebrae of the highly mobile cervical spine, which permits approximately 160° of head rotation, most of which occurs between the skull and the C3 vertebra. Approximately 90° of this rotation occurs between the axis and the atlas at the level of the atlantoaxial loop of the vertebral artery. One study showed occlusion of the vertebral artery when the head is placed in full extension and rotated 90° to the side opposite of the occluded vertebral artery.[9] It is not surprising that vertebral artery occlusion and resultant posterior circulation distribution strokes can occur as a result of a variety of athletic injuries and therapeutic "techniques," such as chiropractic manipulation.[10]

The spinal canal houses the spinal cord and the proximal portion of the cervical roots. Although lumbar canal stenosis produces only radiculopathy because the tip of the conus medullaris is at the level of L1-L2, cervical canal stenosis can produce a sometimes complex picture of cervical myelopathy and radiculopathy. The midsagittal diameter of the cervical canal from C1 to C3 is usually about 21 mm (range 16 to 30 mm) and from C4 to C7 about 18 mm (range 14 to 23 mm).[1] The midsagittal diameter of the spinal cord is 11 mm at C1 and 10 mm from C2 to C6 and 7 to 9 mm below C6.[1] The midsagittal diameter of the cervical cord normally occupies about 40% of the midsagittal diameter of the cervical canal in a healthy individual. The cervical canal midsagittal diameter is decreased by 2 to 3 mm with normal head and neck extension.[1] These anatomic relationships are of clinical importance in the context of head and neck hyperextension injuries in individuals with a congenitally narrow spinal canal, especially in individuals with additional narrowing because of cervical spondylosis. The result can be acute cervical myelopathy.

In addition to the major ligaments of the spine discussed in the article on low back pain, there are several important ligaments unique to the cervical spine. The occipital vertebral ligaments are dense, broad, extremely strong ligaments that connect the occiput to the atlas. These permit 30° of flexion and extension around the atlanto-occipital joint. The stability of the atlantoaxial joint depends almost entirely on ligaments. In this regard, the transverse ligament is the most important, permitting the atlas to rotate around the odontonid process. A tear in this ligament has the same effect as a fractured odontoid process.

With regard to the relationship between the cervical roots and the cervical vertebrae, each numbered cervical root passes through the foramen above the numbered cervical vertebra (ie, the C6 spinal nerve exits through the foramen between the C5 and C6 vertebrae). In the lumbar spine, each numbered root exits below the numbered vertebra (L5 root exits through the foramen between the L5 and S1 vertebrae). This can be a point of confusion, particularly when reviewing MRI reports. With regard to the paraspinous musculature in the neck, there are separate extensors and flexors of the head and the cervical spine, making for a complex muscular arrangement that is in all likelihood a common generator of neck pain.

WHAT ARE THE ESSENTIALS IN THE HISTORY THAT HELP TO DEFINE THE NATURE OF NECK PAIN?

Although the approach to history taking for neck pain is similar in many respects to that for low back pain there are enough differences to warrant a separate discussion (see also the article on low back pain elsewhere in this issue). Patients with cervical disorders of one type or another may present with lower extremity and bladder or bowel symptoms often with only minimal neck pain. It is important in patients with suspected neck disorders to ask about symptoms referable to lower extremities as well as bladder and bowel functions. This can include questions about the presence of paresthesia in the lower extremities, weakness of the lower extremities, gait disorders, impotence in men, and anorgasmia in women along with bladder disturbances. Sometimes differentiating a peripheral neuropathy, cauda equina syndrome, and cervical myelopathy on the basis of the history is more difficult that one might suspect.

WHAT ARE THE ESSENTIALS OF THE PHYSICAL EXAMINATION?

On inspection of the head and neck, findings of reduced spontaneous head movement, head tilt, and neck deformity all raise the possibility of an underlying vertebral column disorder or deformity. Palpation and percussion of the neck/cervical spine, as with low back pain, have a low yield with regard to identifying a specific process. However, paracervical tenderness or other changes such as palpation of a mass do offer support for the diagnosis of a vertebral column disorder.

A gait assessment looking for evidence of bilateral lower extremity weakness and possibly spasticity is important and often easily done. Watching the patient rise from a chair and walk to the examining table often suffices. The traditional neurologic examination including individual muscle group testing of the upper and lower extremities; a sensory examination concentrating on the dermatomes of the upper extremities; and a check of deep tendon reflexes searching for absent reflexes in the upper extremities and possibly heightened reflexes and Babinski signs in the lower extremities can further define and localize the problem to the cervical spine.

In patients presenting with shoulder and upper extremity pain, careful questioning is important. The presence of paresthesia with shoulder and upper extremity pain, with or without a complaint of upper extremity weakness, rules against a diagnosis of shoulder arthropathy and rotator cuff injury. Patients with brachial plexopathy can present with shoulder and upper extremity pain and weakness and paresthesia of the upper extremities. These patients frequently do not have evidence of neck pain or a history of modulation of the pain with head/neck movement. On the basis of the history alone, it can be difficult to distinguish brachial plexopathy from cervical radiculopathy. The primary care physician may reach this differential based on the history (and subsequent physical examination) and be unable to go any further. Diagnostic testing, particularly electromyography and nerve conduction study, is often necessary for ultimate localization. The essentials of the examination can be done in several minutes.

Several neuromuscular tests are particularly helpful in evaluating a patient with neck pain:[1]

- Spurling's maneuver (test): The head is inclined toward the side of the painful upper extremity and then compressed downward by the examiner. If this induces radiating pain and paresthesia into the symptomatic extremity, it strongly suggests nerve root compression, usually secondary to disk herniation. It should be noted that lateral head movement away from the symptomatic extremity sometimes can accentuate pain and paresthesia in the symptomatic upper extremity secondary to stretching of a compressed nerve root.
- Traction "distraction" test: Lifting "traction" on the head may relieve cervical spinal nerve compression reducing upper extremity pain and paresthesia.
- Valsalva test: As with low back pain/sciatica, the Valsalva maneuver with resultant increased intrathecal pressure can sometimes accentuate neck and upper extremity symptoms when due to an underlying cervical radiculopathy.
- Lhermitte's test: In patients with myelopathy that affects the posterior columns, neck flexion can produce paresthesia, usually in the back, but sometimes into the extremities. The Lhermitte's sign is most commonly associated with an inflammatory process such as multiple sclerosis, but it is sometimes noted with spinal cord compression.
- Adson's and hyperabduction tests: Long used in the evaluation of suspected thoracic outlet syndrome, these tests are nonspecific and unreliable. With the patient sitting erect, the upper extremities at the side (Adson) or symptomatic upper extremity abducted and extended (hyperabduction), the radial pulse is palpated. Each test is positive if the pulse disappears and paresthesia develops in the hand of the symptomatic extremity.

WHAT IS THE CAUSE AND WHAT IS THE BEST TREATMENT APPROACH FOR PATIENTS WHO PRESENT WITH NONRADIATING NECK PAIN?

The causes and treatment approach to neck pain are similar to the causes and treatment approach to low back pain (see article on low back pain). Patients presenting with acute and chronic neck pain generally also complain of neck stiffness and reduced mobility. The pain typically is reduced when the patient is recumbent. As with low back pain, if the pain is not reduced by recumbency, vertebral column infections and metastatic cancer should be considered.[1,11,12]

The precise generator of pain usually cannot be identified. The inability to identify a specific etiology is confirmed in part by the lack of precision and specificity of the terms used to describe the syndrome—neck strain, musculoskeletal pain syndrome, neck spasms, myofascial pain syndrome, and in the case of chronic and more widespread pain, fibromyalgia. Tendons, ligaments, paracervical muscles, and facet joints all have been implicated as a source of pain, and all may be. However, none can be determined easily in any given patient.

In these patients, diagnostic testing has a low yield, although chronic neck pain patients frequently undergo more than one battery of tests during the course of pain. Although testing has a low yield in a patient with persistent nonradiating neck pain, after several weeks of pain, diagnostic testing may prove necessary to rule out the unexpected, such as congenital malformations of the vertebral column (eg, Klippel-Feil deformity). Although spinal radiographs almost always show spondylotic changes in older patients with nonradiating neck pain, the correlation between symptoms and radiographs is poor.[13] Even if ultimately an MRI of the cervical spine is obtained, results can be misleading because asymptomatic herniated discs are common and may be seen particularly in older patients with unrelated nonradiating neck and low back pain.[14–16]

As with treatment of low back pain, common sense and conservatism are the cornerstones of management. Treatment of acute nonradiating neck pain is largely empiric and may include the following:[1]

- Relative quiescence/pain avoidance, which, if necessary, may include a short period of bed rest. A cervical pillow or towel rolled up and placed under the neck in bed may help. Long-term bed rest is to be avoided.
- Medications including acetaminophen, nonsteroid anti-inflammatory drugs (NSAIDs), pain medication when necessary, and possibly muscle relaxants.
- Local application of heat or cold, although not scientifically validated, can be tried and then continued if the patient finds either beneficial.
- Bracing (controversial). Short-term use of a soft cervical collar maybe of value situationally, particularly during the performing of certain necessary activities of daily living such as driving. Long-term, regular use of a collar may actually aggravate the problem by leading to paracervical muscle disuse atrophy.

The treatment of chronic nonradiating neck pain is virtually identical to the treatment of chronic low back pain and shares much in common with the treatment of other chronic pain syndromes.[1] Physical therapy, as in the case of treatment of low back pain, is particularly important. A variety of scientifically unvalidated treatments for chronic neck pain are best avoided. They include traction, spinal manipulation/manual therapy, trigger point injections, botulinum toxin injections, transcutaneous electrical nerve stimulation (TENS) therapy, electromagnetic therapy, and acupuncture.

In the case of chronic neck pain, as with any chronic pain syndrome, it is crucial to avoid the regular use of reactive pain medications, particularly potentially addictive analgesics. The overuse of analgesics, even nonaddictive analgesics, may lead to analgesic rebound pain.

HOW COMMON ARE CERVICAL RADICULOPATHIES, AND HOW DO THEY PRESENT?

Although there are many causes of cervical radiculopathy, the most common is intervertebral disk herniation and cervical spondylosis.[17] People in their 40s and 50s are particularly at risk for disk herniation. According to one study, the annual incidence of disk herniation is 83.2 per 100,000, an incidence substantially lower than lumbosacral disk herniation.[18] Risk factors include heavy manual jobs, operation of vibrating equipment, lifting heavy objects, frequent automobile travel, smoking, and coughing. There is an antecedent history of trauma in 14.8% of cases and a past history of lumbar radiculopathy in 41%.[1] Despite these recognized risk factors, most patients wake up with the pain in the morning with no recall of a specific trigger for the pain. A significant percentage of these patients have a prior history of episodes of neck discomfort. The level of disk herniation/radiculopathy is as follows:[18]

- C6–C7 compressing the C7 root: 45% to 60%
- C5–C6 compressing the C6 root: 20% to 25%
- C8–T1 compressing the C8 root: approximately 10%
- C4–C5 compressing the C5 root: approximately 10%

Initial symptoms after disk herniation with radiculopathy are generally neck pain and stiffness. The pain tends to radiate quickly into the shoulder or scapular region and upper extremity; the exact distribution depends on the particular root involved (**Table 1**). Other symptoms include paresthesia, hyperesthesia, and weakness.

Table 1
Symptoms and signs associated with cervical radiculopathy

Root	Pain Distribution	Dermatomal Sensory Distribution	Weakness	Affected Reflex
C4	Upper neck	"Cape" distribution shoulder/arm	None	None
C5	Neck, scapula, shoulder, anterior arm	Lateral aspect of arm	Shoulder abduction Forearm flexion	Biceps Brachioradialis
C6	Neck, scapula, shoulder, lateral arm and forearm into first and second digits	Lateral aspect forearm And hand and 1st and 2nd digits	Shoulder abduction Forearm flexion	Biceps Brachioradialis
C7	Neck, shoulder, lateral arm, medial scapula, extensor surface forearm	3rd digit	Elbow extension Finger extension	Triceps
C8	Neck, medial scapula, medial aspect arm and forearm into 4th, 5th digits	Distal medial forearm to hand and digits 4 and 5	Finger: abduction adduction flexors	Finger flexors

From Levin KH, Covington EC, Devereaux MW, et al. Neck and low back pain. Continuum (NY) 2001;7:1–205; with permission.

Paresthesia and hyperesthesia are generally dermatomal in distribution, with the greatest involvement often centered in the distal portion of the involved dermatome.

HOW DO PATIENTS WITH CERVICAL CANAL STENOSIS PRESENT?

Cervical stenosis may be clinically silent for long periods, sometimes throughout life. Although cervical stenosis and resultant myelopathy can be caused by many pathologic processes, including trauma with resultant hyperextension in the presence of congenital stenosis (a concern in contact sports) and central disk herniation, the most common cause is spondylosis (degeneration).[19] About 80% of people by age 50 and virtually 100% of people by age 70 have cervical spondylosis to some degree.[1]

About a midcervical canal sagittal diameter of 12 mm or less generally is associated with the development of myelopathy; larger dimensions do not rule out the possibility of developing myelopathy under some circumstances. Degenerative change with resultant osteophytes, bulging disks, facet joint hypertrophy, and thickened ligamentum flavuum, in combination with intermittent flexion-extension–mediated injury, can produce cervical myelopathy in the absence of dramatic cervical canal stenosis. In addition to myelopathy as a result of direct cord compression, there can be a compromise of perfusion in the distribution of the anterior spinal artery with resultant ischemic myelopathy.[20] Crandall and colleagues[21] described five distinct cord syndromes representing relatively advanced disease, as follows:

- Brown-Séquard syndrome (as a result of hemicord injury)
- Central cord syndrome, with motor and sensory deficits more marked in the upper extremities than the lower extremities
- Motor system syndrome resembling amyotrophic lateral sclerosis by virtue of lower motor neuron changes in the upper extremities and upper motor neuron changes in the lower extremities in the absence of significant sensory deficit

- Brachialgia and cord syndrome, characterized by upper extremity radicular distribution pain and an admixture of upper and lower motor neuron weakness in the extremities
- Transverse myelopathy, the most common, appearing suddenly or evolving from one of the preceding syndromes; all ascending and descending tracts are involved and sphincter involvement is common

These syndromes generally are not defined clearly early in the course of cervical myelopathy. Symptoms and signs often are subtle early on. Hyperreflexia and extensor plantar responses (Babinski sign), minimal weakness in the lower extremities, and a subtle gait disturbance are common early signs.[19] Occipital headache and cervicalgia commonly are associated with cervical spondylosis, but the cause-and-effect relationship remains uncertain because cervical spondylotic myelopathy often occurs in the absence of head and neck pain. Leg discomfort, including burning paresthesia, can occur and may be confused with sciatica. Combined cervical and lumbar spondylosis can produce overlapping symptoms and signs of cervical myelopathy and cauda equina syndrome/lumbosacral radiculopathy, leading to difficulties in diagnosis. Lhermitte's symptom/sign may be observed early in some patients. Subtle clumsiness and paresthesia in the hands may be the only initial symptoms and can be confused with median and ulnar mononeuropathies.[22] Vertebral basilar transient ischemic events may occur in association with head rotation and resultant vertebral artery compromise.[9]

The differential diagnosis of cervical spondylotic myelopathy includes multiple sclerosis, transverse myelitis, progressive motor neuron disease, subacute combined degeneration, syringomyelia, and cord tumors. Generally speaking, these diagnostic possibilities can be distinguished from each other by the history, physical/neurologic examination, and selected diagnostic tests (MRI, electromyography, and nerve conduction study). "The hard part" is the initial early recognition of an evolving myelopathy.

WHAT IS WHIPLASH AND HOW SHOULD IT BE TREATED?

There are few spinal disorders that are more controversial and contentious than whiplash. Approximately 1 million whiplash (flexion-extension) neck injuries occur annually in the United States, 85% of which are the result of rear-end automobile collisions.[1,23] In contrast to most other injuries, there is a female preponderance of 2:1.[1,23] Some authors have speculated that this gender difference reflects a woman's smaller, less muscular, neck.[1,23]

Whiplash can result in a variety of symptoms and neurologic signs based in part on the velocity of the impact and in part on the presence or absence of underlying cervical spine disease. Myelopathy, radiculopathy, brachial plexopathy, and upper extremity motor neuropathy all can occur. Most patients presenting for evaluation at some point after injury have less specific symptoms, however, and few "hard" signs on examination. Localized neck pain, neck stiffness, occipital headache, dizziness in all of its forms, malaise, and fatigue are common whiplash symptoms.[1,24] Localized paracervical tenderness to palpation, reduced range of neck motion, and weakness of the upper extremities secondary to guarding are common findings.

Although most patients with myofascial symptoms recover in several months, 20% to 40% complain of debilitating symptoms for extended periods, sometimes years.[1] This "late" or chronic whiplash syndrome defined as pain beyond 6 months postinjury, often is mired in litigation.

Mechanisms suggested for chronic whiplash syndrome include subtle lesions of cervical facet joints,[25] cervical ligament strain,[26] disk protrusions, disturbance of vestibular brain stem function, and reduced cerebral perfusion.[24] Some studies suggest psychosocial factors, including litigation, play a major role in chronic whiplash.[1,27,28] A prospective control study from Lithuania, where there is no legal tort system, revealed that late whiplash syndrome does not exist.[29]

Extensive diagnostic testing generally is not necessary in patients with acute whiplash injury. Most patients receive cervical spine x-rays, particularly if taken to an emergency department after the accident. The yield from diagnostic testing for patients with chronic whiplash injury is low, and testing should be avoided in the absence of neurologic findings.

Conservative treatment for acute whiplash injury is the treatment of choice.[30] Rest, avoidance of pain, NSAIDs, perhaps muscle relaxants, and a short course of pain medication all can be helpful. A soft cervical collar for acute whiplash injury can be helpful; however, continuous long-term usage should be avoided.

Treatment for chronic whiplash syndrome also should be conservative. Medications used in the treatment of chronic pain, including serotonin reuptake inhibitors, may have a role. As with any chronic pain syndrome, the persistent use of reactive pain medication is to be avoided. In a subset of late whiplash patients who had facet joint–generated pain as determined by diagnostic blocks with a local anesthetic, percutaneous radiofrequency neurotomy proved beneficial.[31,32]

WHAT IS THE ROLE OF THE FACET JOINT IN NECK (SPINE) PAIN?

The role of the facet (zygapophyseal) joint in the pathogenesis of neck (and low back) pain is controversial.[1,33–35] The lack of localizing specificity of neck pain from the history and physical examination can contribute to this confusion. Although degeneration of the facet joint probably produces pain in some, every clinician is aware of the patient with severe degenerative spine/facet joint disease with no associated pain. Nonetheless, there still is considerable clinical evidence supporting the existence of the facet syndrome. Certainly, degenerative changes in the facet joint can contribute to spinal stenosis and resultant radiculopathy and in the case of the cervical spine, myelopathy. Traumatic capsular tears and age-related degenerative changes are thought to be the most common causes of facet joint–mediated pain.[35] Facet joint disruption may also be at the basis of pain for at least some patients with a whiplash injury.[36] The pain of the facet joint syndrome is generally localized over the affected joint. It is aggravated by extension of the spine. Although the pain is often relatively localized, on occasion it may radiate into the ipsilateral upper extremity. Therefore, the facet joint syndrome is included in the differential diagnosis of radiculopathy. A diagnostic block into the facet joint with a local anesthetic may help to isolate the source of pain. The value of therapeutic facet joint injection remains controversial.[37,38] However, following a diagnostic block with an anesthetic, percutaneous radiofrequency neurotomy of the medial branch of the cervical posterior ramus that innervates the facet joint has been offered as a useful treatment for patients with suspect facet joint arthritis.[32]

CAN FIBROMYALGIA PRESENT AS NECK AND SHOULDER PAIN?

Fibromyalgia is a chronic widespread musculoskeletal pain syndrome of unknown etiology, present by definition for at least 3 months. At its zenith, it usually is generalized to such a degree that it is not confused easily with pain secondary to a localized spine disorder. Early in the evolution of fibromyalgia, however, neck, shoulder, and low back pain may predominate. In addition to aching pain, symptoms include depression, fatigue, malaise, stiffness, disturbed sleep, headache, paresthesia, and irritable bowel.[35]

There is a considerable debate as to whether fibromyalgia is a specific entity or a manifestation of an underlying psychologic disorder including stress and depression.[1] Studies have shown, however, several chemical and physiologic changes suggesting a possible biologic basis, which include increased levels of substance P in serum and cerebrospinal fluid, decreased cerebrospinal fluid tryptophan level, and decreased serum and platelet serotonin levels.[39] The sleep electroencephalogram/ polysomnogram in these patients often reveals an alpha delta sleep pattern (as also can be seen in depression), indicating reduction of the deep sleep phase during which muscle restoration ordinarily occurs.

Examination of patients with fibromyalgia shows widely distributed tender points to light palpation. Diagnosis, according to criteria established by the American College of Rheumatology, requires 11 such tender points. Fibromyalgia is a diagnosis of exclusion. Specific rheumatologic conditions, such as the spondyloarthropathies and polymyalgia rheumatica, need to be considered. Treatment options include tricyclic antidepressants, NSAIDs, a program of regular exercise, periods of rest, massage, and possibly at times the application of local heat.

HOW IS AN ACUTE CERVICAL RADICULOPATHY CAUSED BY DISK HERNIATION/SPONDYLOSIS BEST MANAGED?

Treatment approaches to cervical radiculopathy are similar to lumbar radiculopathy (see the article on low back pain elsewhere in this issue). As with nonspecific acute spine pain, acute radiculopathy is often a self-limiting disorder with recovery expected over a period of weeks.[40,41] The initial management of acute radiculopathy need not differ from the treatment of acute nonradiating neck pain. This is particularly true in the absence of significant weakness. In this setting, relative quiescence with avoidance of activities that increase pain, medications (NSAIDs and pain medication), and the use of a soft cervical collar situationally (I often recommend wearing it reversed to allow for neck flexion and more comfort) can help. Some authors advocate a brief course of oral corticosteroids. Corticosteroids and NSAIDs should not be used in combination.

If the patient has significant weakness within a given cervical myotome, a prompt workup is usually indicated, including MRI of the cervical spine and possibly electromyography and nerve conduction study of the symptomatic upper extremity and ipsilateral paracervical muscles. Spontaneous recovery without surgery can be expected in 75% to 80% of all patients with cervical disk herniation.[42] Spontaneous recovery is in part a result of the absorption and shrinkage of the displaced disk material with resultant reduction of nerve root impingement.[16,42]

As with lumbar radiculopathies, determining when a patient should undergo surgical treatment for a disk herniation causing a radiculopathy is often challenging. There are no hard and fast rules. As discussed in the management of lumbosacral radiculopathies, an important indicator for surgery is the presence of significant weakness in a group of muscles (myotome) innervated by the impinged nerve root. In addition, if there is evidence of cervical myelopathy in a patient with cervical radiculopathy, immediate surgical decompression may be appropriate.

As with the management of lumbar radiculopathy, there are many widely used treatments that are not fully scientifically validated, including oral glucocorticoids, epidural blocks, selected nerve blocks, and acupuncture. Cervical manipulation, chiropractic or otherwise, is to be avoided.

IS CHIROPRACTIC MANIPULATION USEFUL IN TREATMENT OF NECK PAIN?

Chiropractic manipulation for the treatment of spine symptoms including neck pain is a common practice in the United States. Chiropractic treatment is approved by many insurance companies. Chiropractic is the invention of Daniel David Palmer in 1895. At that time, he was a dry goods grocer and part-time magnetotherapist. Chiropractic is based on a theory that all disease is a result of interference with the body's "innate intelligence" by misaligned vertebrae. Some studies have shown marginal benefit for low back symptoms.[17,19,21] However, with regard to chiropractic manipulation of the cervical spine, there is risk with little if any reward.[1,10,43–45] Risks include cervical myelopathy, cervical radiculopathy, and vertebrobasilar artery distribution strokes. Neck manipulation, particularly when it includes a combination of rotation and tilting, stretches the contralateral vertebral artery, producing a sheering force on the segment of the artery at the level of the atlantoaxial joint.[9] This force may result in dissection of the vertebral artery, with resultant potential occlusion of the lumen, thrombus formation, and embolization. The frequency of vertebrobasilar artery distribution strokes is argued, but it is probably more common than reported.[10] Given the risk of complications in the absence of well-documented benefit, chiropractic cervical manipulation should be avoided.[10,46]

ARE THERE ANY OTHER COMPLEMENTARY AND ALTERNATIVE MEDICAL TREATMENTS THAT MIGHT BE OF VALUE FOR PATIENTS WITH NECK PAIN?

There are a variety of complementary and alternative medical (CAM) treatments available for most medical/neurologic conditions. With regard to the treatment of neck pain, the most common CAM treatments, other than chiropractic manipulation, are massage therapy and acupuncture. There is some evidence to suggest that therapeutic massage may be of value in patients with neck pain, in particular nonradiating neck pain.[47] Although scientific validation is limited, massage is safe and appears to reduce pain in at least some patients.

The effectiveness of acupuncture remains controversial. Some studies demonstrated that acupuncture may be more effective than no treatment or sham treatment.[47]

Both massage therapy and acupuncture are generally safe.

Although there is controversy, I generally recommend massage relatively early in the course of neck pain if the patient is not improving. I generally do not recommend acupuncture.

REFERENCES

1. Levin KH, Covington EC, Devereaux MW, et al. Neck and low back pain. Continuum (NY) 2001;7:1–205.
2. Rubin DI. Epidemiology and risk factors for spine pain. Neurol Clin 2007;25: 353–71.
3. Cote P, Cassidy JD, Carroll L, et al. The Saskatchewan health and back pain survey: the prevalence of neck pain and related disability in Saskatchewan adults. Spine 1998;1689–98.
4. Croft PR, Lewis M, Papgeogiou AC, et al. Risk factors for neck pain: a longitudinal study in the general population. Pain 2001;93:317–25.
5. Anderson G. The epidemiolgy of spinal disorders. In: Frymoyer JW, editor. The adult spine: principles and practices. New York: Raven Press; 1991. p. 107–46.

6. Cote P, Cassidy JD, Carrole J, et al. The factors associated with neck pain and its related disability in the Saskatchewan population. Spine 2000;25:1109–17.
7. Cassidy JD, Cote P, Carroll L, et al. The prevalence of neck pain and associated factors: a population-based study from North American. Denmark: E.C.U. Convention; 1999. p. 17–8.
8. Harder S, Veilleux M, Suissa S, et al. The effect of socio-demographic and crash-related factors on the prognosis of whiplash. J Clin Epidemiol 1998;51:377–84.
9. Brown B, Tatlow W. Radiographic studies of the vertebral arteries in cadavers: effects of position and traction on the head. Neuroradiology 1963;81:80–8.
10. Devereaux MW. The neuro ophthalmologic complications of cervical manipulations. J Neuroophthalmol 2000;20:236–9.
11. Deyo RA, Cherkin D, Conrad D, et al. Cost, controversy, crisis: low back pain and the health of the pubic. Annu Rev Public Health 1992;12:141–55.
12. Anonymous. Scientific approach to the assessment and management of activity-related spinal disorders: a monograph for clinicians. Report of the Quebec task force on spinal disorders. Spine 1987;12:S1–59.
13. Deyo RA. Plain roentgenography for low-back pain: finding needles in a hay stack. Arch Intern Med 1989;150:1125–8.
14. Boden SD, Davis DO, Dina TS, et al. Abnormal magnetic resonance scans of the lumbar spine in asymptomatic subjects: a prospective investigation. J Bone Joint Surg Am 1990;72:403–8.
15. Jensen M, Brant-Zawadzki M, Obuchowski N, et al. Magnetic resonance imaging of the lumbar spine in people without back pain. N Engl J Med 1994;331:69–73.
16. Ahmed M, Modic MT. Neck and low back pain: neuroimaging. Neurol Clin 2007; 25:439–71.
17. Algren B, Garfen S. Cervical radiculopathy. Orthop Clin North Am 1996;27: 253–63.
18. Radhakrishnan K, Litchy W, O'Fallon W, et al. Epidemiology of cervical radiculopathy: a population-based study from Rochester, Minnesota, 1976 through 1990. Brain 1994;117:325–35.
19. McCormack B, Weinstein P. Cervical spondylosis: an update. West J Med 1996; 165:43–51.
20. Fehlings M, Skaf G. A review of the pathophysiology of cervical spondylotic myelopathy with insights for potential novel mechanisms drawn from traumatic spinal cord injury. Spine 1998;23:2730–7.
21. Crandall P, Batzdorf U, Conrad D, et al. Cervical spondylotic myelopathy. J Neurosurg 1996;25:57–66.
22. Voskuhl R, Hinton R. Sensory impairment in the hands secondary to spondylotic compression of the cervical spinal cord. Arch Neurol 1990;47:309–11.
23. Evans R. Some observations. Neurol Clin 1992;10:975–97.
24. Kasch H, Bech FW, Stengaard-Pedersen K, et al. Development pain and neurologic complaints after whiplash. Neurology 2003;60:743–61.
25. Winkelstein BA, Nightingale RW, Richardson WJ, et al. The cervical facet capsule and its role in whiplash injury: a biomechanical investigation. Spine 2000;25:1238–46.
26. Ivancic PC, Pearson AM, Pajabi MM, et al. Injury of the anterior longitudinal ligament during whiplash simulation. Eur Spine J 2004;13:61–8.
27. Peterson D. A study of 249 patients with litigated claims of injury. Neurologist 1998;4:131–7.
28. Cassidy JD, Carol LJ, Coté P, et al. Effect of eliminating compensation for pain and suffering on the outcome of insurance claims for whiplash injury. N Engl J Med 2000;342:1179–86.

29. Obelieiene D, Schrader H, Bovim G, et al. Pain after whiplash: a prospective controlled inception cohort study. J Neurol Neurosurg Psychiatr 1999;66:279–82.

30. Carette S. Whiplash injury and chronic neck pain [editorial]. N Engl J Med 1994; 330:1083–4.

31. Barnsley L, Lord SM, Wallis BJ, et al. Lack of effect of intraarticular corticosteroids for chronic pain in the cervical zygapophyseal joints. N Engl J Med 1994;330: 1047–50.

32. Lord S, Barnsley L, Wallis BJ, et al. Percutaneous radio-frequency neurotomy for chronic cervical zygapophyseal-joint pain. N Engl J Med 1996;335:1721–6.

33. Jackson R. The facet syndrome: myth or reality? Clin Orthop 1992;279:110–21.

34. Schwarzer AC, Aprill CN, Derby R, et al. Clinical features of patients with pain stemming from the lumbar zygapophyseal joints: is the lumbar facet syndrome a clinical entity? Spine 1994;19:1132–7.

35. Meleger AL, Krivickas LS. Neck and back pain: musculoskeletal disorders. Neurol Clin 2007;25:419–38.

36. Lord SM, Barnsley L, Wallis BJ, et al. Chronic cervical zygapophyseal joint pain after whiplash: a placebo-controlled prevalence study. Spine 1996;21:1737–45.

37. Nelemens PJ, Bie RA, de Vet HCW, et al. Injection therapy for subacute and chronic benign low back pain. Cochrane Database Syst Rev 2000;2:CD001824.

38. Niemisto L, Kalso E, Malmivaara A, et al. Cochrane Collaboration Back Review Group. Radio frequency denervation for neck and back pain: a systematic review within the framework of the Cochrane Collaboration Back Review Group. Spine 2003;28:1877–88.

39. Russell I. Advances in fibromyalgia: possible role for central neurochemicals. Am J Med Sci 1998;316:377–84.

40. Persson J, Moritz W, Brandt L, et al. Cervical radiculopathy: pain, muscle weakness and sensory loss in patients with cervical radiculopathy treated with surgery, physiotherapy or cervical collar: a prospective controlled study. Eur Spine J 1997; 6:256–66.

41. Deyo RA, Weinstein JN. Low back pain. N Engl J Med 2001;344:363–9.

42. Fager CA. Observations on spontaneous recovery from intervertebral disc herniation. Surg Neurol 1994;42:282–6.

43. Hurwitz EL, Aker PD, Adams AH, et al. Manipulation and mobilization of the cervical spine. Spine 1996;21:1746–60.

44. Gross AR, Hoving JL, Haines TA, et al. Cervical overview group. Manipulation and mobilization for mechanical neck disorders. Cochrane Database Syst Rev 2006;3.

45. Ernst E, Canter PH. A systematic review of spinal manipulation. J R Soc Med 2006;99:192–6.

46. Barr J. Point of view. Spine 1996;21:1759–60.

47. Cherkin DC, Sherman KJ, Deyo RA, et al. A review of the evidence for the effectiveness, safety, and cost of acupuncture, massage therapy, and spinal manipulation for back pain. Ann Intern Med 2003;138:898–906.

Entrapment and Compressive Neuropathies

Barbara E. Shapiro, MD, PhD*, David C. Preston, MD

KEYWORDS

• Entrapment neuropathy • Compressive neuropathy

Entrapment and compressive neuropathies of the upper and lower extremities are frequently encountered disorders in the office.[1–3] Early in their course, they may be mistaken for more proximal lesions of the plexus or nerve roots, orthopedic disorders, or occasionally central nervous system disorders. Certain clinical clues in the history and examination, however, often will suggest the correct diagnosis, aided by appropriate electrodiagnostic (EDX) and imaging studies when indicated. Some of the more common neuropathies are discussed, along with suggestions regarding testing and treatment.

UPPER EXTREMITY
Carpal Tunnel Syndrome

Case vignette
A 34-year-old right-handed woman described intermittent pain of the right hand and wrist with tingling of the index and middle fingers. Symptoms had been present for 6 months, often awakening her from sleep at night. She also noted aching in her arm extending into the shoulder. Symptoms worsened while holding a telephone or book, or driving. Shaking out her hand or placing it under warm running water offered minimal relief of symptoms. She had difficulty buttoning her shirt and opening jars, and reported dropping things from her hands. Neurologic examination showed decreased light touch sensation over the finger pads of the right index and middle fingers, with slight weakness of thumb abduction. There was a Tinel's sign at the wrist, and Phalen's maneuver produced paresthesias in the right middle finger after 30 seconds of wrist flexion.

What is carpal tunnel syndrome, and what are its clinical manifestations?
Carpal tunnel syndrome (CTS), or median neuropathy across the wrist, is the most common entrapment neuropathy in the upper extremity. It is more prevalent in women

Neurological Institute, University Hospitals Case Medical Center, 11100 Euclid Avenue, Cleveland, OH 44106-5040, USA
* Corresponding author.
E-mail address: bes002@aol.com (B.E. Shapiro).

Med Clin N Am 93 (2009) 285–315
doi:10.1016/j.mcna.2008.09.009
0025-7125/08/$ – see front matter © 2009 Elsevier Inc. All rights reserved.

than men.[4] Although symptoms are usually bilateral, they are almost without exception more prominent in the dominant hand, as in this patient. Paresthesias are frequently present in the distribution of the median nerve, including the medial thumb, index, middle and lateral fourth fingers. Sensory loss may be noted in the same distribution, notably sparing the thenar eminence, which is supplied by the palmar cutaneous sensory branch of the median nerve that comes off proximal to the carpal tunnel (**Fig. 1**). Although sensory symptoms predominate, in more advanced cases, thenar wasting with weakness of thumb abduction and opposition may be present, both mediated by the distal median nerve. Tinel's sign (paresthesias radiating into the fingers with tapping over the median nerve at the wrist) is present in over half the cases, although this is a nonspecific sign. In contrast, paresthesias produced with the Phalen's maneuver (holding the wrist in a flexed position) are more sensitive than the Tinel's sign, and more specific to CTS, commonly producing paresthesias in the middle or index fingers after 1 or 2 minutes of wrist flexion.[5]

Neurologic examination may show decreased light touch sensation over the finger pads of the index and middle fingers, with slight weakness of thumb abduction. There may be a Tinel's sign at the wrist, and Phalen's maneuver may produce paresthesias in the median innervated fingers after several seconds of wrist flexion.

Symptoms often are provoked during sleep, when persistent wrist flexion or extension leads to increased pressure in the carpal tunnel, resulting in nerve ischemia and paresthesias. Patients often have difficulty buttoning their shirt or opening jars, or describe suddenly dropping things from their hand. Intermittent wrist pain and paresthesias affecting the index and middle fingers, worsened by movements that involve wrist flexion or extension, such as holding a book or telephone, or driving a car, are suggestive of CTS.[3] Arm discomfort extending into the shoulder is not uncommon, although neck pain should not be seen unless there is a superimposed problem, such as cervical radiculopathy.

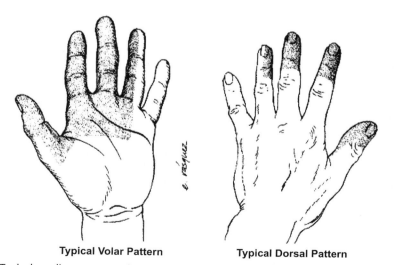

Typical Volar Pattern   **Typical Dorsal Pattern**

Fig. 1. Typical median nerve territory sensory loss pattern in carpal tunnel syndrome. Note that the thenar eminence is spared, supplied by the palmar cutaneous sensory branch of the median nerve. (*From* Stopford JSB. The variation in distribution of the cutaneous nerves of the hand and digits. J Anat 1918;53:14–25.)

What are the causes and pathophysiology of carpal tunnel syndrome?
Most cases of CTS are idiopathic, a result of repeated stress to connective tissue. Patients often report activities that involve repetitive hand use, such as typing on a keyboard.[6] Individuals with a narrow carpal canal are more prone to entrapment.[7] Other medical conditions that predispose to CTS include hypothyroidism, rheumatoid arthritis, diabetes,[8] and various inflammatory, infectious, and systemic disorders such as Lyme disease, sarcoid, and amyloidosis. Routine blood screening for these disorders in patients who have CTS is generally unrevealing, however, unless other symptoms suggestive of systemic disease are present. Pregnancy and hemodialysis also are associated with an increased risk for CTS. Rarely, mass or infiltrating lesions of the carpal tunnel can be seen, such as ganglion cysts, neurofibromas, schwannomas, or arteriovenous malformations.

What is the differential diagnosis of carpal tunnel syndrome?
The differential diagnosis of CTS includes C6-C7 radiculopathy, brachial plexopathy, and proximal median neuropathy. Cervical radiculopathy generally is accompanied by neck pain, and in C6 or C7 radiculopathy, biceps or triceps reflexes are hypoactive or absent. Brachial plexopathy may be accompanied by weakness outside of the median nerve distribution, and reflex changes also may be present. Proximal median neuropathy is rare, accompanied by sensory loss over the thenar eminence, which is not seen in CTS, and weakness of proximal median innervated muscles, such as the long flexors of the thumb, index and middle fingers, and in some cases, arm pronation.

How is Carpal Tunnel Syndrome Diagnosed?

If CTS is suspected clinically, EDX studies, including nerve conduction studies (NCSs) and electromyography (EMG), are helpful in confirming the diagnosis and evaluating for other disorders such as cervical radiculopathy, brachial plexopathy, or proximal median neuropathy that can mimic CTS.[3,9,10] In most cases of CTS, EDX studies easily demonstrate demyelination of the median nerve in the form of conduction velocity slowing across the wrist, resulting in prolonged distal median motor and sensory latencies. If there is secondary axonal loss, median sensory and motor amplitudes are reduced or absent. In mild cases of CTS, however, routine median motor and sensory NCSs may be normal, and the diagnosis may be missed in up to 25% of patients. Referral to an EDX laboratory where sensitive internal comparison studies can be done substantially increases the yield in making the diagnosis of CTS. In these studies, the distal latency of the median nerve is compared with that of an adjacent nerve of similar length and caliber, stimulating and recording across the carpal tunnel. Any significant difference in latency implies a demyelinating lesion along the median nerve. Common internal comparison studies include median versus ulnar palmar mixed nerve studies; median versus ulnar distal motor latencies recording the second lumbrical and interossei respectively; median versus ulnar digit four sensory latencies; and median versus radial digit one sensory latencies.[11–14]

Imaging studies, especially high resolution sonography,[15–17] have been proposed as sensitive diagnostic tools in clinically suspected CTS, although EDX studies remain the gold standard.

Mass lesions, however, especially should be evaluated in the rare patient who presents with prominent symptoms in the nondominant hand, with a palpable mass in the wrist or palm, or with a slowly progressive syndrome that does not wax and wane. In such cases, imaging with MRI or CT scan of the wrist is indicated to look for a structural lesion.

How is carpal tunnel syndrome treated?

Mild CTS often responds to conservative therapy, including removing causative factors, such as repetitive hand use, and applying a neutral wrist splint to the symptomatic hand, especially during sleep. A 1- to 2-week course of nonsteroidal anti-inflammatory medications may help reduce symptoms if there is no medical contraindication. If these measures do not reduce symptoms, a local corticosteroid injection adjacent to the carpal tunnel may be helpful.[18] Repeated injections beyond two to three injections may damage the flexor tendons, and are not recommended. Steroid injections are most useful only in mild cases, or as a temporizing measure, such as during pregnancy, or while treating a reversible medical condition, such as hypothyroidism. Surgical decompression is indicated in those patients who have severe wasting and weakness of the thumb abductors, persistent numbness or paresthesias, or in patients who have failed conservative measures or have ongoing denervation in the abductor pollicis brevis on EMG studies. Those patients who have more functional upper extremity limitation preoperatively may not do as well postoperatively.[19] Of course surgery also is indicated if a mass lesion is present, or in cases of acute CTS following local trauma. Surgery entails sectioning of the transverse carpal ligament to decompress the median nerve, either through a longitudinal incision from the wrist to the palm, or through endoscopic release. Endoscopic release affords a shorter recovery time,[20] yet the transverse carpal ligament is not visualized directly using this technique, which might result in an incomplete section or damage to the median nerve or other nearby structures.[21]

Ulnar Neuropathy at the Elbow

Case vignette

A 65-year-old man was referred for slowly progressive weakness of hand grip, accompanied by numbness and tingling of the right fourth and fifth fingers. He described pain in his arm and elbow. There was no neck or shoulder pain. Examination showed decreased light touch and pinprick sensation in the right fifth finger and medial hand, with moderate weakness of the intrinsic hand muscles. Deep tendon reflexes were normal. There was tenderness of the right ulnar nerve in the groove.

What is ulnar neuropathy at the elbow and what are its clinical manifestations?

Ulnar neuropathy at the elbow is the second most common entrapment of the upper extremity.[22] The most common cause of ulnar neuropathy at the elbow is chronic compression or stretch of the ulnar nerve in the elbow, either at the ulnar groove or more distally in the cubital tunnel.[4,22,23,24] Both present in a similar manner, with the slow progression of intrinsic hand muscle weakness, loss of grip and pinch strength, and wasting of the thenar and hypothenar eminences. In contrast to CTS, in which sensory symptoms predominate, patients may experience no sensory symptoms, despite sensory loss on examination. Elbow pain is common, in some patients radiating down the medial forearm and wrist. The ulnar nerve may be palpably enlarged and tender in the groove. Paresthesias may be provoked by flexing the elbow or applying pressure to the ulnar groove. Weakness of hand grip is common, because of weakness of the ulnar innervated intrinsic hand muscles. Thumb abduction, innervated by the median and radial nerves, is spared. Asking the patient to make a fist may reveal his or her inability to bury digits four and five in the palm, because of weakness of the ulnar innervated flexor digitorum profundus to digits four and five (**Fig. 2**). Sensory disturbance, when present, involves the dorsal and volar fifth finger, medial fourth finger, and dorsal and volar aspects of the medial hand. Sensory loss may extend just beyond the wrist crease. If there is altered sensation beyond the wrist crease into

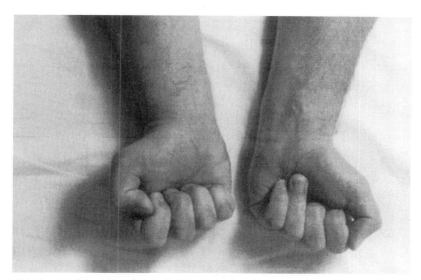

Fig. 2. Weakness of the ulnar flexor digitorum profundus. In ulnar neuropathy at the elbow, making a fist may result in the inability to completely flex the distal phalanx of the fourth and fifth digits because of weakness of the flexor digitorum profundus to digits four and five. The median-innervated flexor digitorum profundus to digits two and three is normal (affected hand shown at right.) (*From* Preston DC, Shapiro BE. Electromyography and neuromuscular disorders. 2nd edition. Philadelphia: Elsevier Butterworth Heinemann; 2005; with permission.)

the medial forearm, however, a more proximal lesion such as in the brachial plexus or C8-T1 nerve roots should be investigated.

Several classic hand postures may occur with ulnar neuropathy at the elbow. The most common, the Benediction posture, results in clawing of the fourth and fifth fingers, (hyperextension of the metacarpophalangeal joints and flexion of the interphalangeal joints of the second and third fingers **Fig. 3**, top). The fingers and thumb are held slightly abducted because of weakness of the interossei and adductor pollicis. The Wartenberg's sign results in abduction of the little finger with the hand at rest (**Fig. 3**, middle), making it difficult for patients to put their hand in their pocket without the little finger getting caught outside. The Froment's sign occurs when the patient is asked to use the thumb and index finger to pinch an object (**Fig. 3**, bottom). Patients flex the thumb and index fingers (median innervated), akin to an "OK" sign, because of weakness of the ulnar intrinsic hand muscles that does not allow them to extend the proximal and distal interphalangeal joints of the thumb and index fingers.

What are the causes and pathophysiology of ulnar neuropathy at the elbow?

Ulnar neuropathy at the elbow usually occurs as a result of chronic mechanical compression or stretch, either at the groove or at the cubital tunnel. The underlying pathophysiology may be demyelination or axonal loss. At the groove, most cases are caused by external compression and repeated trauma, although rare cases of ulnar neuropathy at the groove are caused by ganglia, tumors, fibrous bands, or accessory muscles. So-called tardy ulnar palsy may be seen as a result of elbow fracture, often years before, with subsequent arthritic changes of the elbow joint. In addition, chronic minor trauma and compression, such as chronic leaning on the elbow, can exacerbate or cause ulnar neuropathy at the groove. Ulnar neuropathy at

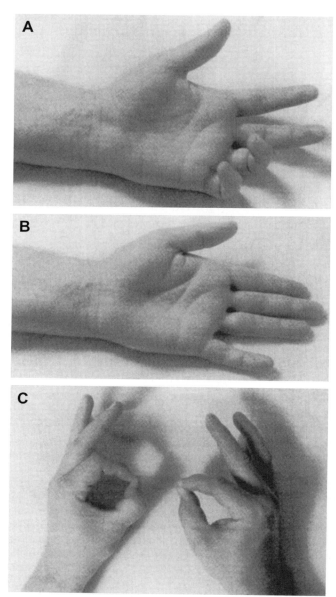

Fig. 3. The Benediction posture results in clawing of the fourth and fifth fingers (*A*), while the fingers and thumb are held slightly abducted because of weakness of the interossei and adductor pollicis. The Wartenberg' sign (*B*) results in abduction of the little finger with the hand at rest, because of preferential weakness of the third palmar interosseous muscle, making it difficult to adduct the little finger. The Froment's sign (*C*) occurs when the patient is asked to use the thumb and index finger to pinch an object. Because of weakness of the ulnar intrinsic hand muscles, patients cannot extend the proximal and distal interphalangeal joints of the thumb and index fingers, and flex the thumb and index fingers (median innervated) to compensate, akin to an "OK" sign. (*From* Preston DC, Shapiro BE. Electromyography and neuromuscular disorders. 2nd edition. Philadelphia: Elsevier Butterworth Heinemann; 2005; with permission.)

the groove also can be seen in patients who have been immobilized because of surgery or who sustain compression during anesthesia or coma. Some contend that repeated subluxation of the ulnar nerve out of the groove, such as during elbow flexion, also leads to ulnar neuropathy.

The cubital tunnel, which is just distal to the groove, is the other major site of compression of the ulnar nerve in the region of the elbow. Although some use the term cubital tunnel syndrome to refer to all lesions of the ulnar nerve around the elbow, it more properly denotes compression of the ulnar nerve under the humeral–ulnar aponeurosis. Some individuals have congenitally tight cubital tunnels that predispose them to compression. Repeated and persistent flexion stretches the ulnar nerve and increases the pressure in the cubital tunnel, leading to subsequent ulnar neuropathy.

What is the differential diagnosis of ulnar neuropathy at the elbow?

The differential diagnosis of ulnar neuropathy at the elbow includes C8-T1 radiculopathy, lower trunk or medial cord brachial plexopathy, or rare cases of ulnar nerve entrapment in the forearm or wrist. Patients who have cervical radiculopathy generally report neck pain radiating into the arm, with sensory disturbance. In both cervical radiculopathy and lower trunk/medial cord brachial plexopathies, which are far less common, weakness is seen in ulnar and nonulnar innervated muscles, such as the thumb abductors (median innervated) and finger extensors (radial innervated), with sensory changes that extend into the medial forearm.

How is ulnar neuropathy at the elbow diagnosed?

In suspected ulnar neuropathy at the elbow, EDX studies can help confirm the diagnosis, and exclude other diagnoses such as cervical radiculopathy or brachial plexopathy. Motor NCSs may demonstrate focal demyelination in the form of conduction block or conduction velocity slowing across the elbow, yielding a definitive diagnosis of ulnar neuropathy at the elbow.[25] If these are not seen, short segmental stimulation studies on the ulnar nerve across the elbow may help localize the lesion either at the groove or the cubital tunnel, which may have implications for the best surgical approach.[22] Sensory and mixed ulnar NCSs across the elbow also may increase the yield of identifying focal slowing in some patients. In many patients who have ulnar neuropathy at the elbow, focal slowing or conduction block cannot be demonstrated, because the underlying pathophysiology is axonal loss. In such cases, findings on needle EMG can localize only the lesion to at or above the take off to the most proximal muscle affected on EMG, although in practical terms the lesion is nearly always at the elbow, either in the groove or the cubital tunnel. EDX studies also are used to look for evidence of a C8-T1 radiculopathy or lower trunk/medial cord brachial plexopathy.

How is ulnar neuropathy at the elbow treated?

Conservative measures are tried first.[26] Activities that require repetitive or sustained elbow flexion should be discontinued, and the patient should be advised to avoid leaning on the elbow. A simple elbow pad may be helpful, or an elbow splint can be applied to prevent sustained elbow flexion.[27] If there is no improvement with conservative measures, especially in a patient who has progressive weakness and wasting of the hand, surgery is indicated.[28,29] Surgical options include decompression of the cubital tunnel, submuscular transposition of the ulnar nerve, and medial epicondylectomy.[30] Although submuscular transposition has the best success rate, it also has the greatest morbidity,[31] including the risk of nerve devascularization. If the lesion is localized to the ulnar groove, transposition generally is indicated. If the lesion can be localized precisely to the cubital tunnel, however, some believe that simple decompression may be optimal.[31–33] Some studies have shown more favorable outcomes in patients who have demyelination, either conduction block or conduction velocity slowing across the elbow.[34] Prognosis is poorest in older individuals, those who have exacerbating medical conditions such as diabetes, or in those in whom symptoms have been present for over a year.[30]

Ulnar Neuropathy at the Wrist

Case vignette

A 24-year-old right-handed man complained of progressive wasting and loss of grip strength of the right hand. He was an avid bicyclist, often bicycling over 20 miles a day. Examination revealed atrophy of the intrinsic hand muscles, most marked in the first dorsal interosseous, with weakness of the abductor digiti minimi and interossei muscles on the right. The thumb abductors and long flexors of digits four and five were strong. There was no tenderness of the ulnar nerve in the groove. Deep tendon reflexes and sensation in the upper extremities were normal.

What is ulnar neuropathy at the wrist and what are its clinical manifestations?

Four clinical presentations of ulnar neuropathy at the wrist are described, depending on the location of the lesion.[35] The first two subtypes are purely motor. In the first subtype, muscles innervated by the deep palmar motor branch are involved, including the interossei, adductor pollicis, and third and fourth lumbricals. In the second subtype, the lesion involves the deep palmar motor branch and the hypothenar muscles. These purely motor subtypes are the most common, accounting for over 75% of all cases of ulnar neuropathy at the wrist. Because of the lack of sensory findings, these patients often are confused with early amyotrophic lateral sclerosis. In the third subtype, there is weakness of hypothenar and deep palmar motor innervated muscles and sensory loss in the medial fourth and volar fifth digits. The fourth subtype presents with isolated sensory loss over the medial fourth and volar fifth digits. Thus, if sensory loss is present, it spares the dorsal medial hand, innervated by the dorsal ulnar cutaneous sensory branch, which arises several centimeters proximal to the wrist.

What are the causes and pathophysiology of ulnar neuropathy at the wrist?

Activities or occupations that involve repetitive movement or force against the ulnar aspect of the wrist predispose to lesions here. This is especially true for bikers, or manual laborers who use tools that cause repetitive pressure against the hypothenar eminence. In these patients, the hypothenar area may become calloused at the compression site. Other risk factors include wrist fracture, trauma, distal musculotendinous fibrous arch, thrombosed ulnar artery, and mass lesions, often a ganglion cyst, within Guyon's canal.[36]

What is the differential diagnosis of ulnar neuropathy at the wrist?

Progressive weakness and wasting of the ulnar intrinsic hand muscles, sparing the median and proximal ulnar innervated muscles, are consistent with ulnar neuropathy at the wrist.

This is a rare condition, yet important to recognize, because it often is confused with early amyotrophic lateral sclerosis, especially in an older patient. In most cases, there are no sensory findings, although there may be sensory loss in digits four and five. Other disorders to consider in the differential diagnosis of ulnar neuropathy at the wrist include C8-T1 radiculopathy, lower trunk or medial cord brachial plexopathy, or rare cases of ulnar nerve entrapment in the forearm. Patients who have cervical radiculopathy generally report neck pain radiating into the arm, with sensory disturbance. In both cervical radiculopathy and lower trunk/medial cord brachial plexopathies, which are far less common, weakness is seen in ulnar and nonulnar innervated muscles, such as the thumb abductors (median innervated) and finger extensors (radial inner-vated), with sensory changes that extend into the medial forearm.

How is ulnar neuropathy at the wrist diagnosed?

If there is a strong suspicion of ulnar neuropathy at the wrist, MRI or CT scan of the wrist and hand are done to look for a structural lesion such as ganglion cyst or tumor. Referral for EDX testing is often instrumental in clarifying the diagnosis, while exclud-ing other disorders.[35] Testing should include ulnar motor NCSs recording both the ab-ductor digiti minimi and the first dorsal interosseous, because the pattern of abnormalities that emerges can help localize the lesion and determine which branches of the ulnar nerve are affected. The other helpful NCS to perform is the lumbrical–in-terossei distal latency comparison. Because the ulnar interossei are innervated by the deep palmar motor branch, this test may identify differential ulnar slowing at the wrist in lesions that involve the deep palmar motor branch.[37] Likewise, short segmen-tal inching studies of the ulnar nerve across the wrist, recording the first dorsal inter-osseous, can be extremely helpful in detecting abrupt changes in latency and amplitude, which help localize the lesion at the wrist.[38] Routine ulnar sensory NCSs recording the fifth digit and the dorsal ulnar cutaneous sensory NCS are done to help determine the level of the lesion. The needle EMG examination of suspected ulnar neuropathy at the wrist entails sampling deep palmar motor and hypothenar inner-vated muscles, proximal ulnar innervated muscles, and median and radial C8-T1 in-nervated muscles to confirm that the abnormalities are limited to ulnar muscles distal to the wrist and to exclude a cervical root or motor neuron lesion. In pure ulnar motor lesions, however, it remains difficult to exclude early amyotrophic lateral scle-rosis. Clinical correlation, questioning for possible risk factors for ulnar neuropathy at the wrist, and serial follow-up remain important.

How is ulnar neuropathy at the wrist treated?

Conservative treatment is usually successful in those patients who have an obvious risk factor, such as bicyclists and those who have work-related risk factors such as manual laborers. In mild cases, symptoms often improve simply by stopping the of-fending activity. Surgical exploration is indicated for any mass lesion in the canal, and in cases where symptoms are progressive or severe, or do not resolve when the offending activity is discontinued.[39]

Radial Neuropathy at the Spiral Groove

Case vignette

A 56-year-old man was referred for a right wrist drop. He awoke from a heavy sleep 4 weeks ago with complete inability to extend his right wrist or fingers, and numbness over the back of his hand between the thumb and index finger. There was no arm, neck, or shoulder pain. Neurologic examination showed complete paralysis of the right wrist and finger extensors. Finger abduction was normal strength when tested with the hand passively extended to the neutral position. Wrist and finger flexion and elbow flexion and extension were normal strength. Light touch sensation was reduced over the first dorsal web space between the thumb and index fingers, and extending into the proximal phalanges of the index, middle, and ring fingers. The right brachior-adialis reflex was absent.

What is radial neuropathy at the spiral groove, and what are its clinical manifestations?

The presentation of a complete wrist and finger drop, with numbness in the lateral dor-sal aspect of the hand, is most consistent with proximal radial neuropathy. The most common site of compression is at the spiral groove. Patients who have radial neuropathy at the spiral groove, also known as Saturday night palsy, present with the acute onset of a marked wrist and finger drop, accompanied by mild weakness of supination and elbow flexion from involvement of the supinator and brachioradialis muscles, respectively. As in this case, the weakness is accompanied by numbness in the lateral dorsal aspect of the hand. Elbow extension remains strong, because the branch to the triceps muscle comes off proximal to the spiral groove. Median and ulnar innervated muscles are also normal. Finger abduction should be tested with the hand held passively extended, by placing the hand on a flat surface, or it may appear to be weak.[40] There is altered sensation over the lateral dorsal hand and dorsal aspects of digits one through four, in the distribution of the superficial radial sensory nerve (**Fig. 4**). The triceps reflex remains intact, and the brachioradialis reflex is depressed or absent.

What are the causes and pathophysiology of radial neuropathy at the spiral groove?
At the spiral groove, the radial nerve lies juxtaposed to the humerus, making it prone to compression, especially following prolonged immobilization. This usually occurs when a person falls into a deep sleep with their arm draped over a chair or bench, such as while intoxicated. The prolonged immobilization leads to compression and demyelination of the radial nerve at the spiral groove. Less commonly, radial neuropathy at the

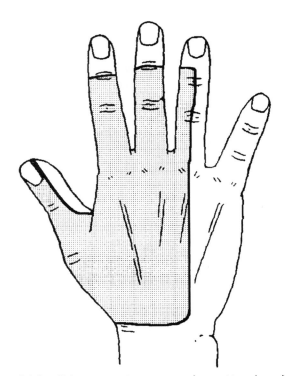

Fig. 4. Typical superficial radial nerve territory sensory loss pattern in radial neuropathy at the spiral groove. The superficial radial sensory nerve supplies sensation over the lateral dorsum of the hand and part of the thumb and dorsal proximal phalanges of the index, middle, and ring fingers. (*From* Preston DC, Shapiro BE. Electromyography and neuromuscular disorders. 2nd edition. Philadelphia: Elsevier Butterworth Heinemann; 2005; with permission.)

spiral groove occurs secondary to a humeral fracture, nerve infarction such as from vasculitis, or strenuous muscular effort.

What is the differential diagnosis of radial neuropathy at the spiral groove?
Radial neuropathies with resultant wrist drop can be caused by compression at other sites, including the axilla, or by entrapment of the posterior interosseous nerve branch of the radial nerve.[3,4,41] Radial neuropathy from prolonged compression may occur in the axilla, for example, in patients who use crutches incorrectly, applying prolonged pressure to the axilla. In this case, there is weakness of arm extension from involvement of the triceps; the triceps reflex is depressed or absent, and sensory disturbance extends from the lateral dorsal hand up into the posterior forearm and arm. None of these are seen in radial neuropathy at the spiral groove.

Other diagnoses that should be considered in a patient who has wrist and finger drop include posterior interosseous neuropathy (PIN), a lesion of the posterior cord of the brachial plexus, an unusual C7 radiculopathy, or a central lesion. These, however, usually can be excluded based on key clinical clues. For example, patients with PIN have a characteristic response to attempted wrist extension. The wrist deviates radially in extension because of the relative preservation of the extensor carpi radialis, which comes off proximal to the PIN, compared with the weak extensor carpi ulnaris, which comes off distal to the lesion. Furthermore, there is no reflex loss or cutaneous sensory loss in PIN, although there may be pain in the forearm from dysfunction of the deep sensory fibers supplying the interosseous membrane and joint capsules. A lesion in the posterior cord of the brachial plexus results in weakness of the deltoid and latissimus dorsi, in addition to radial innervated muscles. In C7 radiculopathy, radial and nonradial innervated C7 muscles are weak, including arm pronation and wrist flexion. Although a central lesion such as stroke can cause arm weakness with wrist and finger drop, there should be accompanying upper motor neuron signs such as spasticity and brisk reflexes.

How is radial neuropathy at the spiral groove diagnosed?
NCSs and EMG are useful for evaluating a patient who has a wrist and finger drop to identify a radial neuropathy, localize the lesion, assess its severity, and establish a prognosis by defining the underlying pathophysiology. EDX evaluation includes a radial motor study looking for evidence of a focal conduction block at the spiral groove or axonal loss. The superficial radial sensory nerve also is examined to look for evidence of axonal loss. If the clinical examination suggests weakness beyond the radial distribution, investigation for a more widespread neuropathy or brachial plexopathy is indicated. If a focal conduction block at the spiral groove cannot be demonstrated, the needle EMG examination may be helpful in distinguishing between PIN, radial neuropathy at the spiral groove, radial neuropathy in the axilla, a lesion of the posterior cord of the brachial plexus, or a C7 radiculopathy.

How is radial neuropathy at the spiral groove treated?
Radial neuropathies from external compression can be managed conservatively in nearly all cases. Most cases at the spiral groove occur from prolonged compression from a one-time episode. In patients who have a significant finger or wrist drop, a cock-up wrist splint is used to keep the wrist and fingers extended. Any offending factors are eliminated, such as improper use of crutches. Length of recovery depends on whether the compression results in demyelination or axonal loss. Patients who have demyelinative lesions usually recover well after several weeks. If the lesion involves axonal loss, recovery may take several months to over a year. Decisions regarding surgical treatment are more controversial. In patients who have progressive

symptoms, or those who have not responded to conservative treatment such as splinting and anti-inflammatory agents, surgical exploration may be advisable to exclude a structural lesion (eg, nerve sheath tumor, lipoma) or release a fibrous band.[42,43]

Suprascapular Neuropathy

Case vignette

A 32-year-old woman noted progressive atrophy of the left posterior shoulder. She described deep pain in her left posterior shoulder with progressive wasting over the scapula for the past year, giving the appearance of a hole in the scapular area. She frequently lifted weights at the gym, and was aware that lifting and external rotation of her left shoulder had become more difficult. There was no numbness, previous episodes of pain or weakness, or family history of similar problems. Examination showed prominent atrophy of the left posterior inferior scapular area, scapular winging, mild weakness of shoulder abduction, and moderate weakness of external rotation of the shoulder. Deep tendon reflexes and sensation were intact.

What is suprascapular neuropathy, and what are its clinical manifestations?

The classic presentation of suprascapular neuropathy is that of insidious onset of muscle wasting over the scapula with reduced ability to externally rotate or abduct the shoulder, and pain in the posterior shoulder. There often appears to be an indentation or hole in the suprascapular area (**Fig. 5**). Weight lifters are particularly prone to this entrapment, because of the repetitive movements about the shoulder. The most common site of suprascapular entrapment is at the suprascapular notch, beneath the transverse scapular ligament (**Fig. 6**). Because the suprascapular nerve is relatively immobile at the suprascapular notch and at its origin at the upper trunk, while the shoulder and scapula are quite mobile, repetitive movements about the shoulder

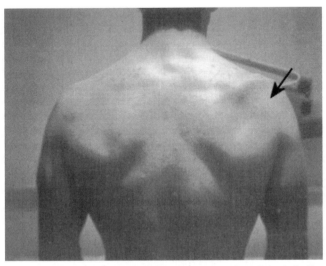

Fig. 5. Suprascapular neuropathy. Note the prominent atrophy of the inferior scapular area on the right. Suprascapular neuropathy results in weakness of shoulder abduction and external rotation, without any cutaneous sensory loss. (*From* Preston DC, Shapiro BE. Electromyography and neuromuscular disorders. 2nd edition. Philadelphia: Elsevier Butterworth Heinemann; 2005; with permission.)

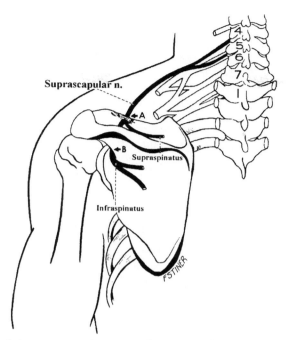

Fig. 6. Anatomy of the suprascapular nerve. The suprascapular nerve first runs under the suprascapular notch (A) to innervate the supraspinatus muscle. Sensory fibers then are given to the shoulder joint before the nerve wraps around the spinoglenoid notch (B) to supply the infraspinatus muscle. (*Adapted from* Haymaker W, Woodhal B. Peripheral nerve injuries. Philadelphia: W.B. Saunders; 1953; with permission.)

result in stretch and nerve injury. Less commonly, the nerve becomes entrapped more distally at the spinoglenoid notch (see **Fig. 6**).

Symptoms and signs depend on the site of nerve entrapment. Entrapment at the suprascapular notch results in prominent shoulder pain because of involvement of the deep sensory fibers to the glenoacromial and acromioclavicular joints. Patients describe deep, boring pain along the superior scapula radiating to the shoulder, exacerbated by shoulder movements, especially adduction of the extended arm. There may be tenderness at the suprascapular notch. Atrophy is recognized most easily over the infraspinatus, which is not covered by the trapezius. There is weakness of shoulder abduction and external rotation. Because other muscles also can perform abduction and external rotation of the shoulder, however, the patient may not notice these limitations. If the entrapment occurs more distally at the spinoglenoid notch, the syndrome is isolated to atrophy and weakness of the infraspinatus muscle.[44] Unlike the more proximal lesions, pain is absent, because the deep sensory fibers to the shoulder joint exit proximal to the motor branch to the infraspinatus.

What are the causes and pathophysiology of suprascapular neuropathy?
People working in certain professions, including professional volleyball players, baseball pitchers, and dancers, and activities that require repetitive movements about the shoulder, such as weight lifting, are associated with a high incidence of suprascapular nerve entrapment, likely as a consequence of repetitive movement of the scapular

that involves shoulder abduction and protraction.[45–50] In these professions, the clinical and EDX findings most often suggest a distal lesion at the spinoglenoid notch. Occasionally, the suprascapular nerve becomes entrapped because of mass lesions, including ganglion cysts (especially at the spinoglenoid notch), sarcomas, and metastatic carcinomas. Certain positions also are associated with suprascapular entrapment, such as positioning during surgical procedures, whereby patients are placed in a knee chest position with the scapula protracted. Other etiologic causes include direct trauma to the shoulder. Brachial neuritis may result in suprascapular neuropathy, although in this case weakness usually is not isolated to the suprascapular nerve, and the reflexes may be depressed.

What is the differential diagnosis of suprascapular neuropathy?

Shoulder weakness also can be caused by C5-C6 radiculopathy, brachial plexopathy, or a lesion of one of the nerves that comes off the upper trunk, or lateral or posterior cord of the brachial plexus. Cervical radiculopathy, however, usually is accompanied by neck pain, and in C5-C6 radiculopathy, one should see a depressed biceps and brachioradialis reflex, along with weakness in other C5-C6 innervated muscles, and sensory complaints. An upper brachial plexopathy, or neuropathy involving one of the nerves that comes off the upper trunk, or lateral or posterior cord, likewise should result in weakness beyond the distribution of the suprascapular nerve, and in some cases reflex and sensory changes. Other conditions that should be considered include rotator cuff injuries and other orthopedic conditions. Local orthopedic conditions may be difficult to differentiate clinically from suprascapular neuropathy. Although weakness should not be present, pain often prevents full muscle activation. Exacerbation of pain by palpation (other than at the suprascapular notch) or by passive shoulder movement (other than abduction and protraction of the shoulder) is unusual for suprascapular entrapment, and suggests an orthopedic problem.

How is suprascapular neuropathy diagnosed?

EDX testing is extremely useful to determine if abnormalities are restricted to the suprascapular innervated muscles, and evaluate for C5-C6 radiculopathy and brachial plexopathy. Motor NCSs of the suprascapular nerve may show reduced amplitudes, as these lesions typically involve axonal loss rather than demyelination. The needle EMG, however, easily demonstrates axonal loss. Both the supraspinatus and infraspinatus muscles should be sampled. In lesions at the suprascapular notch, both are abnormal. With spinoglenoid lesions, however, only the infraspinatus is involved. Other C5-C6 innervated muscles and the cervical paraspinal muscles are also sampled, to exclude a cervical radiculopathy or more widespread brachial plexus lesion. Because the suprascapular nerve has no cutaneous distribution, there is no corresponding sensory nerve to be recorded. Studies of the sensory nerves that pass through the upper trunk of the brachial plexus are performed to help exclude a more widespread plexus lesion. Imaging studies including CT or MRI scan of the shoulder should be done, especially in those patients who have no risk factors for developing a suprascapular neuropathy, to evaluate for a mass lesion.

How is suprascapular neuropathy treated?

Treatment often begins with a trial of conservative therapy, such as rest, physical therapy, and eliminating offending activities such as weightlifting. In one prospective series, lesions caused by traction or repetitive overuse responded equally well to nonoperative and surgical management.[51] Those who do not respond to conservative measures likely will require surgical exploration, especially those who have a ganglion cyst or other known compressive lesion.[24,46] Surgery entails exploration of the suprascapular notch or spinoglenoid notch, depending on results obtained with EDX and imaging studies,[51] with the goal being to decompress and release the nerve from the notch. One series found equally good results with open and arthroscopic treatment of ganglion cysts at the spinoglenoid notch.[51] Surgery is not indicated in those patients with suprascapular neuropathy secondary to brachial neuritis, who improve without surgery.

LOWER EXTREMITY
Peroneal Neuropathy at the Fibular Neck

Case vignette
A 20-year-old man developed a right foot drop after leaving a movie theater. He was unable to dorsiflex the right foot and toes, and described tingling over the top of the foot. He tended to slap the right foot when walking. Examination showed a thin young man who had severe weakness of the right ankle and toe dorsiflexors and ankle evertors. Ankle inversion appeared slightly weak. The remainder of his strength was normal, including ankle and toe plantar flexors, knee flexors and extensors, and proximal muscles around the hip. Deep tendon reflexes were intact throughout, including the ankle reflexes. There was decreased pinprick and cold over the dorsum of the right foot extending up to the lateral calf to just below the knee. There was no pain or Tinel's sign palpating the peroneal nerve across the fibular neck.

What is peroneal neuropathy at the fibular neck, and what are its clinical manifestations?
The classic presentation of a peroneal neuropathy at the fibular neck usually involves both the deep and superficial peroneal nerves (common peroneal neuropathy). This combination of deep and superficial peroneal neuropathy results in weakness of toe and ankle dorsiflexion, ankle eversion, and sensory disturbance over the dorsum of the foot and the lateral calf below the knee.[52–55] There may be pain and a Tinel's sign over the lateral fibular neck. Ankle inversion is spared, which is innervated by the tibial nerve. Ankle inversion, however, must be tested with the ankle in a dorsiflexed position, to avoid the mistaken impression that the tibialis posterior is weak.

What are the causes and pathophysiology of peroneal neuropathy at the fibular neck?
Peroneal neuropathy has several etiologies.[4] Habitual leg crossing may cause repetitive injury to the peroneal nerve because of its superficial location at the fibular neck.[56] Similarly, repetitive stretch from squatting, such as in gardeners, has been associated with peroneal neuropathy. Patients who are thin or have recently lost a great deal of weight are prone to peroneal palsy, probably from the lack of protective supporting adipose tissue at the fibular neck.[57–59] Slowly progressive lesions often suggest a mass lesion, such as a ganglion cyst or nerve sheath tumor.[60] Entrapment of the peroneal nerve at the fibular tunnel, although uncommon, also may present in a progressive manner. Acute peroneal neuropathy may follow trauma, stretch injury such as when the ankle is forcibly inverted, or compression from prolonged immobilization. In the hospital, this occurs most often postoperatively in patients who have received anesthesia or heavy sedation.

What is the differential diagnosis of peroneal neuropathy at the fibular neck?
Other conditions that should be considered in a patient who presents with a foot drop and numbness over the dorsum of the foot include high sciatic neuropathy,[61] lower lumbosacral plexopathy, and L5 radiculopathy. These conditions, however, result in weakness of ankle inversion and sensory loss that extends to the lateral knee, sole

of the foot, or lateral foot, none of which is seen in peroneal neuropathy at the fibular neck. Other signs of a more proximal lesion include a depressed or absent ankle reflex or weakness of hip abduction, extension, or internal rotation.

How is peroneal neuropathy at the fibular neck diagnosed?

EDX studies are especially helpful for evaluating peroneal neuropathy at the fibular neck[52,53,62] and differentiating this from a more proximal lesion. In demyelinating lesions, the peroneal motor NCS can be used to localize the lesion if focal slowing or conduction block is demonstrated across the fibular neck. The yield of finding a demyelinating lesion is increased when the peroneal motor NCS is performed recording the extensor digitorum brevis and the tibialis anterior.[63] In purely demyelinating lesions at the fibular neck, the distal superficial peroneal sensory response remains normal. The presence of a predominantly demyelinating lesion has important prognostic implications. As the underlying axons remain intact, the prognosis for full recovery over a relatively short period is excellent, provided that the cause of the entrapment is no longer present.

If the lesion is primarily axonal loss, peroneal motor and superficial peroneal sensory amplitudes are reduced or absent in common peroneal neuropathy, and one cannot localize the lesion. The degree of axonal loss can be estimated by comparing the distal motor amplitude on the involved side with that on the asymptomatic side, to determine prognosis. Note that in an isolated deep peroneal neuropathy, the superficial peroneal sensory potential remains normal, making it difficult to differentiate from sciatic neuropathy, lumbosacral plexopathy, and L5 radiculopathy. Tibial motor and sural sensory NCSs should be performed to evaluate lesions of the sciatic nerve, lumbosacral plexus, and lumbosacral nerve roots.

The needle EMG is used to confirm the localization, assess the severity of the lesion, and exclude a more proximal lesion. In addition to peroneal innervated muscles, nonperoneal innervated L5 muscles are sampled to exclude a sciatic neuropathy, lumbosacral plexopathy, or radiculopathy. Even if the lesion is localized to the peroneal nerve at the fibular neck by the NCSs, nonperoneal innervated L5 muscles should be sampled to exclude a superimposed lesion. In slowly progressive lesions, MRI scan of the leg and thigh should be done to evaluate for a mass lesion.

How is peroneal neuropathy at the fibular neck treated?

EDX studies are useful in determining the prognosis and treatment options. Those who have predominantly demyelinating lesions at the fibular neck generally have a good prognosis, with good recovery in the first 3 months, once offending factors are eliminated. These patients usually can be managed conservatively, with an ankle foot orthosis to prevent falls and ankle sprains if the foot drop is severe enough to interfere with the patient's gait. Physical therapy exercises are used to prevent contractures. Exacerbating factors, such as habitual leg crossing, should be eliminated. Patients who have lost a great deal of weight recently may benefit from protective padding over the fibular neck. Patients who have axonal loss lesions based on EDX studies (either primary or secondary) have a longer time to recovery and a poorer prognosis. Rarely, surgical exploration is warranted, usually in cases of severe trauma or stretch where the nerve has been so severely damaged that there is no evidence of continuity or reinnervation based on EDX studies after 2 to 6 months, or if there is little to no recovery based on the clinical examination after this time period.[64–68] Some patients may obtain benefit from surgical decompression as far as a year out after their original nerve injury.[67] Surgical exploration also is indicated in slowly progressive lesions when a mass lesion is suspected or seen on the MRI scan.

Meralgia Paresthetica

Case vignette

A 53-year-old woman was referred for burning, pain, and numbness over the right anterolateral thigh, of 3 months' duration. She had a 3-year history of diabetes mellitus, and had recently gained 20 pounds. Strength testing and deep tendon reflexes were normal in the upper and lower extremities. There was an oval-shaped patch of decreased light touch and pinprick sensation over the right anterolateral thigh, and a Tinel's sign at the inguinal ligament on the right side.

What is meralgia paresthetica, and what are its clinical manifestations?

The classic clinical presentation of lateral femoral cutaneous neuropathy, also known as meralgia paresthetica, is burning pain and numbness over the anterolateral thigh, without weakness of reflex changes.[69] The lateral femoral cutaneous nerve of the thigh is a pure sensory nerve that runs directly off the L2-L3 roots around the pelvic brim, and it passes under the inguinal ligament to supply an oval-shaped area of skin over the anterolateral thigh. Entrapment of the nerve may occur as it passes under the inguinal ligament, resulting in a painful, burning, numb patch of skin that can be delineated over the anterolateral thigh (**Fig. 7**). Many patients report hypersensitivity of the numb area. Symptoms are worsened with standing and walking, and relieved by flexing the hip. Because there is no muscular innervation from this nerve, there is no associated muscle atrophy, weakness, or loss of reflexes.

What are the causes and pathophysiology of meralgia paresthetica?

Most cases of meralgia paresthetica are idiopathic, occurring most commonly in patients who are obese; wear tight underwear, pantyhose, or pants; or have diabetes mellitus. Certain occupations also can predispose to compression of the lateral femoral cutaneous nerve, such as workers who wear heavy tool belts. It also can be precipitated by pregnancy. Although most cases are caused by entrapment at the inguinal ligament, some cases have resulted from tumors and other mass lesions such as abdominal aortic aneurysms compressing the upper lumbar plexus more proximally. Compression also may occur perioperatively or postoperatively following hernia repair, renal transplant, hip replacement surgery, iliac crest bone graft harvesting, gastric bypass surgery, and after aortic valve and coronary artery bypass surgery.[70–72] Rare lesions are caused by direct trauma.

What is the differential diagnosis of meralgia paresthetica?

The differential diagnosis includes femoral neuropathy, lumbar plexopathy, and high lumbar radiculopathy. Lumbar radiculopathy usually is accompanied by back pain, and the sensory loss generally is ill defined, in contrast to the fairly well demarcated sensory loss in meralgia paresthetica. In femoral neuropathy and lumbar plexopathy, the sensory loss usually involves the entire anterior thigh, and extends into the medial thigh and leg. Finally, lumbar radiculopathy, plexopathy, and femoral neuropathy may be accompanied by weakness and a depressed knee jerk, which are not seen in meralgia paresthetica.

How is meralgia paresthetica diagnosed?

The diagnosis often is recognized based on the patient's classic clinical presentation of burning pain and numbness restricted to the anterolateral thigh, unaccompanied by back pain, weakness, or reflex changes. Unfortunately, the lateral femoral cutaneous sensory potential is not recorded easily in the EMG laboratory, even in healthy asymptomatic individuals, and especially in obese or older individuals. If the sensory potential is recordable on the asymptomatic side, however, then a low or absent

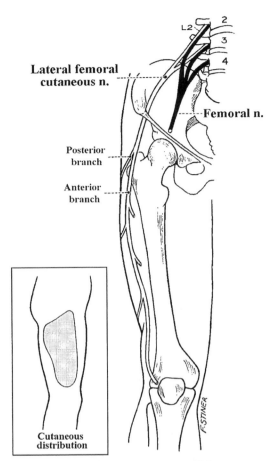

Fig. 7. Anatomy of the lateral femoral cutaneous nerve. This pure sensory nerve comes directly off the L2-L3 roots, and runs under the inguinal ligament, where it may be injured or entrapped. The lateral femoral cutaneous nerve supplies sensation to a large oval area of skin over the lateral and anterior thigh. (*Adapted from* Haymaker W, Woodhal B. Peripheral nerve injuries. Philadelphia: W.B. Saunders; 1953; with permission.)

potential on the symptomatic side is certainly consistent with a diagnosis of lateral femoral cutaneous neuropathy.[73] EDX testing is probably most useful in excluding a femoral neuropathy, lumbosacral plexopathy, or lumbar radiculopathy, if the diagnosis is in question. In this case, femoral and peroneal motor NCSs, and superficial peroneal and saphenous sensory NCSs can be performed, in addition to lateral femoral cutaneous sensory NCS. Note, however, that the saphenous sensory potential may be absent in healthy, asymptomatic individuals, especially in the older population, and both the symptomatic and asymptomatic side must be tested. Needle EMG examination of L3-L4 innervated muscles should be entirely normal in lateral femoral cutaneous neuropathy, being a purely sensory nerve, while denervating changes might be found in lumbar radiculopathy, plexopathy, and in femoral innervated muscles in femoral neuropathy. Imaging with CT or MRI scan of the abdomen and pelvis generally is not recommended unless there is suspicion of a mass lesion, such as in a patient who has known or suspected cancer, or abdominal aortic aneurysm.

How is meralgia paresthetica treated?

In most patients, meralgia paresthetica is time-limited, and conservative therapy is warranted, including removing causative factors. Eliminating tight clothing may be sufficient. Symptoms in obese patients usually resolve with weight loss, and pregnant women after childbirth. In some patients, however, symptoms persist or become intolerable, and medical treatment should be initiated. This is especially true for diabetics, in whom improvement may take months to years. Because the area of discomfort is well demarcated, local treatment such as lidoderm patch, capsaicin, or lidocaine cream may be sufficient to alleviate the discomfort.[74] If this fails, systemic treatment can be tried if there is no contraindication.[75] Typical agents used to treat neuropathic pain include tricyclic or atypical antidepressants such as duloxetine, or anticonvulsants such as gabapentin, pregabalin, or carbamazepine, starting at a low dose and tapering up as tolerated. In refractory cases, patients may receive temporary benefit from local steroid injections, especially if surgical decompression is considered. It remains controversial whether neurolysis with transposition of the lateral femoral cutaneous nerve versus transection of the nerve (neurectomy) is more effective in those patients who ultimately require surgical management, although many believe that transection is the treatment of choice.[69,76–78]

Tarsal Tunnel Syndrome

Case vignette

A 45-year-old woman described persistent foot pain after sustaining a nondisplaced fracture of the ankle 3 months previously, which required 4 weeks of casting. The pain worsened with walking. Examination showed mild atrophy of the right intrinsic foot muscles, with tenderness over the medial ankle. Toe and ankle plantar flexion and dorsiflexion were normal. Light touch and pinprick sensation were decreased over the medial sole of the right foot, and intact over the lateral foot and the dorsum of the foot. Deep tendon reflexes were intact and symmetric throughout, including the ankle jerks.

What is tarsal tunnel syndrome, and what are its clinical manifestations?

Most patients report the gradual onset of burning pain in the ankle and sole of the foot, with numbness and tingling in the heel or sole, depending on which branches are involved. Symptoms are generally unilateral, occur more commonly in women than men, and are worsened with weight bearing. Although there may be wasting of the intrinsic foot muscles, strength testing is usually normal, because proximal muscles also subserve these functions. There may be a Tinel's sign at the tarsal tunnel, although this is a nonspecific sign.

The history and examination are most consistent with distal tibial neuropathy across the tarsal tunnel, also known as tarsal tunnel syndrome (TTS).[79,80]

What are the causes and pathophysiology of tarsal tunnel syndrome?

TTS results from entrapment of the distal tibial nerve under the flexor retinaculum at the medial ankle posteriorly. TTS is probably quite rare, although its incidence is a matter of debate. Although some podiatrists feel that TTS is common, most neurologists believe that it is quite rare. As the distal tibial nerve runs under the flexor retinaculum through the tarsal tunnel at the medial malleolus, it divides into the calcaneal sensory nerves and the medial and lateral plantar nerves (**Fig. 8**). The calcaneal nerves provide sensation to the heel of the sole. The medial and lateral plantar nerves are mixed nerves that innervate the intrinsic foot muscles. The medial plantar nerve supplies sensation to the first three toes and the medial fourth toe, while the lateral plantar nerve supplies the little toe and the lateral fourth toe. One or more of the three nerve branches (calcaneal, medial, and lateral plantar) may be involved in TTS.

Most cases of TTS are idiopathic, with no clear precipitating event. Trauma, such as ankle sprain or fracture, however, also accounts for a large proportion of TTS.[81] Degenerative bone disease, connective tissue disorders such as rheumatoid arthritis, some systemic disorders such as diabetes mellitus and hypothyroidism, and some foot deformities, also may predispose to TTS. Rare cases are caused by varicose veins or other unusual mass lesions such as schwannoma or ganglion cyst in the tarsal tunnel.[82] Occupations or activities that involve repetitive weight bearing, such as jogging, increase the risk for TTS.

What is the differential diagnosis of tarsal tunnel syndrome?
Local orthopedic problems such as plantar fasciitis or bursitis may mimic TTS, although sensory loss and foot weakness should not be seen. Other conditions that may cause numbness or burning of the sole with intrinsic foot muscle wasting include L5-S1 radiculopathy, lumbosacral plexopathy, sciatic neuropathy, proximal tibial neuropathy, or peripheral neuropathy. None of these conditions result in local foot pain,

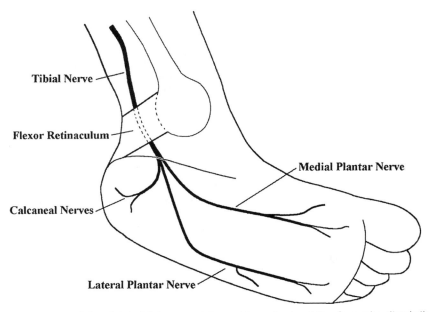

Fig. 8. Anatomy of the distal tibial nerve at the ankle and sole of the foot. The distal tibial nerve runs posterior to the medial malleolus under the flexor retinaculum on the medial side of the ankle (the tarsal tunnel), before dividing into the medial plantar, lateral plantar, and calcaneal nerves. The calcaneal nerves are purely sensory and provide sensation to heel of the sole. The medial and lateral plantar branches both contain motor fibers to supply the foot intrinsics, and sensory fibers to supply the medial and lateral sole, respectively. (*From* Preston DC, Shapiro BE. Electromyography and neuromuscular disorders. 2nd edition. Philadelphia: Elsevier Butterworth Heinemann; 2005; with permission.)

however. In S1 radiculopathy, sciatic neuropathy, and proximal tibial neuropathy, the ankle jerk is reduced or absent, and there may be weakness of proximally innervated muscles, neither of which is seen in TTS. It may be difficult to distinguish early mild peripheral neuropathy from TTS. Peripheral polyneuropathy, however, usually begins in both feet simultaneously, while TTS is most often unilateral. Although TTS involves the sole of the foot, peripheral neuropathy often involves the sole and dorsum of the foot.

How is tarsal tunnel syndrome diagnosed?

The diagnosis of TTS often is made on the basis of typical symptoms and signs and response to treatment. Diagnosis in the EMG laboratory can be quite difficult, partly because of the absence of good evidence-based studies on the validity of electrodiagnostic techniques in TTS.[24,83] Because the medial and lateral plantar sensory and mixed nerve potentials are quite small, they are often unobtainable even in normal subjects, especially in middle-aged or older subjects. Use of near-nerve recording may increase the yield of obtaining a potential.[84] Unless a clear side- to-side difference is seen, however, an absent or low amplitude potential cannot be considered abnormal. Although tibial motor NCSs may reveal a prolonged distal latency if there is demyelination across the tarsal tunnel, this rarely is seen. In axonal loss lesions, the tibial motor amplitudes will be reduced, but this is a nonspecific finding that can be seen in proximal tibial or sciatic neuropathy, lumbosacral plexopathy, S1 radiculopathy, or peripheral neuropathy. Thus, other NCSs are done to exclude a proximal lesion, including peroneal motor and sural sensory NCSs. If the sural sensory response is abnormal, any abnormalities in the plantar nerves are likely secondary to either a polyneuropathy, sciatic neuropathy, or lumbosacral plexus lesion. The H reflex study may be helpful, being normal in TTS, but often abnormal in peripheral neuropathy, proximal tibial neuropathy, sciatic and lumbosacral plexus lesions, and S1 radiculopathy, all of which may cause sensory abnormalities over the sole of the foot.

Many patients find needle EMG of the intrinsic foot muscles painful and difficult to tolerate, and it is difficult to activate these muscles. Furthermore, these muscles often show increased insertional activity and occasionally denervation, even in normal patients. Thus, abnormalities seen in these muscles must be fairly marked, and asymmetric compared with the contralateral side. In addition to the intrinsic foot muscles, more proximal tibial and peroneal innervated muscles should be sampled to exclude a more proximal lesion.

If there are no precipitating factors such as ankle fracture or sprain, or connective tissue disorder, MRI scan of the ankle may be useful to identify a mass lesion such as ganglion cyst or tumor in the tarsal tunnel. If the diagnosis of TTS cannot be confirmed with EDX testing, which is often the case, then radiographs of the foot can be done to look for other causes of foot pain such as spurs, hairline fracture, or arthritis.

How is tarsal tunnel syndrome treated?

Conservative therapy is tried first, including eliminating exacerbating factors, such as tight shoes, and minimizing ankle swelling. The use of insoles and nonsteroidal anti-inflammatory medications may help reduce symptoms. Local corticosteroid injections also may be helpful in alleviating symptoms. If symptoms persist, or if a mass lesion is identified by imaging studies, surgical release of the flexor retinaculum is indicated.[85–87] In one study, those patients with no history of trauma, or with a known mass such as tumor or ganglion cyst, or a short duration of symptoms, had the best prognosis with surgical intervention.[88] Some evidence indicates that combining neurovascular decompression with surgical release of the flexor retinaculum may be effective in idiopathic cases of TTS.[89] In one small series, eight patients who had TTS diagnosed by classical clinical presentation and abnormal EDX studies and who had failed conservative therapy, underwent endoscopic tarsal tunnel release with good to excellent results. Other studies also have shown good results with endoscopic tarsal tunnel release.[90]

Piriformis Syndrome

Case vignette
A 26-year-old woman complained of months of pain in the right buttock, radiating down the leg. Pain was worse with sitting, and relieved with standing or walking. She denied back pain. Neurologic examination was entirely normal, including strength testing, sensation, and deep tendon reflexes.

What is piriformis syndrome, and what are its clinical manifestations?
The typical presentation of piriformis syndrome consists of pain and tenderness in the buttock at the sciatic notch, often radiating down the leg, with the notable absence of back pain. It is more common in women than men, especially following minor trauma to the buttock.[91,92] Some patients report paresthesias in the buttocks radiating down the back or side of the leg into the calf. Weakness of sciatic innervated muscles (gastrocnemius, hamstrings, tibialis anterior) is uncommon. Rarely, concurrent entrapment of the inferior gluteal nerve results in weakness of the gluteal muscles. Symptoms often are worsened during activities that require prolonged sitting, especially on a hard surface, or stooping or bending at the waist. Deep palpation of the sciatic notch may reproduce symptoms. Adduction and internal rotation of the hip may exacerbate symptoms, while standing or walking, or holding the leg externally rotated, may relieve symptoms.

What are the causes and pathophysiology of piriformis syndrome?
Sciatic-type symptoms in the absence of back pain, weakness, sensory loss, or reflex changes are consistent with proximal sciatic neuropathy. As the sciatic nerve leaves the pelvis, it runs under or through the piriformis muscle. Theoretically, a hypertrophied piriformis muscle or associated fibrous bands could compress the sciatic nerve at the pelvic outlet as it runs beneath or through the piriformis muscle in the buttock, resulting in signs and symptoms of proximal sciatic nerve dysfunction, also known as piriformis syndrome.

Robinson coined the term "Pyriformis Syndrome" in 1947,[93] although it had been previously described by others as early as the late 1920s and 1930s.[94,95] Since its original description, the syndrome has fallen in and out of favor as a genuine entity over the years.[96–99] Indeed, most cases that comprised the original descriptions of piriformis syndrome in the 1930s probably would be diagnosed now as lumbosacral radiculopathy, with the advent of the MRI scan and CT/myelogram. Nevertheless, there remains a small group of patients who have buttock pain and tenderness, and sciatic type symptoms, with no demonstrable lesion on MRI scan or CT/myelogram of the lumbosacral spine, and no other discernible structural cause for sciatic symptoms.[100] It is this group of patients for whom the diagnosis of piriformis syndrome is entertained.[101] Criteria for a definitive diagnosis of piriformis syndrome include:

Symptoms of sciatic neuropathy clinically, usually without weakness, sensory loss, or reflex changes

EDX evidence of sciatic neuropathy with no evidence of paraspinal involvement

Imaging studies of the lumbosacral nerve roots, spine, and pelvis that show no evidence of radiculopathy, plexus infiltration or damage, or mass lesions

Surgical exploration showing entrapment of the sciatic nerve within a hypertrophied piriformis muscle

Relief of symptoms following surgical decompression[99]

What is the differential diagnosis of piriformis syndrome?

The major disorder commonly confused with piriformis syndrome is L5-S1 radiculopathy. Both may present with tenderness in the sciatic notch, and pain radiating down the leg. In both disorders, symptoms may be exacerbated with sitting. Back pain, however, is common in radiculopathy, and is not seen in piriformis syndrome. Furthermore, the symptoms in radiculopathy are made worse, not better, with standing or walking. Other disorders confused with piriformis syndrome include lumbosacral plexopathy and sciatic neuropathy caused by a mass lesion, either in the pelvis or thigh, which may be difficult to differentiate from piriformis syndrome. Findings on the clinical examination and EDX testing should help differentiate these.

How is piriformis syndrome diagnosed?

The diagnosis of piriformis syndrome usually is based on a typical history and clinical findings, in the absence of back pain or abnormalities of the lumbosacral nerve roots, plexus, or sciatic nerve seen on imaging studies. EDX studies in piriformis syndrome are invariably normal, or show only minor denervation or reinnervation in sciatic innervated muscles on needle EMG, with normal NCSs. Although sciatic nerve compression distal to the dorsal root ganglion theoretically should result in a low or absent sural or superficial peroneal sensory potential, this generally is not seen in piriformis syndrome. MRI imaging of the buttocks may reveal a fibrous band or anomalous vessel, or a hypertrophied piriformis muscle, compressing the sciatic nerve. This is a nonspecific finding, however, seen with the same frequency in asymptomatic patients, or on the asymptomatic side of symptomatic patients (personal communication, Dr. Cheryl Petersilge). EDX and imaging studies are most useful in excluding lumbosacral root lesions or mass lesions compressing sciatic innervated fibers in the buttocks, pelvis, or thigh.

How is piriformis syndrome treated?

Conservative therapy is tried initially.[102] This consists of physical therapy exercises, including stretching of the piriformis muscle. If this is unsuccessful, then a sciatic nerve block at the sciatic notch, or a local corticosteroid injection into the piriformis muscle, can be done, usually under CT guidance.[103] Indeed, some consider relief of symptoms with sciatic nerve block to be diagnostic of piriformis syndrome, although it is equally true that patients who have lumbosacral radiculopathy also obtain relief with sciatic nerve block. Botulinum toxin injection into the piriformis muscle, under EMG guidance, produced clinical improvement in most patients in a few reported studies.[104,105] Patients who fail conservative therapy, or who respond to local corticosteroid injection initially but with return of symptoms, may be referred for surgical exploration of the sciatic nerve.[102] Surgery consists of sectioning of the piriformis muscle if hypertrophied, or sectioning of fibrous bands or removal of vessels that may be compressing the sciatic nerve in the buttock.[91,100,106] The success of surgery is debated, although those who have compressive fibrous bands or vessels, or abnormal EDX findings, may have a better surgical outcome.

Interdigital Neuropathy (Morton's Neuroma)

Case vignette

A 56-year-old woman described sharp, shooting pain in the ball of the right foot, in the web space between the third and fourth toes. The pain began approximately 6 months previously, and more recently she had noted numbness in the third and fourth toes. Standing and walking made her symptoms worse. Her pain radiated into the third and fourth toes, and occasionally posteriorly to the ankle. Neurologic examination revealed decreased light touch and pain sensation between the third and fourth toes of the right foot. Strength and deep tendon reflexes were intact throughout, and there was no wasting of the intrinsic foot muscles. There was tenderness over the third metatarsal head on the right, and compression of this area produced increased pain and paresthesias in the third and fourth toes.

What is interdigital neuropathy (Morton's neuroma), and what are its clinical manifestations?

The finding of local pain in the ball of the foot between the third and fourth toes, worsened with weight bearing, and accompanied by numbness of the third and fourth toes, is a classic presentation of interdigital neuropathy, also known as Morton's neuroma. It occurs most often between the third and fourth toes, although it can occur between the other toes. The pain often is accompanied by numbness of the third and fourth toes, although if the neuropathy occurs between other toes, then those toes may become numb. It is considerably more prevalent among women than men, especially middle-aged women.

What are the causes and pathophysiology of interdigital neuropathy (Morton's neuroma)?

The likely etiology of Morton's neuroma is chronic repetitive compression of the common plantar digital nerve between the third and fourth metatarsal heads, against the transverse metatarsal ligament.[107] Hyperextension of the metatarsophalangeal joints, for example from wearing high-heeled or pointed shoes, exacerbates the compression. Other predisposing disorders include congenital foot deformities, foot dystonias, spasticity that results in hyperextension of the metatarsophalangeal joints, and rheumatoid arthritis.

What is the differential diagnosis of interdigital neuropathy (Morton's neuroma)?

The differential diagnosis of Morton's neuroma includes other causes of foot pain such as TTS, plantar fasciitis, or arthritis. TTS may be particularly difficult to differentiate, as the pain and numbness usually are limited to one side of the sole of the foot. In TTS, however, the numbness involves the sole of the foot, which distinguishes it from Morton's neuroma. Although plantar fasciitis and arthritis can cause foot pain, especially in the ball of the foot, there is no numbness or sensory loss associated with these conditions unless there is an associated neuropathy. Furthermore, compression of the web space between the metatarsal heads usually does not reproduce the symptoms.

How is interdigital neuropathy (Morton's neuroma) diagnosed?

The diagnosis of Morton's neuroma generally is based on the typical clinical history of pain in the ball of the foot, usually between the third and fourth toes, worsened with weight bearing, and often accompanied by numbness of the corresponding toes. Compression of the web space between the metatarsal heads, by squeezing this area between the examiner's thumb and index finger, often reproduces the pain, and is quite specific for Morton's neuroma.[108] A Tinel's sign may be seen here on occasion.

EDX testing is most useful in excluding other peripheral nerve or nerve root disorders that may result in foot pain, especially TTS, sciatic neuropathy, or lumbosacral radiculopathy laboratory. Sensory NCSs of the interdigital nerves themselves can be done, using near-nerve needle electrodes, looking for a reduction in amplitude or slowing of conduction velocity in the involved interdigital nerve. This technique, however, is somewhat more painful to perform than standard sensory NCSs, and must be done in an EDX laboratory that is equipped to perform such studies.[109,110] Thus, they are not generally part of the standard testing in the diagnosis of Morton's neuroma.

Both MRI scan and ultrasound have been used in the evaluation of patients with suspected Morton's neuroma, each with advantages and disadvantages.[111] The sensitivity and specificity of the MRI scan is particularly dependent on the field of view, type of coil, and sequences used.[112–115] Newer techniques have resulted in greater sensitivity and specificity. The MRI scan is particularly useful for preoperative localization and determining the size of the neuroma. The finding of a neuroma on MRI scan, however, does not necessarily imply a clinically relevant lesion, and clinical correlation is warranted, especially before consideration of surgical treatment.[112,114–116] Although ultrasound is sensitive in detecting abnormalities in the intermetatarsal web space, is more widely available than MRI scan, and also predicts the size of the neuroma accurately, results differ concerning its specificity in distinguishing neuroma from other inflammatory or mass lesions.[87,111]

How is interdigital neuropathy (Morton's neuroma) treated?

The initial treatment consists of conservative measures, including physical therapy, foot orthotics, and eliminating offending factors such as high-heeled shoes.[27,117–119] Local interdigital anesthetic block, often in conjunction with corticosteroids, may be very helpful in relieving symptoms in a significant number of patients.[120] Repeated injections are often necessary, although a positive treatment response to the block does not necessarily predict a positive outcome if surgery is subsequently performed.[121–123] Patients who fail conservative therapy, or have a return of symptoms after a combination of local blocks and conservative therapy such as physical therapy, orthotics, and removal of offending factors, are referred for surgery. In one study, those patients who had a presurgical MRI scan showing a neuroma measuring greater than 5 mm in transverse measurement had a significantly higher good surgical outcome with neurectomy than those who had a neuroma measuring 5 mm or less.[116] Some debate exists as to the best surgical approach, neurolysis of the interdigital nerve versus surgical excision of the neuroma (neurectomy). Both approaches often afford complete relief of symptoms.[27,107,108,118,121,124,125] Some favor neurolysis over neurectomy, because of the real potential of developing a recurrent neuroma in the nerve stump after neurectomy,[126–128] or permanent numbness of the toes.[129] Despite the multitude of published reports, however, there is incomplete evidence from well-designed randomized controlled trials to assess the long-term effectiveness of surgical versus nonsurgical treatments for Morton's neuroma.[130]

REFERENCES

1. Katirji B. Compressive and entrapment neuropathies of the lower extremity. In: Katirji B, Kaminski H, Preston DC, et al, editors. Neuromuscular disorders in clinical practice. Woburn (MA): Butterworth-Heinemann; 2002. p. 774–819.
2. Preston DC. Compressive and entrapment neuropathies of the upper extremity. In: Katirji B, Kaminski H, Preston DC, et al, editors. Neuromuscular disorders in clinical practice. Woburn (MA): Butterworth-Heinemann; 2002. p. 744–73.

3. Preston DC, Shapiro BE. Electromyography and neuromuscular disorders. 2nd edition. Philadelphia: Elsevier Butterworth Heinemann; 2005.
4. Dawson DM, Hallet M, Wilbourn A. Entrapment neuropathies. 3rd edition. Lippincott Raven; 1999.
5. Kuschner SH, Ebramzadeh E, Johnson D, et al. Tinel's sign and Phalen's test in carpal tunnel syndrome. Orthopedics 1992;15(11):1297–302.
6. O'Neil BA, Forsythe ME, Stanish WD. Chronic occupational repetitive strain injury. Can Fam Physician 2001;47:311–6.
7. Bleecker ML, Bohlman M, Moreland R, et al. Carpal tunnel syndrome: role of carpal canal size. Neurology 1985;35:1599–604.
8. Stevens JC, Beard M, O'Fallon WM, et al. Conditions associated with carpal tunnel syndrome. Mayo Clin Proc 1992;67(6):541–8.
9. Jablecki CK, Andary MT, So YT, et al. Literature review of the usefulness of nerve conduction studies and electromyography for the evaluation of patients with carpal tunnel syndrome. Muscle Nerve 1993;16:1392–414.
10. Robinson LR. Electrodiagnosis of carpal tunnel syndrome. Physical Medicine & Rehabilitation Clinics of North America 2007;18(4):733–46.
11. Daube JR. Per cutaneous palmar median nerve stimulation for carpal tunnel syndrome. Electroencephalogr Clin Neurophysiol 1977;43:139–40.
12. Pease WS, Cannell CD, Johnson EW. Median to radial latency difference test in mild carpal tunnel syndrome. Muscle Nerve 1989;12(11):905–9.
13. Preston DC, Logigian EL. Lumbrical and interossei recording in carpal tunnel syndrome. Muscle Nerve 1992;15:1253–7.
14. Uncini A, Lange DJ, Solomon M, et al. Ring finger testing in carpal tunnel syndrome: a comparative study of diagnostic utility. Muscle Nerve 1989;12(9): 735–41.
15. Kwon BC, Jung KI, Baek GH. Comparison of sonography and electrodiagnostic testing in the diagnosis of carpal tunnel syndrome. J Hand Surg [Am] 2008; 33(1):65–71.
16. Visser LH, Smidt MH, Lee ML. High-resolution sonography versus EMG in the diagnosis of carpal tunnel syndrome. J Neurol Neurosurg Psychiatr 2008; 79(1):63–7.
17. Yesildag A, Kutluhan S, Sengul N, et al. The role of ultrasonographic measurements of the median nerve in the diagnosis of carpal tunnel syndrome. Clin Radiol 2008;59(10):910–5.
18. Dammers JW, Veering MM, Vermeulen M. Injection with methylprednisolone proximal to the carpal tunnel: randomised double-blind trial. BMJ 1999; 319(7214):884–6.
19. Katz JN, Losina E, Amick BC 3rd, et al. Predictors of outcomes in carpal tunnel release. Arthritis Rheum 2001;44(5):1184–93.
20. Scholten RJ, Mink van der Molen A, Uitdehaag BM, et al. Surgical treatment options for carpal tunnel syndrome. Cochrane Database Syst Rev The Cochrane Library vol. 2, 2008.
21. Trumble TE, Gilbert M, McCallister WV. Endoscopic versus open surgical treatment of carpal tunnel syndrome. Neurosurg Clin N Am 2001;12(2):255–66.
22. Bradshaw DY, Shefner JM. Ulnar neuropathy at the elbow. Neurologic Clinics 1999;17(3):447–61.
23. Campbell WW, Pridgeon RM, Riaz G, et al. Variations in anatomy of the ulnar nerve at the cubital tunnel: pitfalls in the diagnosis of ulnar neuropathy at the elbow. Muscle Nerve 1991;14(8):733–8.

24. Miller RG. AAEM Case report #1. Ulnar neuropathy at the elbow. Muscle Nerve 1991;14:97–101.
25. Kincaid JC. AAEE minimonograph #31: the electrodiagnosis of ulnar neuropathy at the elbow. Muscle Nerve 1988;11:1005–15.
26. Dellon AL, Hament W, Gittelshon A. Nonoperative management of cubital tunnel syndrome: an 8-year prospective study. Neurology 1993;43:1673–7.
27. Gaynor R, Hake D, Spinner SM, et al. A comparative analysis of conservative versus surgical treatment of Morton's neuroma. J Am Podiatr Med Assoc 1989;79:27–30.
28. Elhassan B, Steinmann SP. Entrapment neuropathy of the ulnar nerve. J Am Acad Orthop Surg 2007;15(11):672–81.
29. Smith T, Nielsen KD, Poulsgaard L. Ulnar neuropathy at the elbow: clinical and electrophysiological outcome of surgical and conservative treatment. Scand J Plast Reconstr Surg Hand Surg 2000;34(2):145–8.
30. Osterman AL, Davis CA. Subcutaneous transposition of the ulnar nerve for treatment of cubital tunnel syndrome. Hand Clin 1996;12(2):421–33.
31. Bartels RH, Verhagen WI, van der Wilt GJ, et al. Prospective randomized controlled study comparing simple decompression versus anterior subcutaneous transposition for idiopathic neuropathy of the ulnar nerve at the elbow: part 1. Neurosurgery 2005;56(3):522–30.
32. Campbell WW, Sahni SK, Pridgeon RM, et al. Intraoperative electroneurography: management of ulnar neuropathy at the elbow. Muscle Nerve 1988;11:75–81.
33. Steiner HH, von Haken MS, Steiner-Milz HG. Entrapment neuropathy at the cubital tunnel: simple decompression is the method of choice. Acta Neurochir 1996;138(3):308–13.
34. Beekman R, Wokke JHJ, Schoemaker MC, et al. Ulnar neuropathy at the elbow: follow-up and prognostic factors determining outcome. Neurology 2004;63: 1675–80.
35. Kothari MJ. Ulnar neuropathy at the wrist. Neurologic Clinics 1999;17(3):463–76.
36. Shu N, Uchio Y, Ryoke K, et al. Atypical compression of the deep branch of the ulnar nerve in Guyon's canal by a ganglion. Case report. Scand J Plast Reconstr Surg Hand Surg 2000;34(2):181–3.
37. Kothari MJ, Preston DC, Logigian EL. Lumbrical–interossei motor studies localize ulnar neuropathy at the wrist. Muscle & Nerve 1996;19(2):170–4.
38. McIntosh KA, Preston DC, Logigian EL. Short-segment incremental studies to localize ulnar nerve entrapment at the wrist. Neurology 1998;50(1):303–6.
39. Padua L, Insola A, LoMonaco M, et al. A case of Guyon syndrome with neuroapraxic block resolved after surgical decompression. Electroencephalogr Clin Neurophysiol 1998;109(2):191–3.
40. Labosky DA, Waggy CA. Apparent weakness of median and ulnar motors in radial nerve palsy. J Hand Surg 1986;11A:528–33.
41. Brown WF, Watson BV. AAEM case report #27: acute retrohumeral radial neuropathies. Muscle & Nerve 1993;16(7):706–11.
42. Kaplan PE. Posterior interosseous neuropathies: natural history. Arch Phys Med Rehabil 1984;65:399.
43. Plate AM, Green SM. Compressive radial neuropathies. Instr Course Lect 2000;49: 295–304.
44. Van Zandijcke M, Casselman J. Suprascapular nerve entrapment at the spinoglenoid notch due to a ganglion cyst. J Neurol Neurosurg Psychiatr 1999; 66(2):245.

45. Callahan JD, Scully TB, Shapiro SA, et al. Suprascapular nerve entrapment. A series of 27 cases. J Neurosurg 1991;74(6):893–6.
46. Fehrman DA, Orwin JF, Jennings RM. Suprascapular nerve entrapment by ganglion cysts: a report of six cases with arthroscopic findings and review of the literature. Arthroscopy 1995;11:727–34.
47. Ferretti A, Cerullo G, Russo G. Suprascapular neuropathy in volleyball players. J Bone Joint Surg 1987;69(2):260–3.
48. Hadley MN, Sonntag VKH, Pittman HW. Suprascapular nerve entrapment. A summary of seven cases. J Neurosurg 1986;64(6):843–8.
49. Holzgraefe M, Kukowski B, Eggert S. Prevalence of latency and manifest suprascapular neuropathy in high-performance volleyball players. Br J Sports Med 1994;28:177–9.
50. Hong CZ, Long HA, Kanakamedala RV, et al. Splinting and local steroid injection for the treatment of ulnar neuropathy at the elbow: clinical and electrophysiological evaluation. Arch Phys Med Rehabil 1996;77(6):573–7.
51. Antoniou J, Tae SK, Williams GR, et al. Suprascapular neuropathy: variability in the diagnosis, treatment, and outcome. Clin Orthop Relat Res 2001;1(386): 131–8.
52. Katirji B. Peroneal neuropathy. Neurol Clin 1999;17:567–91.
53. Katirji MB, Wilbourn AJ. Common peroneal mononeuropathy: a clinical and electrophysiologic study of 116 lesions. Neurology 1988;38:1723–8.
54. Sourkes M, Stewart JD. Common peroneal neuropathy: a study of selective motor and sensory involvement. Neurology 1991;41:1029–33.
55. Wilbourn AJ. Common peroneal mononeuropathy at the fibular head. Muscle Nerve 1986;9:825–36.
56. Nagler SH, Rangell L. Peroneal palsy caused by crossing the legs. JAMA 1947; 133:755–61.
57. Cruz-Martinez A, Arpa J, Palau F. Peroneal neuropathy after weight loss. J Peripher Nerv Syst 2000;5(2):101–5.
58. Harrison MJ. Peroneal neuropathy during weight reduction. J Neurol Neurosurg Psychiatr 1984;47:1260.
59. Streib E. Weight loss and foot drop. Iowa Med 1993;83(6):224–5.
60. Fransen P, Thauvoy C, Sindic CJM, et al. Intraneural ganglionic cyst of the common peroneal nerve, case report and review of the literature. Acta Neurol Belg 1991;91:231–5.
61. Katirji MB, Wilbourn AJ. High sciatic lesions mimicking peroneal neuropathy at the fibular head. J Neurol Sci 1994;121:172–5.
62. Singh N, Behse F, Buchthal F. Electrophysiological study of peroneal palsy. J Neurol Neurosurg Psychiatr 1974;37:1202–13.
63. Devi S, Lovelace RE, Duarte N. Proximal peroneal nerve conduction velocity: recording from anterior tibial and peroneus brevis muscle. Ann Neurol 1977;2: 116–9.
64. Kim DH, Kline DG. Management and results of peroneal nerve lesions. Neurosurgery 1996;39:312–9.
65. Mont MA, Dellon AL, Chen F, et al. The operative treatment of peroneal nerve palsy. J Bone Joint Surg Am 1996;78:863–9.
66. Moore TP, Fritts HM, Quick DC, et al. Suprascapular nerve entrapment caused by supraglenoid cyst compression. J Shoulder Elbow Surg 1997;6:455–62.
67. Thoma A, Fawcett S, Ginty M, et al. Decompression of the common peroneal nerve: experience with 20 consecutive cases. Plast Reconstr Surg 2001; 107(5):1183–9.

68. Vastamaki M. Decompression for peroneal nerve entrapment. Acta Orthop Scand 1986;57(6):551–4.
69. Grossman MG, Ducey SA, Nadler SS, et al. Meralgia paresthetica: diagnosis and treatment. J Am Acad Orthop Surg 2001;9(5):336–44.
70. Ahsan MR, Curtin J. Meralgia paresthetica following total hip replacement. Ir J Med Sci 2001;170(2):149.
71. Antunes PE, Antunes MJ. Meralgia paresthetica after aortic valve surgery. J Heart Valve Dis 1997;6(6):589–90.
72. Eubanks S, Newman L 3rd, Goehring L, et al. Meralgia paresthetica: a complication of laparoscopic herniorrhaphy. Surg Laparosc Endosc & Percutaneous Techniques 1993;3(5):381–5.
73. Seror P. Lateral femoral cutaneous nerve conduction v somatosensory evoked potentials for electrodiagnosis of meralgia paresthetica. Am J Phys Med Rehabil 1999;78(4):313–6.
74. Devers A, Galer BS. Topical lidocaine patch relieves a variety of neuropathic pain conditions: an open-label study. Clin J Pain 2000;16(3):205–8.
75. Dureja GP, Gulaya V, Jayalakshmi TS, et al. Management of meralgia paresthetica: a multimodality regimen. Anesth Analg 1995;80(5):1060–1.
76. Ivins GK. Meralgia paresthetica, the elusive diagnosis: clinical experience with 14 adult patients. Ann Surg 2000;232(2):281–6.
77. Nahabedian MY, Dellon AL. Meralgia paresthetica: etiology, diagnosis, and outcome of surgical decompression. Ann Plast Surg 1995;35(6):590–4.
78. van Eerten PV, Polder TW, Broere CA. Operative treatment of meralgia paresthetica: transection versus neurolysis. Neurosurgery 1995;37(1):63–5.
79. Cimino WR. Tarsal tunnel syndrome: review of the literature. Foot Ankle 1990;11:47.
80. Keck C. The tarsal tunnel syndrome. J Bone Joint Surg 1962;44:180.
81. Lau JT, Daniels TR. Tarsal tunnel syndrome: a review of the literature. Foot Ankle Int 1999;20(3):201–9.
82. Nagaoka M, Satou K. Tarsal tunnel syndrome caused by ganglia. J Bone Joint Surg Br 1999;81(4):607–10.
83. Patel AT, Gaines K, Malamut R, et al. Usefulness of electrodiagnostic techniques in the evaluation of suspected tarsal tunnel syndrome: an evidence-based review. Muscle Nerve 2005;32:236–40.
84. Oh SJ, Kwon KH, Hah JS, et al. Lateral plantar neuropathy. Muscle Nerve 1999; 22(9):1234–8.
85. Oh SJ, Arnold TW, Park KH, et al. Electrophysiologic improvement following decompression surgery in tarsal tunnel syndrome. Muscle Nerve 1991; 14(5)(14):407–10.
86. Oh SJ, Sarala PK, Kuba T, et al. Tarsal tunnel syndrome: electrophysiological study. Ann Neurol 1979;5:327–30.
87. Reade BM, Longo DC, Keller MC. Tarsal tunnel syndrome. Clin Podiatr Med Surg 2001;18(3):395–408.
88. Baba H, Wada M, Annen S, et al. The tarsal tunnel syndrome: evaluation of surgical results using multivariate analysis. Int Orthop 1997;21(2):67–71.
89. Kohno M, Takahashi H, Segawa H, et al. Neurovascular decompression for idiopathic tarsal tunnel syndrome: technical note. J Neurol Neurosurg Psychiatr 2000;69(1):87–90.
90. Krishnan KG, Pinzer T, Schackert G. A novel endoscopic technique in treating single nerve entrapment syndromes with special attention to ulnar nerve transposition and tarsal tunnel release: clinical application. Neurosurgery 2006;59(Suppl.1):89–100.

91. Benson ER, Schutzer SF. Post-traumatic piriformis syndrome: diagnosis and results of operative treatment. Patient Care Manag 1999;81(7):941–9.

92. Parziale JR, Hudgins TH, Fishman LM. The piriformis syndrome. Am J Orthop 1996;25(12):819–23.

93. Robinson DR. Piriformis syndrome in relation to sciatic pain. Am J Surg 1947;73: 355–8.

94. Freiberg AH. Sciatic pain and its relief by operations on muscle and fascia. Arch Surg 1937;34:337–50.

95. Yeoman W. The relation of arthritis of the sacroiliac joint to sciatica, with an analysis of 100 cases. Lancet 1928;2:1119–22.

96. Fishman LM, Schaefer MP. The piriformis syndrome is underdiagnosed. Muscle Nerve 2003;28:646–9.

97. McCrory P. The "piriformis syndrome"–myth or reality? Br J Sports Med 2001; 35(4):209–10.

98. Silver JK, Leadbetter WB. Piriformis syndrome: assessment of current practice and literature review. Orthopedics 1998;21:1133–5.

99. Stewart J. The piriformis syndrome is overdiagnosed. Muscle Nerve 2003;28: 644–5.

100. Rodrigue T, Hardy RW. Diagnosis and treatment of piriformis syndrome. Neurosurg Clin N Am 2001;12(2):311–9.

101. Steiner C, Staubs C, Ganon M, et al. Piriformis syndrome: pathogenesis, diagnosis, and treatment. J Am Osteopath Assoc 1987;87:318–23.

102. Barton PM. Piriformis syndrome: a rational approach to management. Pain 1991;47(3):345–52.

103. Wyant GM. Chronic pain syndromes and their treatment. III. The piriformis syndrome. Can Anaesth Soc J 1979;26:305–8.

104. Fishman LM, Konnoth C, Rozner B. Botulinum neurotoxin type B and physical therapy in the treatment of piriformis syndrome: a dose-finding study. Am J Phys Med Rehabil 2004;83:442–50.

105. Lang A. Botulinum toxin type B in piriformis syndrome. Am J Phys Med Rehabil 2004;83:198–202.

106. Sayson SC, Ducey JP, Maybrey JB, et al. Sciatic entrapment neuropathy associated with an anomalous piriformis muscle. Pain 1994;59(1):149–52.

107. Dellon AL. Treatment of Morton's neuroma as a nerve compression. The role for neurolysis. J Am Podiatr Med Assoc 1992;82:399–402.

108. Wu KK. Morton neuroma and metatarsalgia. Curr Opin Rheumatol 2000;12: 131–42.

109. Falck B, Hurme M, Hakkarainen S, et al. Sensory conduction velocity of plantar digital nerves in Morton's metatarsalgia. Neurology 1984;34(5):698–701.

110. Oh SJ, Kim HS, Ahmad BK. Electrophysiological diagnosis of the interdigital nerve of the foot. Muscle Nerve 1984;7:224.

111. Kaminsky S, Griffin L, Milsap J, et al. Is ultrasonography a reliable way to confirm the diagnosis of Morton's neuroma? Orthopedics 1997;20:37–9.

112. Bencardino J, Rosenberg ZS, Beltran J, et al. Morton's neuroma: is it always symptomatic? Am J Roentgenol 2000;175(3):649–53.

113. Terk MR, Kwong PK, Suthar M, et al. Morton neuroma: evaluation with MR imaging performed with contrast enhancement and fat suppression. Radiology 1993;189:239–41.

114. Williams JW, Meaney J, Whitehouse GH, et al. MRI in the investigation of Morton's neuroma: which sequences? Clin Radiol 1997;52:46–9.

115. Zanetti M, Ledermann T, Zollinger H, et al. Efficacy of MR imaging in patients suspected of having Morton's neuroma. Am J Roentgenol 1997;168(2):529–32.
116. Biasca N, Zanetti M, Zollinger H. Outcomes after partial neurectomy of Morton's neuroma related to preoperative case histories, clinical findings, and findings on magnetic resonance imaging scans. Foot Ankle Int 1999;20(9):568–75.
117. Brantingham JW, Snyder WR, Michaud T. Morton's neuroma. J Manipulative Physiol Ther 1991;14(5):317–22.
118. Nunan PJ, Giesy BD. Management of Morton's neuroma in athletes. Clin Podiatr Med Surg 1997;14(3):489–501.
119. Wu KK. Morton's interdigital neuroma: a clinical review of its etiology, treatment, and results. J Foot Ankle Surg 1996;35:112–9.
120. Hughes RJ, Alik K, Jones H, et al. Treatment of Morton's neuroma with alcohol injection under sonographic guidance: follow-up of 101 cases. Am J Roentgenol 2007;188(6):1535–9.
121. Greenfield J, Rea J Jr, Il feld FW. Morton's interdigital neuroma. Indications for treatment by local injections versus surgery. Clin Orthop 1984;185:142–4.
122. Strong G, Thomas PS. Conservative treatment of Morton's neuroma. Orthop Rev 1987;16:343–5.
123. Younger AS, Claridge RJ. The role of diagnostic block in the management of Morton's neuroma. Can J Surg 1998;41:127–30.
124. Jarde O, Trinquier JL, Pleyber A, et al. Treatment of Morton neuroma by neurectomy. Apropos of 43 cases. Rev Chir Orthop Reparatrice Appar Mot 1995;81(2):142–6.
125. Keh RA, Ballew KK, Higgins KR, et al. Long-term follow-up of Morton's neuroma. J Foot Surg 1992;31(1):93–5.
126. Amis JA, Siverhus SW, Liwnicz BH. An anatomic basis for recurrence after Morton's neuroma excision. Foot Ankle 1992;13(3):153–6.
127. Gauthier G. Thomas Morton's disease: a nerve entrapment syndrome. A new surgical technique. Clin Orthop 1979;142:90–2.
128. Young G, Lindsey J. Etiology of symptomatic recurrent interdigital neuromas. J Am Podiatr Med Assoc 1993;83(5):255–8.
129. Diebold PF, Daum B, Dang-Vu V, et al. True epineural neurolysis in Morton's neuroma: a 5-year follow-up. Orthopedics 1996;19(5):397–400.
130. Thomson A, Gibson JNA, Martin D. Interventions for the treatment of Morton's neuroma. Cochrane Database Syst Rev 2007;4.

Peripheral Neuropathy

Robert M. Pascuzzi, MD

KEYWORDS

- Peripheral neuropathy • Guillain-Barré syndrome
- Charcot-Marie-Tooth disease • CIDP • POEMS

Patients who have peripheral neuropathy present in a variety of scenarios to the office, to the emergency department, and a times in the setting of other major medical problems. The majority of patients can be diagnosed, classified, and managed based on history and physical examination.

PATIENT ONE: ACUTE PERIPHERAL NEUROPATHY
Question: How to Approach a Patient who Presents with Symptoms of Acute or Rapidly Developing Peripheral Neuropathy?

Case presentation 1

A 31-year-old farmer presents with 48 hours of progressive difficulty described as initial trouble with getting up out of a chair and going up and down stairs with subsequent trouble walking, decline in balance, and heaviness in the arms. The patient noted several days of a febrile illness with abdominal cramps, loose stools, and malaise before the onset of these symptoms. Past medical and family histories are unremarkable.

Examination shows 4/5 strength involving arms and legs with slightly greater weakness proximally than distally. There is reduced position and vibration sense at the toes and ankles. Muscle stretch reflexes are absent throughout. Cranial nerve function is normal and forced vital capacity (FVC) is 5 L.

Discussion

This patient presented with an acute progressive quadriparesis heralded by a gastrointestinal illness. The examination suggests that the weakness likely was at the level of the motor unit (anterior horn cell, roots, peripheral nerve, neuromuscular junction, or muscle). The presence of somewhat more weakness proximally than distally raised the question of a myopathy but the finding of sensory deficit in the feet pointed toward a localization, including sensory and motor function. Thus the likely localization was the sensory motor peripheral nerve and or the roots. As all neurologists have seen, there are patients who present with an acute myelopathy in whom the examination looks more peripheral than central. Patients who have spinal cord infarction or transverse myelitis and even some who have compressive lesions may present with an

Department of Neurology, Indiana University School of Medicine, Emerson Hall 125, 545 Barnhill Drive, Indianapolis, IN 46202, USA
E-mail address: rpascuzz@iupui.edu

Med Clin N Am 93 (2009) 317–342
doi:10.1016/j.mcna.2008.12.001
0025-7125/08/$ – see front matter © 2009 Elsevier Inc. All rights reserved.

acute progressive quadiparesis, reduced stretch reflexes, reduced muscle tone, and variable form of sensory deficit, and it may be challenging to know with certainty that the problem is peripheral rather than a myelopathy. As a general rule, even if patients are experiencing the phenomenon of acute spinal shock with reduced tone and hypoactive muscle stretch reflexes, the majority of such patients display an extensor toe sign in the early phase of their illness. Also, as a general rule, if clinicians are not completely certain that a problem is peripheral, then it behooves them to obtain immediate MRI of the spine.

The presence of proximal weakness more than distal or, in some patients, arm weakness worse than leg can make the diagnosis of peripheral neuropathy less obvious. Many clinicians consider patients who have distal more than proximal and leg more than arm weakness as reflecting the distribution of peripheral neuropathy, but a significant proportion of patients who have acute peripheral neuropathy may present otherwise.

The differential diagnosis for the patient (discussed in Case Presentation 1) is headlined by acute inflammatory demyelintating polyradiculoneuropathy (acute inflammatory neuropathy or Guillain-Barré syndrome [GBS]). The antecedent illness, time course for presentation, and preponderance of motor involvement all are in favor of GBS.

As such, the patient should be admitted to an ICU setting in which he can have meticulous nursing care and vigilant monitoring for respiratory, bulbar, and autonomic dysfunction. For the patient discussed in Case Presentation 1, I would push for an immediate MRI of the entire spine with gadolinium. Routine laboratory tests should be sent off and supplemented with studies (discussed later) for conditions that may mimic GBS depending on the level of certainty of the diagnosis. Tests that can provide evidence to support the GBS diagnosis include a spinal fluid evaluation. I would obtain a cerebrospinal fluid (CSF) examination after looking at the MRI study. Also, blood for GM1 ganglioside antibodies can be useful especially in patients who have a gastrointestinal prodromal illness when looking for *Campylobacter jejuni*–related GBS. Often the establishment of Campylobacter-related illness helps with the long-term prognosis and realistic expectations for the time course of recovery.

What is Known About Guillain-Barré Syndrome and How Should Patient Evaluation and Treatment be Handled?

GBS is considered the prototype "postinfectious" neurologic disorder. The majority of patients describe an antecedent febrile illness, followed in days or weeks by the development of ascending paralysis, which seems to be on the basis of an acute inflammatory peripheral neuropathy. Although most skilled neurologists recognize GBS when they see it, the disorder is heterogeneous and diverse in its antecedent events, clinical presentations, and natural course. Even the name is diverse, with GBS, Landry-Guillain-Barré-Strohl syndrome, acute inflammatory demyelinating polyradiculoneuropathy, and acute inflammatory neuropathy all synonymous.

History of Guillain-Barré syndrome

Octave Landry[1] is credited with the earliest description of what has come to be recognized as GBS. In 1859 Landry reported a condition, which he called *acute ascending paralysis*, describing a patient who had a febrile illness in the springtime, which was followed by the development of sensory symptoms within 2 months. One month later, the patient developed subacute progressive inability to walk due to leg weakness, respiratory failure, and death. Landry pointed out that bowel and bladder function were spared, sensory involvement was mild, and muscles respond to faradic electrical stimulation. The patient had an autopsy, but this apparently did not include the peripheral nerves. Landry reviewed four other cases from his own experience and five from the medical literature. He emphasized the absence of central nervous system symptoms or signs, the occasional presence of muscle cramps, occasional relapsing course, and the tendency for a favorable outcome. He also noted that two of the cases occurred after an acute illness, two were associated with menstrual irregularities, one was post partum, and one possibly associated with syphilis. Westfall, in 1876, referred to this condition as "Landry's ascending paralysis."

Then, in 1916, Guillain and colleagues[2] reported on two soldiers who developed an acute paralysis associated with loss of muscle stretch reflexes. They emphasized the presence of elevated CSF protein concentration with a normal cell count (albuminocytologic dissociation). Their report did not recognize Landry's prior observations. Guillain and colleagues state in their original paper, that the illness

> is characterized by motor difficulties, loss of the deep tendon reflexes with preservation of cutaneous reflexes, paresthesias with slight impairment of objective sensation, muscle tenderness, slight alteration in nerve conduction and electromyographic patterns, and a remarkable increase in cerebrospinal fluid albumin in the absence of a cellular reaction (albumino-cytologic dissociation).

Although the general clinical observations are attributed to Guillain and Barré, Andre Strohl probably was responsible for the electrophysiologic aspects. Guillain and Barré[3] further developed their concept of the disease in subsequent publications, including *Travaux Neurologiques de Guerre* in 1920. Strohl's name largely was eliminated in the subsequent publications by Guillain and Barré. Death from respiratory failure remained a common outcome until the late 1940s when the development of ICUs and mechanical ventilation allowed for an overall reduction in mortality from GBS. Additional landmarks in clinical thinking on GBS include the observation by C. Miller Fisher[4] of a variant associated with ophthalmoplegia, ataxia, and areflexia, published in 1956.

Pathophysiology

In 1949 the classic clinical pathologic correlations were first reported by Haymaker and Kernohan.[5] In 50 cases of what was called Landry-Guillain-Barré syndrome, they noted predominant inflammatory abnormalities in the anterior spinal roots. Because inflammatory cells were not present in more distal segments of peripheral nerves until late in the illness, they described the disorder as a "polyradiculoneuropathy." The subsequent seminal neuropathologic study by Asbury and coworkers in 1969 described findings in 19 patients, noting abundant lymphocytic infiltration in spinal roots and nerves, leading them to conclude, "the pathologic hallmark of idiopathic polyneuritis is a perivascular mononuclear inflammatory infiltrate."[6]

Inflammatory demyelinating neuropathy

The pathology is classically that of a mononuclear inflammatory infiltrate in the endoneurium and myelin sheath. Patchy segmental multifocal demyelination is present along peripheral nerves, including nerve roots, whereas the axons themselves are relatively spared except in more severe cases. Inflammatory infiltrates are comprised of lymphocytes, monocytes, and occasional plasma cells and tend to be perivascular. Less commonly, polymorphonuclear leukocytes are seen. The abnormalities are prominent around ventral roots and in the plexus and proximal nerve trunks but in some cases are present to an equal or greater extent distally along peripheral nerves. Similar inflammatory abnormalities also can be seen in dorsal roots and autonomic ganglia. In occasional patients there is axonal degeneration; in such cases, degeneration of anterior horn cells and dorsal root ganglia cells can be present, suggesting chromatolysis. Although most of the pathology is found in the peripheral nervous system, there are occasional case reports that demonstrate perivascular inflammation in the central nervous system. A few weeks after the onset of demyelination, Schwann's cells are noted to proliferate. Several weeks later, as inflammation resolves, remyelination becomes evident.

Animal models resembling GBS were developed as early as 1955 by Waksman and Adams.[7] Experimental allergic neuritis depends on the sensitivity of the P2 protein of peripheral nerve myelin and closely resembles human GBS in terms of clinical, electrophysiologic, and pathologic features. In humans, however, there is no clear evidence that the primary inflammatory attack is directed at the P2 protein.[8,9] A second animal model, galactocerebroside neuritis, involving antibodies against galactocerebroside, has been developed in rabbits. This animal model is not as similar pathologically as experimental allergic neuritis, because the cellular component of the nerve attack is not demonstrable. In addition, antigalactocerebroside antibodies are not present in human GBS. Although most of the pathologic observations have emphasized lymphocyte-mediated delayed hypersensitivity as a possible mechanism, there also is evidence to suggest the role of circulating autoantibodies directed against the myelin sheath.[8–10] Perhaps GBS is a syndrome with a variety of immunologic mechanisms to account for an acute or subacute peripheral neuropathy.

Campylobacter, Guillain-Barré syndrome, and axonal Guillain-Barré syndrome

In 1984 Kaldor and Speed[11] reported serologic evidence of *Campylobacter jejuni* infection in 38% of a group of patients from Australia who had GBS. Subsequent reports supported this association, including that of Vriesendorp and colleagues,[12] in which 15% of 58 patients who had GBS had evidence of recent Campylobacter infection. Many additional studies confirm the association between Campylobactor infection and subsequent GBS.[13,14] Rees and Hughes[15] found *Campylobacter jejuni* in stool samples of 11% of patients who had GBS, along with serologic abnormalities in an additional 5 of 36 patients. Of the 25% of patients overall who had stool culture or serologic evidence for Campylobacter infection, most had experienced diarrhea as an antecedent illness. In these series, there was a tendency for patients to have predominantly an axonal neuropathy as opposed to a demyelinating neuropathy and the presence of IgG anti-GM1 ganglioside antibodies.

Although GBS typically is a demyelinating neuropathy, there is a subgroup of patients who have clinical, electrophysiologic, and pathologic features indicating primarily an axonal injury as opposed to loss of the myelin sheath. Feasby and colleagues[16,17] in 1986 noted a subgroup of patients who had GBS and who had electrophysiologic findings of axonal degeneration, usually with severe paralysis and slow recovery, and pathologic changes in two cases indicating axonal degeneration without demyelination, and called this variant "axonal GBS." There has been disagreement about whether or not this represents an axonal variant of GBS or whether or not it represents a truly distinct type of peripheral neuropathy.

Griffin and colleagues[18] reported four patients who died 7 to 60 days after the onset of clinically diagnosed GBS. Two of these patients had serologic evidence of recent *Campylobacter jejuni* infection. Autopsy findings in three patients studied 7 to 18 days after onset of symptoms showed ongoing wallerian degeneration of ventral and dorsal root fibers and peripheral nerves with mild demyelination or lymphocytic infiltration. Macrophages were present in the periaxonal space of myelinated internodes, and occasional intra-axonal macrophages also were present. The patients studied 60 days after the onset of symptoms showed extensive loss of large fibers in roots and peripheral nerves and only mild demyelination and remyelination. These carefully studied cases confirm that GBS, as defined clinically, can be associated with a severe sensory-motor neuropathy in which the predominant lesion involves axons of motor and sensory fibers, and that an axonal form of GBS can follow *Campylobacter jejuni* infection.[18–20] A pure motor acute axonal neuropathy, a frequent cause of paralysis in China, also has been associated with antiganglioside antibodies.[20,21]

The prevailing theory for the association between Campylobacter infection and GBS is based on the lipopolysaccharide coat, which is rich in glycoconjugates. This lipopolysaccharide coat has similarities to human glycoconjugates, and it may be that antibodies generated against the lipopolysaccharide coat cross-react with glycoconjugates on peripheral nerves. Therefore, it may be that there is a shared epitope between the Campylobacter organism and human peripheral nerves[18] or so-called molecular mimicry.[22]

Illa and colleagues[23] reported axonal GBS in seven patients that began 5 to 15 days after parenteral injection of gangliosides. These patients had high titers of IgG GM1 antibodies with specificity for motor nerve terminals. Studies by Yuki and colleagues[24–27] indicate that the neuroepitope could be GM1 ganglioside or GD1a ganglioside. The Fisher variant of GBS has been associated with antibodies against GQ1b gangliosides.[27–29] Therefore, it may be that glycolipids or glycoproteins having epitopes similar to GM1 or GD1a are the immunologic attack site in the axonal forms of GBS.[18]

Guillain-Barré syndrome clinical features

GBS is the most common cause of acute nontraumatic generalized paralysis in young adults, with an annual incidence of 1.2 cases per 100,000 in developed countries. GBS can affect any age group from children to the elderly, although epidemiologic studies suggest that there is a peak in young adults and a second smaller peak in the fifth to seventh decades. It occurs in men slightly more often than in women.

Antecedent events

A variety of antecedent events precede the development of acute ascending paralysis. Roper and colleagues[10,30] prospectively studied patients who had GBS at Massachusetts General Hospital, noting that 49% had a prior upper respiratory tract infection, 10% had a diarrhea illness, and 3% had some form of pneumonia. In 3% of cases, Epstein-Barr virus infection was implicated and cytomegalovirus (CMV) infection occurred in 3%. Generalized malaise was noted in 3%, and another 3% had miscellaneous associated antecedent events, including Hodgkin's disease, surgery, systemic lupus, or vaccination. In 27% of patients, there was no prior identifiable illness or antecedent event.[30] Other reported associations with GBS have included viral hepatitis, mycoplasma, Lyme disease, and sarcoidosis. Reports of GBS in the setting of HIV infection suggest a stronger association than expected by chance occurrence.[31] *Campylobacter jejuni* infection as a cause of an acute diarrhea illness can be associated with subsequent GBS (described previously). Vaccinations occasionally are implicated. Widespread public attention and notoriety occurred with the swine flu vaccination program in 1975 as a result of the suggestion of an increased incidence of GBS associated with the vaccine.

Symptoms and signs

Usually patients experience an acute respiratory or gastrointestinal illness that lasts for several days and then resolves. This is followed in 1 to 2 weeks by the development of ascending paralysis. Typically, the legs are involved initially, and within a few days, the arms. Although described as an ascending paralysis, the weakness usually is approximately as marked in proximal limb muscles as in distal muscles. Patients often present with a complaint of difficulty walking, trouble arising from a chair or going up or down stairs, or simply instability of gait. Weakness tends to progress, usually over a course of 1 to 3 weeks. On occasion, patients have a fulminant rapidly progressive course in which paralysis becomes maximal within 1 or 3 days. Overall, approximately 50% of patients who have GBS reach maximal weakness by 1 week, 70% by 2 weeks, and 80% by 3 weeks into the course of the illness. Although symptoms are predominantly motor, patients commonly have mild paresthesias or mild objective sensory deficits on examination, in particular those involving position and vibration sense. Limb weakness is symmetric, and there is symmetric loss of the muscle stretch reflexes. Approximately one third of patients develop respiratory involvement requiring mechanical ventilation, and 50% develop cranial nerve involvement, most often facial weakness. One half of patients develop oropharyngeal weakness and 10% to 20% a degree of ocular involvement. Approximately 50% of patients develop autonomic dysfunction (including fluctuations of blood pressure, heart rate, ileus, or urinary retention). After the progression of weakness stops, patients tend to plateau for 2 to 4 weeks and then recover slowly. The recovery is such that by 6 months into the course of illness, 85% of patients are ambulatory. In 3% of cases there is recurrence of the paralytic illness, although some of these patients instead may have a chronic inflammatory neuropathy as opposed to recurrent GBS.

Overall, the mortality from the acute illness is reported as from 2% to 5%. Approximately 50% of patients have some degree of long-term residual symptomatic abnormality. Fifteen percent to 20% of patients have residual motor weakness at 1 year, and 5% remain severely disabled. This generally favorable natural history is the standard basis against which any therapeutic modality must be compared.

Laboratory testing

Within the first few days, most patients typically develop an abnormal spinal fluid profile, with high CSF protein concentration in the absence of a pleocytosis (albumino-cytologic dissociation). Glucose concentration is normal as are cultures. The elevation of CSF protein concentration is presumed to result from an increased permeability of the blood-CSF barrier. In the first day or 2, the CSF protein concentration commonly is normal. In Ropper's series, 34% of patients had normal CSF protein concentrations when measured in the first week, whereas in the second week only 18% were normal.[30] Serial CSF studies may be necessary to demonstrate an abnormality. Up to 5% to 10% of patients who have GBS may have a lymphocytic pleocytosis with as many as 100 white blood cells per mm.[3] In patients who have a CSF pleocytosis, the possibility of GBS associated with HIV infection, CMV, Lyme disease, or sarcoidosis should be considered.

Approximately 5% of patients who have GBS have abnormal liver function tests. Occasionally, patients demonstrate increased muscle enzymes, as seen in many forms of acute denervation. In severe or sudden cases of paralysis, stool cultures for *Campylobacter jejuni* may be positive, and many of these patients have associated anti-GM1 antibodies in serum.

Electromyography and nerve conduction studies can document the presence of a peripheral neuropathy that is of a demyelinating type.[32–36] A demyelinating neuropathy tends to produce very slow nerve conduction velocities, dispersed compound muscle action potentials (CMAP), and multifocal conduction block. Early on, the abnormalities on nerve conduction studies may be limited to very prolonged F waves. Because the neuropathy typically is a demyelinating type with sparing of the axons, there usually is little fibrillation on electromyography needle examination. In the first few days, the nerve conduction studies may be normal or only mildly abnormal. The electrophysiologic abnormalities tend to lag behind the clinical examination. Severe reduction in the CMAP amplitude may predict the long-term outcome. Miller and colleagues[37] showed that CMAP amplitudes less than 10% of normal were associated with a less favorable long-term prognosis Similarly, the North American Guillain-Barré Study Group noted worse prognosis associated with CMAP amplitude less than 20% of normal. Such observations are not universally accepted, as Triggs and colleagues found that 50% of patients who had severely reduced CMAP amplitudes were clinically normal at 1 year.[38]

In patients who have an axonal form, the electrophysiologic picture differs in that the nerve conduction studies show low amplitude responses, the conduction velocity is reduced more mildly, and the needle examination shows profuse fibrillation.

Fisher syndrome

In 1956 Fisher[4] reported "an easily recognizable syndrome...characterized among other features by total external ophthalmoplegia, severe ataxia and loss of the tendon reflexes." This well recognized variant of GBS has been given the eponym, Fisher syndrome, and accounts for approximately 5% of the cases of acute GBS in most series. Patients typically present with diplopia followed within several days by ataxia or clumsiness of the limbs. Some patients describe dizziness. Over the first week of neurologic symptoms, patients usually develop hypoactive or absent muscle stretch reflexes. One half of patients describe paresthesias. Occasionally, other cranial nerves are involved, resulting in oropharyngeal or facial weakness. Approximately one third of patients develop associated severe limb weakness with respiratory failure. The ophthalmoplegia evolves over 1 to 3 days and usually is severe or complete and symmetric. Most patients have ptosis. Pupillary function tends to be normal. The presence of ataxia has raised the question of cerebellar involvement. There may be intention tremor, suggesting a cerebellar deficit. Some patients have unsteadiness, lightheadedness, or dizziness. Vertigo, nystagmus, cerebellar dysarthria, and scanning speech, however, usually are absent. Patients who have Fisher syndrome most often have an elevated spinal fluid protein concentration, but they are more likely than those who have typical GBS to have normal CSF. A study comparing elevation of CSF protein with anti-GQ1b antibodies in 123 patients who had Fisher syndrome observed albumino-cytologic dissociation (high CSF protein) 59% during the first 3 weeks of illness compared with serum anti-GQ1b IgG antibody positivity in 85%.[39] The electrophysiologic studies show mild slowing of nerve conduction velocities compared with typical GBS and are more likely to be normal in the limbs than in GBS.

Differential diagnosis of patients who have Guillain-Barré syndrome

The differential diagnosis includes the spectrum of illnesses causing acute or subacute paralysis. Spinal cord compression, transverse myelitis, and spinal cord infarction should be considered. Peripheral neuropathies from a variety of causes can mimic GBS, including critical illness polyneuropathy; various toxins, including nitrofurantoin, chemotherapeutic drugs, and heavy metal poisons, such as arsenic and thallium; autoimmune inflammatory diseases, such as systemic lupus and polyarteritis nodosa; meningoradiculitis, as can be seen with Lyme disease, HIV infection, carcinomatous meningitis, and sarcoidosis; a paraneoplastic acute peripheral neuropathy; acute intermittent porphyria; and diphtheria. Hypokalemic periodic paralysis, myasthenia gravis, botulism, and poliomyelitis also should be considered. Then, presence of an acute or subacute flaccid paralysis in the setting of CNS signs and symptoms (such as encephalitis) should raise the question of West Nile virus infection.

For patients who present with an acute and early-on predominantly sensory neuropathy with distal burning numbness followed in days to weeks by motor involvement, a toxic neuropathy should be considered, as from chemotherapy; nitrofurantoin; heavy metals, such as arsenic and thallium; and the presence of a B vitamin deficiency, in particular thiamine.

Suggested laboratory evaluation for patients who have Guillain-Barré syndrome

Patients who present with an acute or subacute paralytic syndrome resembling GBS should have the following laboratory studies considered in every case:

1. If there is evidence pointing to a focal spinal cord lesion, patients should have emergent MRI scan of the appropriate level of the spine. The presence of focal spinal pain, a discreet sensory level, prominent bladder and bowel dysfunction, paraparesis without arm involvement, or selective areflexia in the legs with normal reflexes in the arms all should mandate careful exclusion of a myelopathy by performing an emergency MRI scan.
2. CSF should be analyzed for evidence of a myelitis and for the albumino-cytologic dissociation typical of GBS. If the spinal fluid is sampled within the first few days and is normal, a repeat study a week or 2 into the illness may be helpful if the diagnosis remains unclear. If there is a significant pleocytosis, consider HIV infection, CMV, Lyme disease, and sarcoidosis.
3. Appropriate blood work includes complete blood cell (CBC) count, electrolytes, and liver and renal function tests. With regard to underlying conditions, which can mimic or be associated with GBS, serum tests for an autoimmune inflammatory disease, such as systemic lupus and polyarteritis nodosa, should be done. All patients should be screened for HIV infection, and selected patients screened for Lyme disease, sarcoidosis, and West Nile virus infection.
4. Urine collection for acute intermittent porphyria is indicated.
5. Tests for hypokalemic periodic paralysis, myasthenia gravis, botulism, poliomyelitis, and diphtheria depend on the clinical evidence and suspicion and are not necessary in every patient.
6. Heavy metal poisoning can produce an acute or subacute peripheral neuropathy. In patients who have a predominantly axonal form of GBS, heavy metal screens should be obtained, particularly for arsenic and thallium. Similarly, patients who have pancytopenia, elevated liver function tests, and a history suggestive of a systemic illness also should be screened carefully for heavy metal poisoning. Patients who have recurrent episodes of acute neuropathy also should be screened carefully for toxins.
7. When the antecedent illness is gastrointestinal syndrome with diarrhea, stool cultures and serologic studies may reveal evidence for Campylobacter jejuni.
8. Screening for infection from Epstein-Barr virus, CMV, hepatitis virus, and Mycoplasma pneumoniae should be considered.
9. A careful review of patients' prior medication lists for any potentially neurotoxic drug, such as nitrofurantoin, may lead to a diagnosis of drug-induced toxic

neuropathy, as might a history of recent cancer chemotherapy. Megadose vitamin exposure, in particular pyridoxine, also should be considered.

Treatment of Guillain-Barré syndrome

All patients who have suspected GBS should be hospitalized for vigilant monitoring resulting from the high risk for respiratory failure and need for intubation and mechanical ventilation. Baseline spirometry, including FVC, and oximetry should be obtained. Indications for intubation include an FVC dropping below 12 mL/kg or, in a normal-sized adult, FVC falling below 1 L. Patients who are subjectively dyspneic or look to be struggling to breathe should be intubated, even if their FVC is above these levels. In general err on the side of early intubation rather than late. A simple bedside estimate of FVC can be made by having patients count out loud. If a patient can take a maximal inspiration and then can count up to 25, the FVC probably is approximately 2 L. A patient who can count up to 10 probably has approximately 1 L FVC.

The cornerstone of treatment is that of meticulous general medical support.[40–42] There should be a low threshold for putting patients in an ICU. All patients who are having progression of their weakness should be in an ICU. The common complications of GBS include respiratory failure, dysautonomia (especially cardiac arrhythmias, which may occur in 5% of cases), pneumonia, bladder dysfunction, pain, depression, phlebitis, pulmonary embolus, and syndrome of inappropriate antidiuretic hormone. Further complications from immobility and bed rest include decubiti; secondary compression neuropathy, such as ulnar neuropathy and peroneal neuropathy; and the psychiatric sequelae associated with a prolonged immobilizing stay in an ICU.[41] Intense back and limb pain improve with corticosteroids and other drugs used for neuropathic pain.

Immunotherapy

Corticosteroids To date there have been no studies that demonstrate the effectiveness of corticosteroids in the treatment of GBS. There have been retrospective nonrandomized studies along with several small prospective randomized studies, which have shown no clear benefit.[43] The use of high-dose intravenous methylprednisolone, as reported by Hughes, also has shown no benefit.[44] The Dutch GBS Study Group recently reported results of a prospective randomized control trial of IV methylprednisolone (500 mg/day for 5 days) versus placebo.[45] All patients also received intravenous immunoglobulin (IVIG). In this large study of 225 patients, there was no significant difference between treatment with methylprednisolone and those receiving placebo.[45] In summary, to date there is no compelling evidence to support the use of corticosteroids in patients who have GBS. The Quality Standards Subcommittee of the American Academy of Neurology published its practice parameter on immunotherapy for GBS syndrome concluding that corticosteroid therapy is not beneficial.[46]

Plasma exchange In 1978, Brettle and colleagues[47] first reported the benefits of plasma exchange (PE) in the treatment of GBS. Several large randomized trials have subsequently demonstrated benefit of PE in treating GBS.[48–52] The North American GBS Study Group,[49,50] the French,[52] and the Swedish[48] studies all have shown comparable benefit. In the North American GBS Study Group, the total volume of exchange was 200 mL/kg over 1 to 2 weeks or approximately 4 to 5 exchanges of 3.5 to 4 L on average.[49] There was no clear difference in the occurrence of complications in the PE versus the control group. The time to improve one clinical grade, which was defined as coming off the ventilator or being able to walk, decreased by 50% in the

PE group (19 days versus 40 days in the untreated group). The percent of patients was improved at 1 month, and the average clinical grade, was approximately 15% to 20% better in the PE group than in the control group. In addition, the time to regain independent walking was decreased by approximately 40% in the PE group (53 days versus 85 days in the untreated patients). No benefit was shown in this study when PE was started later than 2 weeks from onset of symptoms, leading to the suggestion that it be used as early as possible when the diagnosis is made.[49] Approximately 10% of patients are found to "rebound" and they often improve with repeat PE. The American Academy of Neurology practice parameter on immunotherapy for GBS syndrome performed a meta-analysis of all six PE studies, revealing that the proportion of patients on the ventilator 4 weeks after randomization was reduced to 48 of 321 in the PE group compared with 106 of 325 in the control group (relative risk [RR], 0.56; 95% CI, 0.41 to 0.76; $P = .0003$). In a meta-analysis of four studies for which the outcome was available, 135 of 199 PE and 112 of 205 control patients had recovered full muscle strength after 1 year (RR, 1.24 in favor of PE; 95% CI, 1.07 to 1.45; $P = .005$). One class II trial demonstrated a convincing beneficial effect of PE in more mildly affected ambulatory patients. In the meta-analysis, the RR of serious adverse events was similar in the PE and control groups.[46]

The practice parameter recommendation is:[46]

PE is recommended for nonambulant patients within 4 weeks of onset (level A, class II evidence) and for ambulant patients within 2 weeks of onset (level B, limited class II evidence). The effects of PE and IV immunoglobulin (IVIg) are equivalent.[46]

Intravenous immunoglobulin High-dose IVIG initially was reported to be beneficial in GBS by Kleyweg and colleagues[53] in 1988. In 1992, the Dutch GBS Study Group reported a prospective randomized trial comparing IVIG with PE.[54] In their study, IVIG was given at a dose of 0.4 g/kg per day for 5 days and was shown to be as beneficial as PE. The IVIG-treated patients showed a significantly shorter time to improve one disability grade, and somewhat fewer complications occurred in the IVIG group. Smaller series have suggested the greater possibility of clinical worsening during and after IVIG treatment[55] along with an increase in the relapse rate of patients after treatment with IVIG.[55,56] The PE group in the Dutch study had outcome results similar to the control group (untreated group) of the North American Plasma Exchange Trial. Bril and colleagues prospectively compared IVIG with PE in the treatment of 50 patients who had GBS.[57] Standard outcome measures did not differ between the two groups. Overall, 61% of the PE-treated patients and 69% of the IVIG patients improved by one disability grade at 1 month. The complication rate was found somewhat higher in the PE group. They concluded that the efficacy of IVIG in the treatment of GBS is similar to that PE, and that it can be used with safety. There was no difference in the relapse rate between the two therapies. This compares with the Dutch GBS Study Group, which reported 34% improvement of one disability grade within 1 month of receiving PE[54] compared with 53% in those receiving IVIG and the reported 59% improvement rate of the PE-treated patients in the North American trial.[49] Brill and colleagues also noted an increased frequency of complications in the PE group, including pneumonia, venous thrombosis, and line sepsis, compared with the IVIG group (19 versus 5). In the Dutch GBS study, 68 complications were noted in the PE group compared with 39 in the IVIG group. A prospective multicenter trial revealed that PE followed by IVIG showed no significant benefit compared with PE alone in any measured outcome, indicating that combination therapy (PE followed by IVIG) is unlikely to be beneficial.[58] Studies of IVIG in children who have GBS also indicate a beneficial effect.[59]

In general, IVIG is considered safe. Mild side effects, including headache, nausea, myalgia, fever, or chills, are reported in 1% to 15% of patients.[55–57,60–62] There are sporadic anecdotal reports, however, of more severe complications, including transmission of hepatitis C,[63] acute renal failure,[64] nephrotic syndrome,[65,66] stroke,[67,68] myocardial infarction,[69,70] aseptic meningitis,[71–73] and reversible encephalopathy with cerebral vasospasm.[74–91] Toxicity may be a result of sucrose toxicity, allergic phenomena, and effects of the high protein concentration on blood viscosity.

In the American Academy of Neurology practice parameter on immunotherapy for GBS, a meta-analysis of three trials comparing IVIG with PE revealed nonsignificant trends in favor of IVIG. There were no significant differences in the meta-analysis of time until discontinuation of mechanical ventilation and the proportions of patients dead or disabled after 1 year between the IVIG- and PE-treated groups. In each trial, there were more adverse events in the PE group than in the IVIG group. The practice parameter recommendation is:[46]

IVIg is recommended for patients with GBS who require aid to walk within 2 (level A recommendation) or 4 weeks from the onset of neuropathic symptoms (level B recommendation derived from class II evidence concerning PE started within the first 4 weeks and class I evidence concerning the comparisons between PE and IVIg started within the first 2 weeks). The effects of IVIg and PE are equivalent.[46]

Currently, there is evidence to support the use of PE or IVIG early on in the course of GBS. Current data do not provide an indication of one therapy being clearly superior to the other.

PATIENT TWO: CHRONIC SENSORY PERIPHERAL NEUROPATHY
Question: What to do with a Patient who Comes to the Office with Chronic Burning Numbness in the Feet?

Case presentation 2
A 52-year-old man presents with 2 to 3 years of gradual progressive burning, stinging, and tingling in the feet with a lesser extent of tingling in the fingertips bilaterally. He feels as though the feet are on fire and at times as though a blowtorch has been aimed at the soles. Shoes, socks, and even the light touch of bed sheets are very irritating and limit his ability to rest. When he is up on his feet walking around the pain becomes more severe. Intermittently there are sharp stabs or jabs of shooting and electrical shock pain in the feet. The examination shows decreased sensation in a stocking-glove pattern, which is symmetric. Muscle strength is normal. The muscle stretch reflexes are normal in the arms and at the knees but absent at the ankles. The legs are as shown in **Fig. 1.**

Discussion
This patient had a common clinical presentation of a chronic progressive sensory neuropathy with a great deal of burning discomfort. This type of predominantly small fiber sensory neuropathy has three common causes in my practice. The first cause is diabetes, and in the patient in Case Presentation 2, the presence of brown discoloration over the shins is a strong clue toward that as the underlying systemic disease—necrobiosis lipoidica diabeticorum. If a patient has type 1 diabetes, do not pursue any further tests to find the underlying cause. If there is no known history of diabetes and the screening studies are normal, then a glucose tolerance test is indicated. If all tests are normal and documentation of small fiber neuropathy is believed

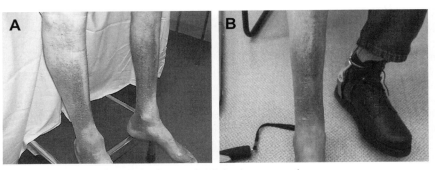

Fig. 1. Necrobiosis lipoidica diabeticorum in diabetic neuropathy.

essential then a skin biopsy should demonstrate loss of the small hypomyelinated fibers, although it will not provide the cause. The second clinical scenario associated with this neuropathy that is common is that of patients who have chronic alcohol overuse (and presumed toxicity to peripheral sensory nerves) or nutritional deficiency and, more specifically, vitamin B deficiency (usually thiamine). Therefore, a malnourished patient or one who has chronic alcohol use and who presents with this scenario is common. The third large group is one that has everything else, a veritable plethora of underlying conditions that can cause progressive burning–small fiber neuropathy. Some of the more serious conditions that can be diagnosed include chronic toxic neuropathies and amyloidosis and even those associated with a systemic vasculitis, such as Sjögren's syndrome, and copper deficiency. Most of the patients in this third group, however, have no identifiable underlying cause that can be found, regardless of the degree of the workup.

In general, if a patient has diabetes or has a strong alcohol or nutritional problem, I do not pursue much additional workup. Otherwise, I do obtain nerve conduction studies and an electromyogram and screen patients not only for diabetes but also for liver and kidney function, thyroid function, vitamin B_{12} level, CBC count, and serum protein electrophoresis to look for for a monoclonal gammopathy. I am more selective in sending studies for HIV, sarcoidosis, heavy metal poisoning, vasculitis, and other uncommon causes.

Approximately one third of the patients in my practice have chronic distal sensory neuropathy with or without pain and no clear cause. The literature provides a name for this condition, cryptogenic sensory neuropathy, and has observations that such patients should be expected to remain stable of slightly progressive over time. In these patients, management is symptomatic. Reflecting old school habits, I prefer starting with tricyclic antidepressant drugs (amitriptyline and nortriptyline); in an otherwise healthy adult, I start with 25 mg before bedtime; if a patient is small, frail, or sensitive to medications, however, I begin with 10 mg every night and increase the dose every week by 10 to 25 mg (**Box 1**). Most patients seem to improve at a dose of 25 to 75 mg at night. Most of my colleagues begin with gabapentin (300 mg at night) and increase weekly (to 300 mg three times a day). Should that fail, the next agents generally used in my universe are pregabalin (beginning at 50 mg at night with gradual increase) and duloxetine (beginning at 20–30 mg at night with gradual increase). Adjunctive pain control can be achieved with use of a mild narcotic (propoxyphene or codeine). For patients who have nutritional problems, vitamin B supplements, more specifically thiamine, may be of value although many patients seem to have residual long-term burning dysesthesias in spite of aggressive replacement therapy.

Box 1

Suggested treatment of neuropathic pain

Trigeminal neuralgia (sharp, stabbing face pain)

Carbamazepine (100 mg three times a day), increased to 200 mg three times a day in 3–4 days, or oxcarbazapine beginning at 150 mg twice a day and increased

Baclofen (10 mg twice a day), increased gradually to maximum 20 mg four times a day

Gabapentin (300 mg at night), increased as needed

Pregabalin (50 mg twice a day) and increased gradually

Limb neuralgia (sharp, stabbing, zinging lightning, bee-sting pain)

1. Phenytoin 100 mg orally two to three times a day

2. Carbamazepine

3. Baclofen

4. Gabapentin

5. Pregabalin

Continuous burning dysesthesias and supersensitivity (as in a diabetic neuropathy patient)

1. Amitriptyline or nortriptyline (10–25 mg orally at night) or duloxetine (30 mg at night) and increased gradually

2. Gabapentin

3. Pregabalin

4. Duloxetine

5. Propoxyphene or acetaminophen with codeine

6. Carbamazepine (or oxcarbazepine) 100 mg (150) twice a day and increased gradually

7. Topical capscasin

8. Mexiletine

PATIENT THREE: SUBACUTE OR CHRONIC PROGRESSIVE MOSTLY MOTOR AND SOME SENSORY NEUROPATHY (THE CHRONIC INFLAMMATORY DEMYELINATING POLYNEUROPATHY SCENARIO)
Question: What to do with a Patient who Comes to the Office with Several Months of Progressive Weakness due to Neuropathy?

Case presentation 3

A 50-year-old man presents with 8 months of slowly progressive trouble with walking and balance and mild numbness and tingling in the feet.

The examination shows mild weakness in the arms at 4+/5 very symmetric and moderate weakness in the legs 3/5 in the forelegs and 4/5 in the hips and thighs. Sensation is clearly reduced in a stocking and glove distribution to light tough and sharp sensation and moderately reduced to vibration and positions sense in the toes. Cranial function is normal. He denies pain. Muscle stretch reflexes are absent throughout and the patient has no other deficits on examination. The scenario is one of predominant and significant motor neuropathy. Of course the patient has sensory involvement but the likely diagnosis is suspected based on the preponderance of motor deficits. Symmetry and absent stretch reflexes are similar to the collage of examination findings seen in GBS but the protracted time course lead to a suspicion of chronic inflammatory demyelinating polyneuropathy (CIDP). It is written that if a patient presents with a GBS disorder and continues to progress beyond 8 weeks that it is by definition CIDP. Keys to establishing the diagnosis include the predominant motor involvement, absent stretch reflexes, elevation of spinal fluid protein, and nerve conduction studies showing marked slowing of velocity. If a patient has preserved muscle stretch reflexes, if the spinal fluid protein is normal, and if the nerve conduction studies do not show evidence for an acquired demyelinating neuropathy, then one should be cautious about making this diagnosis. Like it or not, with the large number of patients who have chronic neuropathy of unclear cause, it has become fashionable to assume they have variants of CIDP. Not only does this tend to derail the pursuit of the correct diagnosis but also all it leads too often to prolonged courses of a variety of immunotherapy. As corticosteroids are indicated for treatment of CIDP it is not unusual for a patient to receive 6 to 12 months of high-dose prednisone with no significant improvement before redirection of the diagnostic workup. Similarly, it is increasingly common for patients who have semiquasi CIDP to be treated with IVIG or subcutaneous immunoglobulin for months or years without a confirmed diagnosis and without significant clinical improvement. A therapeutic trail of prednisone and IVIG is not unreasonable when the diagnosis is murky and there are no other good options (a good option always includes a second opinion at referral subspecialty center). But those therapeutic trials should be with clear understanding of the risk (medical in the case of corticosteroids and financial in the case of IVIG), a fixed time-frame for monitoring, and understanding that there needs to be clear-cut impressive improvement in the patient's clinical status as reported by the patient and as confirmed by the clinician. Patients who have real CIDP do improve and the improvement is impressive. Treatment often is necessary for many years and, in some patients, decades although one should attempt to reduce and if possible withdraw treatment every 2 years or so.

Chronic Inflammatory Demyelinating Polyneuropathy Wannabes

A condition similar to CIDP can be associated with monoclonal gammopathy. A serum protein electrophoresis test (SPEP) should be obtained in every patient in whom CIDP is considered. In some patients who have an associated gammopathy the relationship is coincidental. In others, patients seem to have a chronic neuropathy associated with the gammopathy that otherwise is benign. Alternatively, the detection of a gammopathy may lead to the establishment of amyloidosis, lymphoma, Waldenström's macroglobulinemia, and other serious underlying systemic/hematologic disorders. I propose that every patient who has a CIDP-type presentation and who has a monoclonal gammopathy be evaluated by a hematologist. One of the most striking CIDP-type presentations is the patient who has motor-sensory neuropathy, absent reflexes, elevated CSF protein, and a gammopathy and who has a modest improvement temporarily with immunotherapy. The limited benefit of treatment and the presence of gammopathy should trigger a search for osteosclerotic myeloma and POEMS syndrome. Be suspicious of hair or skin changes. Darkened skin, increased hair-growth, and tight skin similar to scleroderma can be seen. Such patients need a metastatic bone survey and if any sclerotic or lytic lesions are detected then aggressive hematology-oncology consultation ensues. A sclerotic lesion may be solitary or may be one of many and when biopsied the presence of osteosclerotic myeloma can allow for an appropriate treatment program. In patients who have a solitary bone lesion, local radiation not only does cure the malignancy but also results in dramatic improvement in patients' peripheral neuropathy.

PATIENT FOUR: MULTIFOCAL MOTOR AND SENSORY NEUROPATHIES
(MULTIPLE MONONEUROPATHIES)
Question: What to do with a Patient who Comes to the Office with Several
Months of Patchy Asymmetric Weakness and Sensory Loss?

Case presentation 4

A 45-year-old woman presents with a 4-month history of symptoms. She initially had the onset of intense right though pain and sudden onset of foot drop and numbness over the top of the foot. Approximately 3 weeks later she noted numbness and tingling in the ulnar aspect of the left hand along with mild weakness. Two weeks prior to presentation, she developed intense left flank pain and weakness in the thigh. The examination shows the presence of a right foot drop and sensory findings of a peroneal neuropathy, weakness and sensory loss of a left femoral neuropathy, sensory and motor findings of a left ulnar neuropathy, weakness on lifting the right knee (hip flexor) and extending the knee (quadriceps), and weakness of the interosseous muscles of the left hand (finger spreading, ulnar nerve). Muscle stretch reflexes are reduced to normal except for an absent left knee jerk and absent right ankle jerk.

Discussion

This patient had a peripheral neuropathy characterized by patchy multifocal nerve dysfunction. The clinical picture often is referred to as mononeuritis multiplex. If the syndrome develops gradually over many years then the cause can be any one of several chronic predisposing conditions. When it develops over weeks to months, however, and in particular when associated with acute and painful onset of mononeuropathy, the condition becomes a medical emergency. In the patient in Case Presentation 4, it is essential to screen for vasculitis. Vasculitities known to cause mononeuritis multiplex include polyarteritis nodosa, Sjögren syndrome, and necrotizing vasculitis associated with mixed connective tissue disease. This patient needs an immediate serologic and systemic evaluation for vasculitis, including rheumatology consultation. Although the evaluation is in progress, I recommend that such a patient be empirically treated with high-dose corticosteroids (methylprednisolone [1000 mg daily for 3 days] and then reduced) and suggest hospitalization for treatment and expeditious evaluation. The reason for an emergent approach to these patients is that an active vasculitis is likely to produce nerve trunk infarctions resulting from involvement of the vasa nervorum. I have seen patients go on to infarct proximal nerve trunks in 3 to 4 limbs such that they cannot walk or use their arms adequately. Because nerve infarction damages the axon, the recovery phase is slow and incomplete. Axonal regeneration occurs at a snail's pace of an inch per month (a millimeter per day) such that it may take 6 months to 2 years for strength to return—thus, the importance of treating empirically when mononeuritis multiplex is first suspected.

Other causes of mononeuritis multiplex include multiple myeloma, Waldenström's macroglobulinemia, cryoglobulinemia, lymphoma, and sarcoidosis; in some parts of the world, leprosy should be considered. Diabetes mellitus is a known predisposing factor to the development of multiple mononeuropathies.

QUESTION: WHAT ABOUT A PATIENT WHO HAS LIFELONG SYMPTOMS OF TRANSIENT MONONEUROPATHIES?

If patients have a history going back to childhood or teenage years of multiple painless mononeuropathies that gradually recover, then a diagnosis of hereditary neuropathy with liability to pressure palsy should be pursued. This is an underrecognized cause of compressive neuropathies in otherwise healthy individuals.

Approximately 80% of patients have a positive family history and a genetic test is available to confirm the diagnosis. Patients tend to wake up with a foot drop from peroneal neuropathy that resolved over several months, and they wake with an ulnar neuropathy, median neuropathy, or a wrist drop from compressive radial neuropathy. They have defective myelin sheath that predisposes them to compressive nerve dysfunction. They do not have pain. The treatment is prevention with avoiding nerve compression and use of soft sleeping surfaces, such as a waterbed, padding, and so forth. The condition is autosomal dominant. A diagnosis spares a patient unnecessary surgery for carpal tunnel syndrome, ulnar nerve entrapment, a variety of other tests, and treatment that is of no value. The hereditary nature of the condition should be useful for other family members who are being evaluated for various mononeuropathies (**Fig. 2**).

QUESTION: WHAT ABOUT A PATIENT WHO HAS HAD MONTHS TO YEARS OF PURE MOTOR MONONEUROPATHIES?

An important consideration in patients who present with asymmetric painless weakness in the hands and forelegs is multifocal motor neuropathy. The patients come in after a gradual development of hand symptoms going back 6 to 12 months. Usually the symptoms are asymmetric and patients often have atrophy and fasciculation. Because there is no sensory loss and the indolent insidious progression, there often is a suspicion that patients may have amyotrophic lateral sclerosis or motor neuron disease. Patients who have amyotrophic lateral sclerosis, however, usually have upper motor neuron signs (hyper-reflexia) and often they have bulbar symptoms and signs that never occur in multifocal neuropathy. The nerve conduction studies should be central to confirming the presence of multiple motor mononeuropathies with areas of conduction block along the course if the nerve. Additionally, approximately 50% of these patients have anti-GM1 ganglioside antibodies in their serum. When confirmed with either of these studies, patients are treated with high-dose intravenous or subcutaneous gamma globulin and the majority actually improve in the setting of treatment.

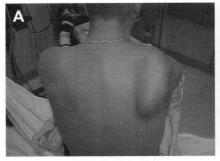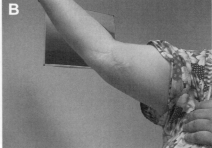

Fig. 2. A 24-year-old man who had long thoracic nerve palsy. At age 12 he had a peroneal neuropathy, and he frequently awakens with tingling and weakness in the limbs. The 44-year-old mother of the patient has had bilateral ulnar nerve surgery, bilateral carpal tunnel release, and surgery for thoracic outlet syndrome. These two patients have hereditary neuropathy with liability to pressure palsy.

PATIENT FIVE: CHARCOT-MARIE-TOOTH DISEASE
Question: When to Suspect a Hereditary Neuropathy?

Case presentation 5

*A 45-year-old man presents with several years several years of gradual decline in running and he has quit playing sports due to twisting his ankles. He feels his balance is poor on uneven ground and when walking in dim light. He has no pain. He notes that his father and aunt had similar symptoms starting in adulthood but neither ever required a wheelchair. The examination shows normal muscle strength and bulk in the hips and thighs. There is mild weakness with foot dorsiflexion bilaterally. He also has mild weakness with extension of the fingers and spreading of the fingers; otherwise the upper extremity strength is normal. Sensory examination shows normal sharp sensation throughout but the patient's vibrations sense is definitely reduced at the toes and to a lesser degree at the ankles. His proprioception also is slightly reduced at the toes. Gait shows the patient to have a mild steppage quality. Muscle stretch reflexes are uniformly absent. The appearance of the legs and feet are similar to those shown in the photos (**Fig. 3**).*

Discussion

This patient has a chronic, predominantly motor, peripheral neuropathy without the typical burning stinging tingling symptoms of patients who have an acquired (diabetic) neuropathy. The predominance of motor involvement, the fact that all the reflexes are absent even though the weakness is restricted to the most distal muscles, and the presence of dimorphic appearance (see **Fig. 3**) all point to a hereditary neuropathy lumped together as Charcot-Marie-Tooth disease [CMT]. The family history in this case adds further certainty to the diagnosis. There are several reasons to make this diagnosis. When made, it spares patients a costly and endless set of future diagnostic

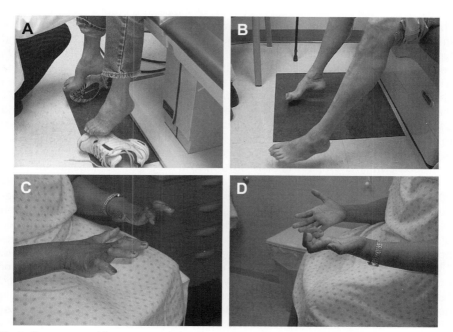

Fig. 3. Pes cavus and hammertoe deformity in CMT. Hand atrophy CMT.

studies. Further, it gives patients an answer. Third, it allows for a clear understanding of prognosis. Extremely slowly progressive, nothing will change overnight—no surprises. Most patients do not require a wheelchair although those affected more severely might. There is no effect on cognition, bladder, bowel, and so forth. Patients feel better with an answer and a prognosis. The fourth reason to make the diagnosis is for family counseling purposes given the hereditary basis for the disease. Although most patients have an autosommal dominant form of CMT, there are a variety of subtypes with differing patterns of inheritance.

Question: What Should be Done in the Way of Laboratory Evaluation for Patient Five?

With some patients I do nothing. As there is no treatment at this juncture that is proved to slow the course of CMT, expensive gene testing for decision making regarding treatment cannot be justified. For general physicians, I suggest that the most cost-effective and useful diagnostic step is consultation with a neuromuscular specialist. Nerve conduction studies typically reveal absent responses in the legs and very slow conduction velocity in the arms. If the study is performed by a physician who has limited understanding of CMT, the report concludes something like, "very severe generalized peripheral neuropathy," when a patient is in this case is really quite strong. The mismatch of abnormalities on the nerve conduction studies and the clinical examination should raise the question of hereditary neuropathy if it has not already been considered. Regarding speed of nerve conduction, we are born with motor nerves having sufficient myelin to provide approximately 25 m per second velocity. During the initial 3 years of life, myelin improves and matures such that by age 3, patients should have an adult range for nerve conduction, approximately 50 m per second speed of conduction. Patients who have CMT have lifelong detectable slow conduction velocity, often in the 20- to 30- m per second range. From age 3 up, the presence of velocities in the 20- to 30-m per second range indicates a problem with the myelin sheath. The other major group of patients who have demyelinating neuropathy (other than CMT) is those who have CIDP. Because CIDP is more rapidly progressive and typically improves with immunotherapy it is important to make the distinction. On nerve conduction studies the CMAP typically is dispersed and choppy in appearance whereas in CMT it typically is smooth. Patients who have CIDP have an elevation spinal fluid protein whereas patients who have CMT do not. Patients who have CMT have a very protracted course (often the history extends back for decades) and patients who have CMT have strikingly distal weakness, whereas CIDP are more likely to also have significant proximal weakness. The dysmorphic features (see **Fig. 3**) are never acquired from CIDP. Approximately 50% of patients who have CMT have a high arch (pes cavus) and approximately 30% have a very flat foot (pes planus). The cocked-up toes (hammertoe deformity) also are seen in most patients. Approximately 20% to 30% of patients have hypertrophic nerves that can be palpated on examination. If there is access to a genetic counselor it is ideal for patients to discuss the various genetic issues. Gene testing is widely available for many but not all subtypes of CMT. Although it seems obvious to run those tests in every patient who has suspected CMT, I suggest waiting until the neuromuscular consultation is completed. The full battery, or panel, of gene tests is extensive and cost is a major problem for patients who have limited resources; many insurance programs do not cover genetic testing. Even the Muscular Dystrophy Association neuromuscular clinic system in general does not cover genetic testing. Benefits must be weighed against the cost of extensive testing. In many patients a good neuromuscular specialist can pinpoint the subtype of CMT with sufficient accuracy so that if gene testing is desired then a single test may suffice instead of a costly panel. The most common abnormalities are CMT1A duplication, Cx32, an dMFN2 mutations. I have cared for patients in whom a battery of gene tests were performed, with patients getting a large bill for out-of-pocket expenses, and because there is no specific proved treatment for any of the CMT conditions, the patients feel like the decision to test was in retrospect faulty. Because forms of CMT cannot be tested for, the patients may invest a small fortune in gene tests and still not have a specific answer.

The treatment is symptomatic. For significant foot drop we use ankle foot orthotics, although one third of our patients try them and conclude they are more comfortable and function better without. For those in whom hand function is affected, occupational therapy for selection of tools for activities of daily living is central to management. If patients have musculoskeletal ankle pain, we use analgesics, and if patients have muscle cramps, we use quinine or gabapentin. I tend to see these patients in long-term follow-up once per year. One important aspect of their follow-up (as they do not change much over 12 months) is to keep them informed and in the loop about new developments and potential clinical trials for treatment.

PATIENT SIX: ACUTE OR SUBACUTE SENSORY NEUROPATHY OR SENSORY ATAXIA
Question: What does it mean if a Patient Presents with Acute or Subacute Pure Sensory Neuropathy?

Case presentation 6
A 30-year-old woman presents with 3 weeks of progressive numbness and tingling in the feet and hands and wobbly ataxic gait. Examination shows markedly decreased position and vibration sense in the toes and fingertips, decreased sensation to pin prick distally in the limbs in symmetric fashion, and reduced muscle stretch reflexes. Muscle strength is normal. The patient has a very wide-based wobbly gait and with eyes closed tends to fall over.

Discussion
This patient has a sensory neuronopathy with the lesion located most likely in the dorsal root ganglia and affecting large sensory fibers, resulting in a profound degree of position and vibratory loss and ataxic gait (sensory ataxia). There are several causes to consider in such a patient. Given the presence of a 3-week history the patient may have an immune-mediated inflammatory sensory neuronopathy, in other words, a sensory form of Guillain-Barré syndrome. Such patients may have an elevated spinal fluid protein and may improve spontaneously or more rapidly with immunotherapy, such as IVIG or plasmapheresis. Alternatively, patients could have vitamin B_{12} deficiency, which causes a sensory neuronopathy with involvement of the large fibers causing difficulty with position and vibration sense. Such patients often have subacute combined systems degeneration, which leads to a combination of dorsal column dysfunction, and descending corticospinal tract deficits, giving the patient some degree of spasticity, stiffness in the legs, and Babinski's signs. Such patients should have a serum vitamin B_{12} level and CBC count to screen for vitamin B_{12} deficiency. Sjögren's syndrome also can be associated with a sensory neuronopathy, and appropriate serologic studies are indicated.

Of great importance for a subacute presentation in otherwise healthy young persons is an occult malignancy leading to a sensory neuronopathy as a remote effect of carcinoma. Patients who have this condition typically have detectable levels of anti-Hu antibodies in serum. This paraneoplastic antibody should be screened in such patients; if positive, an aggressive search for an occult malignancy is indicated. The anti-Hu or antineuronal antibody type 1 can cause not only a sensory neuropathy but also a paraneoplastic encephalomyelitis. The anti-Yo or anti-Purkinje cell antibody is associated with cerebellar degeneration, particularly in women who have ovarian cancer. Other paraneoplastic antibodies include the anti-Ri or antineuronal antibody type 2 which is associated with the opsoclonus/myoclonus syndrome in adults. There is an antibody against amphiphysin, which is seen in patients who have paraneoplastic stiff person syndrome. Those who have anti–voltage-gated calcium channels have Lambert-Eaton syndrome and small cell cancer of the lung.

In patients who have a pure sensory neuropathy as a paraneoplastic disorder, there is selective damage to the dorsal root ganglia associated with some degree of perivasculitic lymphocytic infiltration. There is diffuse distal symmetric symptomatology with early involvement of discriminative modalities, profound impairment of coordination, the presence of pseudoathetosis, uselessness of the limbs, and areflexia in the setting of relative preservation of strength. The underlying malignancies in such patients often are small cell carcinoma, but occasionally breast and prostatic cancer are associated with a pure sensory neuropathy. Patients who have received toxic chemotherapy, such as platinum or vincristine, may have that as the cause of their sensory symptoms. Some of the blood dyscrasias and those receiving megadoses of pyridoxine/vitamin B_6 can have a sensory neuronopathy from dorsal root ganglia involvement. Immunotherapy and successful treatment of an associated malignancy (if the patient has that condition) are the main therapeutic options.

PATIENT SEVEN: POEMS
Question: How to Approach a Patient who has Chronic Neuropathy and Changes in Skin and Hair?

Case presentation 7

*A 55-year-old teacher presented with 6 months of progressive weakness, sensory loss, and change in gait. He has had changes in speech and phonation. He also noted new hair growth (**Fig. 4**) and skin tightness and thickness. The examination shows that he is weak at 4/5 in the limbs and has reduced sensation in distal fashion and absent muscle stretch reflexes throughout. The presence of progressive proximal and distal symmetric weakness, distal sensory loss, and absent reflexes fits best with the CIDP presentation (described previously). His nerve conduction velocities are approximately 25 m per second and spinal fluid protein is elevated at 110 with normal cells. He had screens for diabetes, thyroid, vitamin B_{12}, heavy metals, and vasculitis that were normal. His neurologist believed this fit*

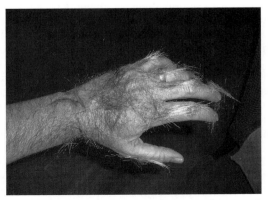

Fig. 4. A 55-year-old teacher with 6 months' progressive weakness and new hair growth.

best with CIDP and treated him with high-dose corticosteroids. He had mild improvement in strength for 2 months but then seemed to progress. Also, he developed a steroid psychosis on prednisone and became dysinhibited, delusional, and at times violent. Because his neuropathy symptoms were not responding well to the treatment and he could not tolerate corticosteroids he was referred for further assessment.

Discussion

The presence of new hair growth and tight thick skin in the setting a peripheral neuropathy should raise the question of *Polyneuropathy, Organomegaly, Endocrinopathy, Monoclonal protein, and Skin changes (POEMS) syndrome. Hair growth, scleroderma-like skin, hyperpigmentation, and whitening the nails all can be seen as the (skin changes seen in POEMS). The neuropathy of POEMS is similar to that seen in CIDP and it is common for patients to initially receive that diagnosis and associated management. They tend not to respond favorably to treatment of the long term, however, and eventually present for progressive neuropathy. The endocrine problems with POEMS may have been another factor in this patient. The key toward a favorable outcome for him is to suspect POEMS and obtain a SPEP, which in every case reveals

---

Box 2
Sensory mononeuropathies 2009

Meralgia paresthetica: lateral femoral cutaneous neuropathy (meros = thigh, algos = pain, paresthetica = tingling)

    Causes: sporadic, diabetes, obesity, pregnancy, pelvic disease, holster, toolbelt, surgical table, familial

Cheiralgia ("hand pain") paresthetica: superficial radial sensory neuropathy

    Handcuffs, IV, blood draws (legal stuff)

Gonyalgia paresthetica: infrapateller branch of the saphenous nerve

    Idiopathic, knee trauma, surgery, "influenza knee"

    Viral, diabetes

Saphenous neuropathy: same differential

Digitalgia paresthetica: digital neuropathy

    Fingers > toes

Notalgia paresthetica: posterior rami of T2-T6 (notos = back)

    Cause unknown but benign tingling, itching, burning

    ? Due to sharp right angle course of the nerve through the multifidus muscle

Intercostal neuropathy

    Mostly thoracic

    Diabetes, herpes zoster, pregnancy

    Radicular pain

Mental nerve neuropathy: numb chin syndrome

    Ominous: 25% malignancy; look for mets at the base of the skull or CSF

Facial sensory neuropathy: trigeminal neuropathy

    Sarcoidosis, Sjögren's syndrome, scleroderma

a monoclonal gammopathy. Then the patient needs a bone survey looking for evidence of osteosclerotic myeloma. If a sclerotic bone lesion is found, then a biopsy secures the diagnosis and provides the justification for treatment. Treatment options include radiation if solitary and chemotherapy if multiple lesions are detected.

Question: Is there any Low-Hanging Fruit in the Management of Patients who have Peripheral Neuropathy?

Regardless of the cause and type of neuropathy, patients are prone to the following common symptoms, although at times the focus is so much on diagnosis and primary treatment that there is failure to methodically address the common symptomatic issues that may benefit patients more than anything else.

1. Mechanical problems from weakness: splints for foot drop and wrist drop can have a major impact on function and in the case of ankle-foot orthotics can reduce the risk for falls and further ankle trauma.
2. Neuropathic "pain" (see **Box 1**).
3. Muscle camps. Cramps can occur with any peripheral nerve of nerve root disorder in which the motor component is affected. Most true muscle cramps are neurogenic and not the result of muscle disease. It helps to ask patients about their cramps and if they want treatment. If treatment is desired then I suggest the following: for patients who have severe muscle cramps, there are several medications that work nicely to control the symptoms. Quinine (260 mg), one tablet each evening, is safe and the most consistently effective. Unfortunately, in 2007, the Food and Drug Administration (FDA) required all but one manufacturer of quinine to remove their respective products from the market, and the FDA also strongly advises that the one remaining available product (Qualaquin [324 mg]) be used only for the treatment of malaria and not for the treatment of muscle cramps (because of concerns over the safety of the quinine). In my opinion, low-dose quinine (260 mg daily) is remarkably safe but these regulatory actions may make quinine more difficult to provide to patients. Quinine is in tonic water but a full glass daily provides only 40 to 50 mg of quinine. If quinine is ineffective or unavailable, then the tendency is to use gabapentin at low doses; baclofen, oxcarbazepine, tizanidine, zinc, or vitamin E may be useful in selected patients.
4. Restless lags syndrome (RLS): there are several conditions that are well established to predisposing to the development of RLS. Anemia, in particular iron deficiency, is associated with RLS. And patients who have peripheral neuropathy for any cause also are predisposed. So it behooves clinicians to explore RLS in all patients who are followed for peripheral neuropathy, as patients are relatively easy to treat with dopaminergic drugs or low-dose opioids.
5. Know the sensory mononeuropathies (**Box 2**).

REFERENCES

1. Landry O. Note sur la paralysie ascendante aigue. Gazette Hebd 1859;6:472–4.
2. Guillain G, Barré JA, Strohl A. Sur un syndrome de radicu-lo-nevrite avec hyper-albuminose du liquide cephalo-rachidien sans reaction cellulaire. Remarques sur les caracteres clinques et graphiques des reflexes tendineux. Bulletins et memories de la societe medicale des hopitaux de Paris. Paris: Masson et Cie 1916;40:1462–70.
3. Guillain G, Barré JA. Travaux neurologiques de guerre. Masson et Cie (Paris), 1920.

4. Fisher CM. An unusual variant of acute idiopathic polyneuritis syndrome of ophthalmoplegia, ataxia and areflexia. N Engl J Med 1956;255:57–65.

5. Haymaker W, Kernohan JW. The Landry-Guillain-Barre syndrome. A clinicopathologic report of fifty fatal cases and a critique of the literature. Medicine 1949;28:59–141.

6. Asbury AK, Arnason BG, Adams RD. The inflammatory lesion in idiopathic polyneuritis. Medicine 1969;48:173–215.

7. Waksman BH, Adams RD. Allergic neuritis: an experimental disease of rabbits induced by the injection of peripheral nervous tissue and adjurants. J Exp Med 1955;102:213–35.

8. Hartung HP, Pollard JD, Harvey GK, et al. Immunopathogenesis and treatment of the Guillain-Barre syndrome—Part I. Muscle Nerve 1995;18:137–53.

9. Hartung HP, Pollard JD, Harvey GK, et al. Immunopathogenesis and treatment of the Guillain-Barre syndrome—Part II. Muscle Nerve 1995;18:154–64.

10. Ropper AH. The Guillain-Barre syndrome. N Engl J Med 1992;326:1130–6.

11. Kaldor J, Speed BR. Guillain-Barré syndrome and Campylobacter jejuni: a serological study. Br Med J 1984;288:1867–70.

12. Vriesendorp FJ, Mishu B, Blaser M, et al. Serum anti-bodies to GM1, peripheral nerve myelin, and *Campylobacter jejuni* in patients with Guillain-Barré syndrome and controls: correlation and prognosis. Ann Neurol 1993;34:130–5.

13. Enders U, Karch H, Toyka KV, et al. The spectrum of immune responses to *Campylobacter jejuni* and glycoconjugates in Guillain-Barré syndrome and in other neuroimmunological disorders. Ann Neurol 1993;34:136–44.

14. Tam CC, Rodrigues LC, O'Brien SJ. Guillain-Barre syndrome associated with Campylobacter jejuni infection in England, 2000–2001. Clin Infect Dis 2003;37:307–10.

15. Rees JH, Hughes RAC. *Campylobacter jejuni* and Guillain-Barré syndrome. Ann Neurol 1994;35(2):248.

16. Feasby TE, Gilbert JJ, Brown WF, et al. An acute axonal form of Guillain-Barré polyneuropathy. Brain 1986;109:1115–26.

17. Feasby TE, Hahn AF, Brown WF, et al. Severe axonal degeneration in acute Guillain-Barré syndrome: evidence of two different mechanism? J Neurol Sci 1993;116:185–92.

18. Griffin JW, Li CY, Ho TW, et al. Pathology of the motor-sensory axonal Guillain-Barre syndrome. Ann Neurol 1996;39:17–28.

19. Griffin JW, Li CY, Ho TW, et al. Guillain-Barré syndrome in northern China: the spectrum of neuropathologic changes in clinically defined cases. Brain 1995;118:577–95.

20. Ho TW, Mishu B, Li CY, et al. Guillain-Barré syndrome in northern China: relationship to *Campylobacter jejuni* infection and anti-glycolipid antibodies. Brain 1995;118:597–605.

21. McKhann GM, Cornblath DR, Griffin JW, et al. Acute motor axonal neuropathy: a frequent cause of acute flaccid paralysis in China. Ann Neurol 1993;33:333–42.

22. Oomes PG, Jacobs BC, Hazenberg MPH, et al. Anti GM1 IgG antibodies and Campylobacter bacteria in Guillain-Barré syndrome: evidence of molecular mimicry. Ann Neurol 1995;38:170–5.

23. Illa I, Ortiz N, Gallard E, et al. Acute axonal Guillain-Barré syndrome with IgG antibodies against motor axons following parenteral gangliosides. Ann Neurol 1995;38:218–24.

24. Yuki N, Taki T, Takahashi M, et al. Penner's serotype 4 of *Campylobacter jejuni* has a lipopolysaccharide that bears a GM1 ganglioside epitope as well as one that bears a GD1a epitope. Infect Immun 1994;62:2101–3.

25. Yuki N, Yamada M, Sato S, et al. Association of IgG anti-GD1a antibody with severe Guillain-Barre syndrome. Muscle Nerve 1993;16:642–7.
26. Yuki N, Yoshino H, Sato S, et al. Acute axonal polyneuropathy associated with anti-GM1 antibodies following *Campylobacter jejuni* enteritis. Neurology 1990;40:1900–2.
27. Willison HJ, Veitch J, Patterson G, et al. Miller Fisher syndrome is associated with serum antibodies to GQ1b ganglioside. J Neurol Neurosurg Psychiatr 1993;56:204–6.
28. Yuki N, Sato S, Tsuji S, et al. Frequent presence of anti-GQ1b antibody in Fisher's syndrome. Neurology 1993;43:414–7.
29. Willison HJ, Veitch J. Immunoglobulin subclass distribution and binding characteristics of anti-GQ1b antibodies in Miller Fisher syndrome. J Neurochem 1994; 50:159–65.
30. Ropper AH, Wijdicks EFM, Truax BT. Guillain-Barré Syndrome. Philadelphia: F.A. Davis, Publishers; 1991.
31. Cornblath DR, McArthur JC, Kennedy PGE, et al. Inflammatory demyelinating peripheral neuropathies associated with HTLV III infection. Ann Neurol 1987;21: 32–40.
32. Albers JW, Donofrio PD, McGonagle TK. Sequential electrodiagnostic abnormalities in acute inflammatory demyelinating polyradiculoneuropathy. Muscle Nerve 1985;8:528–39.
33. Albers JW, Kelly JJ Jr. Acquired inflammatory demyelinating polyneuropathies: clinical and electrodiagnostic features. Muscle Nerve 1989;12:435–51.
34. Eisen A, Humphreys P. The Guillain-Barré syndrome. A clinical and electrodiagnostic study of 25 cases. Arch Neurol 1974;30:438–43.
35. McLeod JG. Electrophysiological studies in the Guillain-Barre syndrome. Ann Neurol 1981;9(Suppl):20–7.
36. Olney RK, Aminoff MJ. Electrodiagnostic features of the Guillain-Barre syndrome: the relative sensitivity of different techniques. Neurology 1990;40:471–5.
37. Miller RG, Peterson GW, Daube JR, et al. Prognostic value of electrodiagnosis in Guillain-Barre syndrome. Muscle Nerve 1988;11:769–74.
38. Triggs WJ, Cros D, Gominak SC, et al. Motor nerve inexcitability in Guillain-Barré syndrome. Brain 1992;115:1291–302.
39. Nishimoto Y, Odaka M, Hirata K, et al. Usefulness of anti-GQ1b IgG antibody testing in Fisher syndrome compared with cerebrospinal fluid examination. J Neuroimmunol 2004;148:200–5.
40. Chalela JA. Pearls and pitfalls in the intensive care management of Guillain-Barre syndrome. Semin Neurol 2001;21:399–405.
41. Henderson RD, Lawn ND, Fletcher DD, et al. The morbidity of Guillain-Barre syndrome admitted to the intensive care unit. Neurology 2003;60:17–21.
42. Kieseier BC, Hartung HP. Therapeutic strategies in the Guillain-Barre syndrome. Semin Neurol 2003;23:159–68.
43. Hughes RAC, Newsom-Davis JM, Perkin GD, et al. Controlled trial of prednisolone in acute polyneuropathy. Lancet 1978;750–3.
44. Guillain-Barre Syndrome Steroid Trial Group. Double-blind trial of intravenous methylprednisolone in Guillain-Barre syndrome. Lancet 1993;341:586–90.
45. van Koningsveld R, Schmitz PI, Meche FG, et al. Dutch GBS study group. Effect of methylprednisolone when added to standard treatment with intravenous immunoglobulin for Guillain-Barre syndrome: randomised trial. Lancet 2004;363:192–6.
46. Hughes RA, Wijdicks EF, Barohn R, et al. Quality Standards Subcommittee of the American Academy of Neurology. Practice parameter: immunotherapy for Guillain-Barre syndrome: report of the Quality Standards Subcommittee of the American Academy of Neurology. Neurology 2003;61:736–40.

47. Brettle RP, Gross M, Legg NJ, et al. Treatment of acute polyneuropathy by plasma exchange. Lancet 1978;2(8099):1100.
48. Osterman PO, Lundemo G, Pirskanen R, et al. Beneficial effects of plasma exchange in acute inflammatory polyradiculoneuropathy. Lancet 1984;2(8415):1296–9.
49. The Guillain-Barre Syndrome Study Group. Plasmapheresis and acute Guillain-Barre syndrome. Neurology 1985;35:1096–104.
50. McKhann GM, Griffin JW, Cornblath DR, et al. Plasmapheresis and Guillain-Barre syndrome: analysis of prognostic factors and the effect of plasmapheresis. Ann Neurol 1988;23:347–53.
51. French Cooperative Group on Plasma Exchange in Guillain-Barre Syndrome. Efficiency of plasma exchange in Guillain-Barre syndrome: role of replacement fluids. Ann Neurol 1987;22:753–61.
52. French Cooperative Group on Plasma Exchange in Guillain-Barre syndrome. Plasma exchange in Guillain-Barre syndrome: one-year follow-up. Ann Neurol 1992;32:94–7.
53. Kleyweg RP, van der Meche FGA, Meulstee J. Treatment of Guillain-Barre syndrome with high-dose gammaglobulin. Neurology 1988;38:1639–41.
54. van der Meche FGA, Schmitz PIM. Dutch Guillain-Barre Study Group: a randomized trial comparing intravenous immune globulin and plasma exchange in Guillain-Barre syndrome. N Engl J Med 1992;326:1123–9.
55. Castro LHM, Ropper AH. Human immune globulin infusion in Guillain-Barre syndrome: worsening during and after treatment. Neurology 1993;43:1034–6.
56. Irani DN, Cornblath DR, Chaudry V, et al. Relapse in Guillain-Barre syndrome after treatment with human immune globulin. Neurology 1993;43:872–5.
57. Bril V, Ilse WK, Pearce R, et al. Pilot trial of immunoglobulin versus plasma exchange in patients with Guillain-Barre' syndrome. Neurology 1996;46:100–3.
58. Plasma Exchange/Sandoglobulin Guillain-Barré Syndrome Trial Group. Randomised trial of plasma exchange, intravenous immunoglobulin, and combined treatments in Guillain-Barré syndrome. Lancet 1997;349:225–30.
59. Koul R, Chacko A, Ahmed R, et al. Ten-year prospective study (clinical spectrum) of childhood Guillain-Barre syndrome in the Arabian peninsula: comparison of outcome in patients in the pre- and post-intravenous immunoglobulin eras. J Child Neurol 2003;18:767–71.
60. Mokrzycki MH, Kaplan AA. Therapeutic plasma exchange: complications and management. Am J Kidney Dis 1994;23:817–27.
61. Rodnitzky RL, Goeken JA. Complications of plasma exchange in neurologic patients. Arch Neurol 1982;39:350–4.
62. Bouget J, Chevret S, et al. Plasma exchange morbidity in Guillain-Barre syndrome: results from the French prospective, double-blind, randomized, multicenter study. Crit Care Med 1993;21:651–8.
63. Thornton CA, Ballow M. Safety of intravenous immunoglobulin. Arch Neurol 1993;50:135–6.
64. Duhem C, Dicato MA, Ries F. Side-effects of intravenous immune globulins. Clin Exp Immunol 1994;97(Suppl 1):79–83.
65. Bjoro K, Froland SS, Yun Z, et al. Hepatitis C infection in patients with primary hypogammaglobulinemia after treatment with contaminated immune globulin. N Engl J Med 1994;331:1607–11.
66. Tan E, Hajinazarian M, Bay W, et al. Acute renal failure resulting from intravenous immunoglobulin therapy. Arch Neurol 1993;50:137–9.
67. Silbert PL, Knezevic WV, Bridge DT. Cerebral infarction complicating intravenous immunoglobulin therapy for polyneuritis cranialis. Neurology 1992;42:257–8.

68. Steg RE, Letkowitz DM. Cerebral infarction following intravenous immunoglobulin therapy for myasthenia gravis. Neurology 1994;44:1180–1.
69. Woodruff RK, Grigg AP, Firkin FC, et al. Fatal thrombotic events during treatment of autoimmune thrombocytopenia with intravenous immunoglobulin in elderly patients. Lancet 1986;328:217–8.
70. Dalakas MC. High-dose intravenous immunoglobulin and serum viscosity: risk of precipitating thromboembolic events. Neurology 1994;44:223–6.
71. Scribner CL, Kapit RM, Phillips ET, et al. Aseptic meningitis and intravenous immunoglobulin therapy. Ann Intern Med 1994;121:305–6.
72. Sekul EA, Cupler EJ, Dalakas MC. Aseptic meningitis associated with high-dose intravenous immunoglobulin therapy: frequency and risk factors. Ann Intern Med 1994;121:259–62.
73. DeVlieghere FC, Peetermans WE, Vermylen J. Aseptic granulocytic meningitis following treatment with intravenous immunoglobulin. Clin Infect Dis 1994;18:1008–10.
74. Voltz R, Rosen FV, Yousry T, et al. Reversible encephalopathy with vasospasm in a Guillain-Barré syndrome patient associated with intravenous immunoglobulin. Neurology 1996;46:250–1.
75. Martin CN, Hughes RAC. Epidemiology of peripheral neuropathy. J Neurol Neurosurg Psychiatr 1997;62:310–8.
76. Boulton AJ, Gries FA, Jervell JA. Guidelines for the diagnosis and outpatient management of diabetic peripheral neuropathy. Diabet Med 1998;15:508–14.
77. Rosenberg NR, Portegies P, deVisser M, et al. Diagnostic investigation of patients with chronic polyneuropathy: evaluation of a clinical guideline. J Neurol Neurosurg Psychiatr 2001;71:205–9.
78. Davies L, Spies JM, Pollard JD, et al. Vasculitis confined to peripheral nerves. Brain 1996;119:1441–8.
79. Dyck PJ, Berstead TJ, Coon DL, et al. Nonsystemic vasculitic neuropathy. Brain 1987;110:843–54.
80. Dyck PJB, Norell JE, Dyck PJ. Microvasculitis and ischemia in diabetic lumbosacral radiculoplexus neuropathy. Neurology 2000;53:2113–21.
81. Saperstein DS, Katz JS, Amato AA, et al. Clinical spectrum of chronic acquired demyelinating polyneuropathies. Muscle Nerve 2001;24:311–24.
82. Russell JW, Feldman EL. Impaired glucose tolerance—does it cause neuropathy. Muscle Nerve 2001;24:1109–12.
83. Gabriel CM, Hughes RAC, Howard R, et al. Prospective study of the usefulness of sural nerve biopsy. J Neurol Neurosurg Psychiatr 2000;68:442–6.
84. Reilly MM. Classification of the hereditary motor and sensory neuropathies. Curr Opin Neurol 2000;13:561–4.
85. Nobile-Orazio E. Multifocal motor neuropathy. J Neuroimmunol 2001;115:4–18.
86. Sindrup SH, Jensen TS. Efficacy of pharmacological treatments of neuropathic pain: an update and effect related to mechanism of drug action. Pain 1999;83:389–400.
87. Felz MW, Smith CD, Swift TR. A six-year-old girl with tic paralysis. N Engl J Med 2000;342:90–4.
88. Wolfe GI, Barohn RJ. Cryptogenic sensory and sensorimotor polyneuropathies. Semin Neurol 1998;18:105–11.
89. Wolfe GI, El-Feky WH, Katz JS, et al. Antibody panels in idiopathic polyneuropathy and motor neuron disease. Muscle Nerve 1997;20:1275–83.
90. Amato AA, Collins MP. Neuropathies associated with malignancy. Semin Neurol 1998;18:125–44.
91. Mauermann ML, Burns TM. The evaluation of chronic axonal polyneuropathies. Semin Neurol 2008;28:133–51.

Seizure Disorders

Steven C. Schachter, MD[a,b],*

KEYWORDS

- Epilepsy • Seizure • Convulsion
- Diagnosis• Antiepileptic drug

Epilepsy is one of the most common neurologic disorders encountered in clinical practice, affecting an estimated 2 to 4 million people in the United States or approximately 1 in 50 children and 1 in 100 adults.[1] Approximately 1 million women of childbearing age in the United States have epilepsy,[2,3] and the incidence increases over the age of 70 years to more than 100 cases per 100,000 persons.[4]

Despite advances in the sensitivity of diagnostic tests, especially neuroimaging studies, less than half of patients with epilepsy have an identifiable etiology such as congenital brain malformations, inborn errors of metabolism, brain trauma, brain tumors, stroke, intracranial infection, vascular malformations, or cerebral degeneration.[5] In elderly patients, cerebrovascular disease, cerebral degeneration, and brain tumors are more common etiologies than in younger patients.[6]

In as much as epilepsy is characterized by recurrent seizures, the goal of treatment is to completely suppress seizures without causing troublesome side effects or serious idiosyncratic reactions. Antiepileptic drugs (AEDs) are the mainstay of therapy. Because patients with epilepsy also face psychosocial problems such as driving limitations, anxiety or depression, social stigma, and difficulty securing or retaining employment, primary care providers (PCPs) may need to refer patients to other specialists as necessary.

This article reviews the clinical evaluation of epilepsy, pharmacologic treatment, the role of the PCP, and considerations needed for women of childbearing potential and the elderly.

EVALUATION OF PATIENTS WITH NEW ONSET SEIZURES

The objective of the initial evaluation of a patient with suspected seizures is to exclude other conditions that mimic seizures (**Box 1**) and to look for an underlying cause. The first consideration in selecting an AED is an assessment of the patient's seizure type,

Dr. Schachter served as editor-in-chief of www.epilepsy.com until October 1, 2008.
[a] Department of Neurology, Harvard Medical School, MA, USA
[b] Department of Neurology, Beth Israel Deaconess Medical Center, 330 Brookline Avenue, Room K-478, Boston, MA 02215, USA
* Corresponding author. Department of Neurology, Beth Israel Deaconess Medical Center, 330 Brookline Ave, Room K-478, Boston, MA 02215.
E-mail address: sschacht@bidmc.harvard.edu

Med Clin N Am 93 (2009) 343–351
doi:10.1016/j.mcna.2008.10.001
0025-7125/08/$ – see front matter © 2009 Elsevier Inc. All rights reserved.

> **Box 1**
> **Differential diagnosis of seizures**
>
> *Neurologic conditions*
>
>   Dementia ("sun downing")
>
>   Migraine (classic, basilar, confusional)
>
>   Movement disorders (tics, Tourette's syndrome, shuddering)
>
>   Periodic paralysis
>
>   Sleep disorders (parasomnias, sleep attacks)
>
>   Syncope
>
>   Transient global amnesia
>
>   Transient ischemic attack
>
> *Psychiatric conditions*
>
>   Conversion disorders
>
>   Disassociation
>
>   Fugue state
>
>   Panic attacks
>
>   Somatization
>
> *Other disorders*
>
>   Breath holding spells
>
>   Cardiac arrhythmia
>
>   Drug intoxication

which, in turn, is based on a seizure description obtained from the patient or witnesses to the seizure. Because the patient may have been unconscious during the seizure, an accurate description of the seizure may only be available from onlookers. Establishing the seizure type also has implications for the likelihood of a cerebral lesion underlying the seizure disorder.

Seizure Types

The seizure type is usually established from a description of the behaviors that occurred before and during the seizure, as well as after the seizure (the postictal period). The two main seizure types are generalized and partial seizures. Generalized seizures affect both sides of the brain simultaneously and are usually not associated with cerebral pathology. Absence seizures and generalized tonic-clonic seizures (described later) are subtypes of generalized seizures. By comparison, partial seizures arise from a localized area of the cerebral cortex and indicate the possibility of an underlying lesion affecting cortical function.

Symptoms that patients experience when the seizure begins are called simple partial seizures, with "simple" meaning that consciousness is not impaired. Patients may refer to these symptoms as auras or warnings. Typical simple partial seizures include nausea, fear, jerking of one side of the body, or a metallic taste, although a wide variety of auras have been described.[7]

Patients who do not have a conscious warning at the start of their seizures abruptly lose consciousness, which they later may describe as a fadeout or blackout. Three seizure types are characterized by loss of consciousness: complex partial seizures (with "complex" meaning that consciousness is impaired), absence seizures, and generalized tonic-clonic seizures. Because patients are unconscious during these types of seizures, they have no memory of what happened, except perhaps for the warning in complex partial seizures that begin as simple partial seizures.

Complex partial seizures (previously known as temporal lobe seizures and psychomotor seizures) are the most common type of seizure in adults with epilepsy. During complex partial seizures, patients appear awake but do not meaningfully interact with people around them or respond normally to instructions or questions. Instead, patients seem to stare off into space and either remain still or demonstrate repetitive nonpurposeful behaviors (called automatisms), such as chewing, lip smacking, repeating words or phrases, aimless walking or running, or undressing. If patients are forcibly restrained or redirected during complex partial seizures, they may lash out or become aggressive.[8] Complex partial seizures typically last less than 3 minutes and may be immediately preceded by a simple partial seizure, which the patient may or may not remember, and which may occur at times in the same patient without progressing to loss of consciousness. After complex partial seizures, patients may appear confused or somnolent and may complain of a migrainous headache, depressed affect, and embarrassment.

Absence seizures, one of the generalized seizure subtypes, are characterized by the sudden onset of staring with impaired consciousness. They typically last between 5 and 10 seconds and may occur hundreds of times a day, particularly in association with boredom and hyperventilation. They begin in childhood, and 90% of patients have a spontaneous remission before adulthood.

Generalized tonic-clonic seizures (also called grand mal seizures or convulsions), also a subtype of generalized seizures, often begin with a loud scream. The extremities then stiffen (tonic phase), the patient falls to the ground, and cyanosis ensues. After 60 to 90 seconds, the extremities start to jerk, eventually in unison, for an additional 1 to 2 minutes (clonic phase). Bloody frothy sputum may be seen coming out of the patient's mouth. The termination of the clonic phase represents the onset of the postictal period. The patient appears to be in a deep sleep and then wakes up gradually over minutes to hours, often complaining of a migrainous headache and possibly pain if an injury occurred.

Seizure Triggers

Some patients have seizures in the setting of strong emotions or stress, intense exercise, flashing lights, or loud music. These triggers are often experienced immediately before the seizure. Other physiologic states, including fever, the premenstrual period, and sleep deprivation, may lower the seizure threshold in individual patients and are important to identify so that patients can avoid exposure.

Diagnostic Studies

Testing is appropriate, especially for patients presenting with their first seizure, to exclude significant metabolic dysfunction, infection of the central nervous system, and a cerebral lesion. Laboratory studies include assays for glucose, calcium, and magnesium, hematology studies, renal function tests, and toxicology screens. Patients presenting with a fever or stiff neck should also undergo a lumbar puncture once a mass lesion has been excluded by CT or MRI.

Electroencephalograms (EEGs) are helpful to support the diagnosis of epilepsy and provide evidence in support of classifying a patient's seizure type as generalized or partial; however, EEGs are not sensitive, and more than half of patients with epilepsy have normal initial findings. If the first EEG is normal, it should be repeated with the patient sleep deprived, although the test may still be normal in patients with definite epilepsy. A normal EEG cannot exclude epilepsy assuming the patient is not having a seizure while the EEG is being recorded.

Brain Imaging Studies

A brain imaging study should be performed in nearly all cases of new onset seizures and especially in patients who present with partial seizures.[9] Brain MRI is more sensitive than CT for most lesions that cause partial seizures. In an emergency, a CT scan is useful to rule out a mass lesion, cerebral hemorrhage, or stroke. As is true for EEGs, nearly half of patients with epilepsy have normal or nonspecifically abnormal studies. MRI scans should be repeated over time if there is progressive worsening of the patient's neurologic examination, cognitive function, or seizure frequency or severity.

GOALS OF THERAPY AND WHICH ANTIEPILEPTIC DRUGS SHOULD BE PRESCRIBED

The goal of treatment is to completely suppress seizures without causing intolerable side effects.[10,11] Initial treatment with an AED achieves these goals in as many as 70% of patients. The prognosis for seizure control in the other 30% is less favorable. These patients may require numerous trials of AEDs, either as monotherapy or combination therapy.[11]

Nearly 20 drugs are available in the United States for the treatment of epilepsy. Pharmacologic characteristics differ significantly from one AED to another (**Table 1**). For example, some AEDs are nearly completely protein bound in the serum (eg, phenytoin and valproate), whereas others are not protein bound at all (gabapentin and levetiracetam). The plasma half-life of AEDs ranges from 12 hours to 4 days, and a steady state is reached after 3 days to 3 weeks depending on the specific AED. Most AEDs are metabolized by the liver and excreted by the kidney; therefore, compromised hepatic function decreases the metabolism of certain AEDs, and impaired renal function reduces the rate of drug clearance of renally excreted AEDs.

The primary side effects associated with AED therapy (**Table 2**) are referable to the central nervous system and include headache, dizziness, drowsiness, ataxia, double vision, slurred speech, and confusion. The severity of these side effects usually parallels the titration rate, the total daily dose, and the number of concomitantly prescribed AEDs (polytherapy). Mild side effects tend to diminish or resolve over time or with dosage adjustment, but more pronounced symptoms may persist and interfere with the patient's cognitive or behavioral functioning. Other common side effects include rash, nausea, vomiting, and weight gain or loss. Idiosyncratic reactions such as symptomatic hyponatremia, pancreatitis, agranulocytosis, hepatic dysfunction or failure, serum sickness, and Stevens-Johnson syndrome are rare but may be serious and even fatal. Screening laboratory studies, including blood counts, and liver and renal function tests should generally be obtained before initiation of treatment to provide a baseline and repeated if clinically indicated.[12]

Selection of AEDs should be based on their Food and Drug Administration (FDA) indication, the patient's seizure type, the pharmacokinetic profile of the drug, the potential for adverse effects and drug-drug interactions, and cost. With the exception of medical emergencies, therapy should be initiated with a low dose and increased

Table 1
Pharmacokinetic profiles of selected AEDs

Drug	Plasma Protein Binding (%)	$t_{1/2}$ (h)[a]	Time to Steady-State Serum Level (Days)	Therapeutic Serum Level (μg/mL)
Carbamazepine	70–80	11–17	3–10	4–12
Ethosuximide	0	40–50	6–12	40–100
Gabapentin	0	5–7	1–2	Not established
Lamotrigine	50–55	10–15	5–15	Not established
Levetiracetam	<10	7–8	2–3	Not established
Oxcarbazepine	40	8–10	3–4	Not established
Phenytoin	90	15–30	5–15	10–20
Pregabalin	0	6	2–3	Not established
Topiramate	9–17	20–24	5	Not established
Valproate	60–95	6–18	2–4	50–150

[a] $t_{1/2}$ = half-life.

slowly until seizures are completely controlled or until bothersome side effects occur that persist. **Table 3** lists the AEDs suggested by a recent survey of epilepsy specialists as first-line therapy. This list differs in some respects from FDA indications; therefore, a comparison with the FDA indications found in package inserts is warranted.[13] If the initial AED fails to control seizures or produces intolerable side effects before an adequate serum concentration is reached, another AED should be tried. The dosage of the first AED should be tapered as the dosage of the substitute AED is titrated upward to a therapeutic level.

Dosing schedules can be found in package inserts and usually are a function of the half-life of the AED.[14] Drugs with long half-lives, such as phenobarbital or extended-release preparations, can be taken once or twice daily, whereas those with relatively short half-lives, such as immediate release carbamazepine, may need to be taken three to four times a day.

KEYS TO MAINTAINING PATIENT COMPLIANCE

Patient compliance with the dosing schedule is crucial to maintaining seizure control without side effects. Noncompliance may result in an increase in seizure frequency or severity, side effects, or higher or lower than usual AED serum concentrations. Noncompliance usually is an indication of a communication barrier in which the importance of regularly taking the medication is not understood by the patient, but other causes include memory lapses, complicated AED regimens, denial of illness, and fixed incomes. Patient education, the use of pill boxes, and engaging members of the patient's support system may be helpful.

THE ROLE OF THE PRIMARY CARE PROVIDER

In many instances, PCPs make the diagnosis of epilepsy, initiate therapy, and schedule regular follow-up visits to assess seizure frequency, side effects, and compliance. PCPs may also refer patients to a neurologist for further diagnostic and therapeutic suggestions, particularly if the diagnosis is in question, if the seizures do not respond to initial therapy, or to assess the feasibility of discontinuing AEDs. For patients whose

Table 2
Adverse effects of selected AEDs

Drug	Systemic Effects	Neurotoxic Effects	Rare Idiosyncratic Reactions
Carbamazepine	Nausea, vomiting, diarrhea, hyponatremia, rash, pruritus, fluid retention	Drowsiness, dizziness, blurred or double vision, lethargy, headache	Agranulocytosis, Stevens-Johnson syndrome,[a] toxic epidermal necrolysis,[a] aplastic anemia, hepatic failure, dermatitis/rash, serum sickness, pancreatitis
Ethosuximide	Nausea, vomiting	Sleep disturbance, drowsiness, hyperactivity	Agranulocytosis, Stevens-Johnson syndrome, hepatic failure, dermatitis/rash, serum sickness
Gabapentin	Fluid retention	Somnolence, dizziness, ataxia	Unknown
Lamotrigine	Rash, nausea	Dizziness, somnolence	Stevens-Johnson syndrome, hypersensitivity syndrome
Levetiracetam	Unknown	Somnolence, dizziness, headache, anorexia, nervousness, irritability	Unknown
Oxcarbazepine	Rash, hyponatremia	Drowsiness, dizziness, headache, diplopia, nausea, vomiting, ataxia	Unknown
Phenytoin	Gingival hypertrophy, body hair increase, rash, lymphadenopathy	Confusion, slurred speech, double vision, ataxia, neuropathy (with chronic use)	Agranulocytosis, Stevens-Johnson syndrome, aplastic anemia, hepatic failure, dermatitis/rash, serum sickness
Pregabalin	Fluid retention	Somnolence, dizziness, asthenia, ataxia, headache	Unknown
Topiramate	Anorexia	Ataxia, poor concentration, confusion, dizziness, fatigue, paresthesia, somnolence, word-finding difficulty, cognitive slowing, depression	Nephrolithiasis, glaucoma, metabolic acidosis
Valproate	Weight gain, nausea, vomiting, hair loss, easy bruising	Tremor	Agranulocytosis, Stevens-Johnson syndrome, aplastic anemia, hepatic failure, dermatitis/rash, serum sickness, pancreatitis

[a] Stevens-Johnson syndrome and toxic epidermal necrolysis are significantly more common in patients with the human leukocyte antigen (HLA) allele, HLA-B*1502, which occurs almost exclusively in patients with ancestry across broad areas of Asia, including South Asian Indians. Patients with ancestry from areas in which HLA-B*1502 is present should be screened for the allele before starting treatment with carbamazepine. If these individuals test positive, carbamazepine should not be started unless the expected benefit clearly outweighs the increased risk of serious skin reactions.

Table 3
Recommended AEDs for adults according to seizure type[13]

Seizure Type	First-Line Therapy (In Alphabetical Order)
Primary generalized tonic-clonic seizures	Valproate, lamotrigine, topiramate
Partial seizures	—
Adult	Carbamazepine, lamotrigine, oxcarbazepine
Elderly	Lamotrigine, levetiracetam
Absence seizures	Valproate, ethosuximide, lamotrigine

seizures do not respond to initial therapy, other AEDs are typically suggested by the neurologist, either alone or in combination with the initial AED. Patients with seizures that are resistant to multiple trials of AEDs may be candidates for nonpharmacologic treatments, including diet-based approaches (ketogenic diet, low glycemic index diet, modified Atkins diet), brain surgery, or vagus nerve stimulation. Patients with epilepsy usually require chronic therapy and follow-up, which is often provided by the PCP.

The care that patients with epilepsy require often goes beyond AEDs because they may have psychosocial problems, cognitive impairments, affective disorders (most commonly depression or anxiety),[8] and educational or vocational needs. The PCP should work in close cooperation with other medical and social services professionals, as well as involve family members as necessary.

ADVICE FOR PATIENTS

First and foremost, the PCP should discuss the diagnosis and the proposed treatment plan, and he or she should go over these details on subsequent visits until the patient clearly understands and is an active partner in the treatment process, particularly with regard to compliance with AED treatment and lifestyle modifications.

Patients should be advised to eat a healthy diet, to obtain regular and sufficient sleep to avoid daytime drowsiness, to avoid illicit drugs and alcohol (other than an occasional glass of beer or wine), and to alert the PCP if there are any changes in their concomitant medications, including over-the-counter drugs, herbs, and vitamin supplements. Patients and those around them should learn how to respond to a seizure and the circumstances that should prompt emergency attention (eg, repeated seizures or injury). Patients whose seizures are caused by specific situations, such as flashing lights or loud music, should plan ahead to minimize their exposure to these forms of stimulation. Helpful Web sites for patients include www.epilepsyfoundation.org and www.epilepsy.com.

CONSIDERATIONS APPLYING TO WOMEN OF CHILDBEARING AGE AND THE ELDERLY
Women of Childbearing Age

Nearly 1 million women of childbearing potential in the United States have epilepsy.[2,15] The issues uniquely faced by women pertain to fertility, contraception, and pregnancy. Fertility may be reduced by the neuroendocrine effects of some AEDs or as a consequence of epilepsy.[16] Likewise, hepatic enzyme-inducing AEDs may lower the potency of hormonal contraceptives, resulting in contraceptive failure.[2]

All AEDs are potentially teratogenic. Data to indicate which AED is associated with the lowest likelihood of birth defects are not currently available. The overall risk of birth defects in the offspring of epileptic women who take AEDs is 5% to 6%, or approximately twice the rate in the general population.[12] The most frequently seen birth defects are neural tube defects (especially in association with valproate and carbamazepine), cleft lip, cleft palate, heart defects, and microcephaly. Therapy with two or more AEDs concomitantly significantly increases the risk of malformations. Preconception treatment with 0.4 to 4 mg/day of folic acid may reduce the risk of fetal malformations in women who become pregnant, although research to support this recommendation is lacking. High resolution level II fetal ultrasonography should be performed at 16 to 18 weeks of gestation to detect neural tube defects, cardiac anomalies, and limb defects.[2] Amniocentesis and serum alpha-fetoprotein levels may also be useful.[2,12]

Seizure frequency increases during pregnancy in approximately one of three patients because of hormonal and metabolic changes, sleep deprivation, stress, and noncompliance (mainly because women may discontinue AEDs out of fear of birth defects).[2] AED serum levels may decline steadily during pregnancy because of physiologic changes that affect AED pharmacokinetics, often requiring dosage increases. Serum levels of these AEDs usually rise postpartum.

Elderly Patients

In older adults, the prevalence of epilepsy steadily increases with age. Within a few decades, it is predicted that nearly half of patients with new onset epilepsy will be aged more than 65 years. Contributing factors are Alzheimer's disease, cerebrovascular disease, brain tumor, head injuries, and alcohol or drug abuse.[17] Seizures in the elderly may be mistaken for dementia, cerebrovascular insufficiency, or cardiac problems.

The pharmacology of AEDs is different in elderly patients than in young adults because of age-related changes in absorption, distribution, water-to-fat ratio, and liver and renal function.[11] In addition, protein binding is lower in elderly patients. The risk of drug-drug interactions is higher in this age group because concomitant drugs are often taken for comorbid medical conditions. The result of these factors is a higher propensity for AED-related side effects. This possibility can be minimized by initiating AED therapy with a lower dose and titrating more slowly than in young adults, aiming for a lower target serum concentration than in younger patients.[11]

SUMMARY

The goal of epilepsy treatment is to eliminate seizures without significant side effects. The large majority of patients achieve these goals. The PCP has a central role in the diagnosis and treatment of epilepsy and may work collaboratively with neurologists and other health care professionals according to the needs of individual patients.

REFERENCES

1. Hauser WA, Hesdorffer DC. Epilepsy: frequency, causes and consequences. New York: Demos; 1990.
2. Devinsky O, Yerby MS. Women with epilepsy: reproduction and effects of pregnancy on epilepsy. Neurol Clin 1994;12:479–95.
3. Morrell MJ. Guidelines for the care of women with epilepsy. Neurology 1998; 51(5 Suppl 4):S21–7.
4. Loiseau J, Loiseau P, Duche B, et al. A survey of epileptic disorders in southwest France: seizures in elderly patients. Ann Neurol 1990;27:232–7.
5. Schachter SC. Iatrogenic seizures. Neurol Clin 1998;16:157–70.
6. Azar NH, Abou-Khalil BW. Epilepsy in the elderly. Semin Neurol 2008;28(3): 305–16.

7. Schachter SC, editor. Epilepsy in our words: personal accounts of living with seizures. Oxford (UK): Oxford University Press; 2008.

8. Marcangelo MJ, Ovsiew F. Psychiatric aspects of epilepsy. Psychiatr Clin North Am 2007;30(4):781–802.

9. Cascino GD. Neuroimaging in epilepsy: diagnostic strategies in partial epilepsy. Semin Neurol 2008;28(4):523–32.

10. Pellock JM, Willmore LJ. A rational guide to routine blood monitoring in patients receiving antiepileptic drugs. Neurology 1991;41:961–4.

11. Elger CE, Schmidt D. Modern management of epilepsy: a practical approach. Epilepsy Behav 2008;12(4):501–39.

12. So EL. Update on epilepsy. Med Clin North Am 1993;77(1):203–14.

13. Karceski S, Morrell M, Carpenter D. The treatment of epilepsy in adults: expert opinion, 2005. Epilepsy Behav 2005;7(Suppl 1):1–64.

14. Wyler AR. Modern management of epilepsy: recommended medical and surgical options. Postgrad Med 1993;94(3):97–8 [103–8].

15. Herzog AG, Schachter SC. Valproate and the polycystic ovarian syndrome: final thoughts. Epilepsia 2001;42(3):311–5.

16. Hamed SA. Neuroendocrine hormonal conditions in epilepsy: relationship to reproductive and sexual functions. Neurologist 2008;14(3):157–69.

17. Hauser WA. Seizure disorders: the changes with age. Epilepsia 1992;33(Suppl 4): S6–14.

Cerebrovascular Disease

Louis R. Caplan, MD[a,b,*], D. Eric Searls, MD[a,b],
Fong Kwong Sonny Hon, FRCP[c]

KEYWORDS

- Cerebrovascular disease • Stroke • Intracerebral hemorrhage
- Subarachnoid hemorrhage • Transient ischemic attack

AIMS AND QUERIES

Effective management of patients who have cerebrovascular disease depends on accurate diagnosis. Outpatient ambulatory visits have advantages and disadvantages over inpatient encounters. The office allows more privacy, room, time, and relative freedom from distractions. Seeing the patient and significant others in their usual attire adds information not obtained from seeing the patient in the hospital. The inpatient setting allows for more rapid diagnostic testing, frequent nursing observation, and the possibility of deploying advanced pharmacologic and mechanical therapies for stroke.

In ambulatory patients, the key questions are as follows: What is the diagnosis (what and where are the vascular and brain lesions)? How urgent is the problem? Should the patient be hospitalized? What tests should be ordered, and how soon? What treatment should be prescribed? What explanations and instructions should be given? These questions must be answered quickly, directly after the outpatient encounter. This article focuses on the first issues—making the diagnosis and planning the evaluation of a patient suspected of having cerebrovascular disease.

Box 1 lists the data the clinician needs to know.[1] Because cerebrovascular disease is so heterogeneous, management of individual patients depends on the type, location, and severity of the cerebrovascular disease and the presence, severity, and location of the resultant brain injury. Diagnosis and acquisition of data are accomplished best by a question-driven approach.

[a] Department of Neurology, Cerebrovascular Division, Beth Israel Deaconess Medical Center, 330 Brookline Avenue, Boston, MA, 02215-5400, USA
[b] Cerebrovascular Division, Department of Neurology, Harvard University, School of Medicine, 127 Palmer, 330 Brookline Avenue, Boston, MA 02215, USA
[c] Department of Medicine, Pamela Youde Nethersole Eastern Hospital, 10 Tai Man Road, Hong Kong, China
* Corresponding author. Cerebrovascular Division, Department of Neurology, Harvard University, School of Medicine, 127 Palmer, 330 Brookline Avenue, Boston, MA 02215.
E-mail address: lcaplan@bidmc.harvard.edu (L.R. Caplan).

Med Clin N Am 93 (2009) 353–369
doi:10.1016/j.mcna.2008.09.004
0025-7125/08/$ – see front matter © 2009 Elsevier Inc. All rights reserved.

medical.theclinics.com

> **Box 1**
> **Data needed to treat a patient with brain ischemia logically**
>
> Stroke mechanism, ischemic or hemorrhagic, and their subtypes
>
> Nature, location, and severity of the causative cardiac-cerebrovascular-hematologic lesions
>
> Pathophysiology of the vascular lesion that caused the brain injury-hemorrhage, hypoperfusion, or embolism
>
> Nature and function of the key cellular and serologic blood components and any disorder of coagulation
>
> State of the brain, whether normal, infarcted, or injured but recoverable
>
> *From* Caplan LR, Hon FK. Clinical diagnosis of patients with cerebrovascular disease. Prim Care 2004;31(1):96; with permission.

Does the Patient have Cerebrovascular Disease or a Mimic?

Many conditions cause clinical findings that closely resemble cerebrovascular disorders. **Table 1** lists the most frequent stroke mimics and whether they tend to produce general or focal neurologic symptoms and signs.[1] Brain tumors occasionally cause sudden-onset symptoms. Seizures, migraine attacks, and faints sometime are difficult to separate from transient ischemic attacks (TIAs). **Table 2** lists the differential diagnostic features of these common stroke mimics.[1] Hypoglycemia, severe hyperglycemia, severe hyponatremia, hypocalcemia, and other toxic and metabolic conditions occasionally can cause focal brain symptoms. Diagnosis is based on the presence of risk factors for vascular disease, the tempo of onset, the presence of concurrent conditions, and the clinical course of development of neurologic symptoms and signs. In many patients, recognition that the disorder is not cerebrovascular is based on the neuroimaging presence of another condition, such as a tumor, subdural hematoma, brain abscess, or hemorrhage. Stroke mimics are also diagnosed by blood and

Table 1
Frequent stroke mimics and their tendency to produce general versus localized nervous system findings

Conditions	Focal Symptoms	Nonfocal Symptoms
Frequent disorders		
Seizures	+ +	+ +
Transient ischemic attacks	+ + + +	Occasionally
Migraine	+ + + +	+ + + +
Syncope	—	+ + + +
Less frequent disorders		
Vestibulopathy	+ +	+ +
Metabolic	+	+ + +
Neoplasm	+ + +	+
Multiple sclerosis	+ + + +	—
Psychiatric	+ +	+ +
Peripheral nerves and roots	+ + + +	—

From Caplan LR, Hon FK. Clinical diagnosis of patients with cerebrovascular disease. Prim Care 2004;31(1):96; with permission.

Table 2
Differential diagnostic features

	Seizures	TIAs	Migraine	Syncope
Demographics	Any age Children are common	Older patients Stroke risk factors present Men>women	Younger age Women>men	Any age Often younger Women>men
Central nervous system symptoms	Aura preceding Positive symptoms: limb jerking, head turning, eye deviation, loss of consciousness Negative symptoms: (weakness) may develop postictally	Negative symptoms: numbness, weakness, aphasia, visual loss, ataxia All sensory modalities affected simultaneously	First positive symptoms, then negative symptoms in same modality Scintillating scotomas and paresthesias most frequent Second sensory modality is involved after the first clears	Light-headed, dim vision, distant noises, decreased alertness Transient loss of consciousness
Timing	20–180 sec Absence, atonic seizures & myoclonic jerks briefer	Usually <1 h	Usually 30 min to several h Intermittent daily, weekly, monthly, or yearly	Usually a few seconds Sporadic attacks during years
Associated symptoms	Tongue biting, incontinence, automatisms Headache, myalgias postictally	—	Headache, vomiting, photophobia, phonophobia	Diaphoresis, pallor, nausea

Adapted from Caplan LR, Hon FK. Clinical diagnosis of patients with cerebrovascular disease. Prim Care 2004;31(1):97; with permission.

cerebrospinal fluid testing that shows a toxic, metabolic, or infectious process and does not show brain infarction or hemorrhage.

Does the Patient have Cerebrovascular Disease or a Seizure?

Differentiating between strokes and seizures is important (although some stroke patients have seizures at the onset of their stroke). Incorrect diagnosis can lead to the wrong management and can have severe, even life-threatening consequences for the patient. **Table 2** lists common features of seizures.[1] Once a seizure has concluded (the postictal period), it can be especially difficult to discern between the two conditions. During the postictal period, the patient may develop headache or muscle soreness. The patient may have focal weakness, such as a monoparesis or hemiparesis (otherwise known as a postictal paresis). This weakness can last from several hours to a day after the seizure's termination. Postictal paresis can easily be mistaken for the effects of a stroke. Although diagnosing a seizure is based on the clinical picture, ancillary testing (electroencephalogram) can be helpful and may confirm the diagnosis.

If the Disorder is Cerebrovascular, is the Problem Hemorrhage or Ischemia?

Differentiation into hemorrhagic and ischemic conditions is an important initial step. These two mechanisms are diametrically opposite. In intracranial hemorrhage, there is leakage or rupture of a blood vessel that results in blood in the brain tissue, ventricles, subarachnoid space, or epidural space, whereas in ischemia, blood cannot perfuse brain tissue. The brain tissue is starved of vital nutrients and energy. For patients who have ischemic brains, the aim is to restore blood flow and thereby increase delivery of oxygen and other nutrients. In hemorrhage patients, however, the aim is to stop the bleeding and prevent further hemorrhages. About 85% of strokes are ischemic, and about 15% are hemorrhagic.[2,3] Separation between bleeding and ischemia is based on the clinical history and examination, but corroboration is always necessary by brain imaging that shows either subarachnoid or intraparenchymatous blood, a brain infarct, or the absence of bleeding without infarction. In some patients, spinal puncture is necessary to document bleeding into the subarachnoid space because brain imaging in these patients sometimes does not show hemorrhage, especially if the hemorrhage was small or occurred days before imaging.[4] The absence of bleeding and important nonvascular pathology on brain neuroimaging in patients with acute-onset focal brain symptoms is usually sufficient evidence that the problem is brain ischemia, especially when the patient has stroke risk factors and cardiac or cerebrovascular lesions shown by vascular imaging and cardiac evaluation.

What if the Problem is Hemorrhage? Is the Bleeding Subarachnoid or Intracerebral?

Hemorrhagic conditions should be separated into subarachnoid hemorrhage (SAH) and intracerebral hemorrhage (ICH). These two subtypes of hemorrhage have different causes, different clinical findings, and different treatment strategies. About 5% of all strokes are due to SAH, and about 10% are due to ICH, depending on age, sex, educational and social status, and racial composition of patients studied.[2,3]

Subarachnoid bleeding usually occurs rapidly over several seconds. In some patients, it is preceded by a "warning headache," or minor bleeding, within days or weeks of the major rupture.[5,6] This warning headache is often misdiagnosed as a migraine, sinusitis, the flu, or tension headache. The major SAH episode presents as the sudden onset of severe, usually diffuse, headache. The vast majority of patients (97%) describe it as the "worst headache of their life."[7] The headache occurs ipsilateral to the site of bleeding in 30% of patients.[7] Vomiting, cessation of activity, and decreased level of consciousness are frequently present. After several hours, the breakdown of blood products in the cerebrospinal fluid (CSF) leads to meningismus, or neck pain, in 74% of patients.[8] As bloody CSF circulates to the lower back, severe low back pain and bilateral radicular pain may result. One third of patients have slight or severe focal motor deficits.[8] Ophthalmologic examination may show subhyaloid hemorrhages in 25% of aneurysmal subarachnoid hemorrhage patients.[9] Subhyaloid hemorrhages are venous hemorrhages that occur between the retina and vitreous membrane, and may be unilateral or bilateral.

Confirming the diagnosis of subarachnoid hemorrhage hinges on the use of brain imaging and CSF examination. CT of the brain is usually performed before lumbar puncture to rule out a large intracranial mass. The presence of a large focal intracranial lesion, including tumor, large intraparenchymal hemorrhage, or abscess, could place the patient at high risk for herniation during a lumbar puncture. Lesions in the posterior fossa are especially dangerous.

CT and MRI of the brain are highly sensitive tests for detecting acute SAH. If performed within the first 2 days of SAH, CT scans have 95% to 100% sensitivity for intracranial hemorrhage.[4,10] This sensitivity diminishes to 85% within 5 days, 50% after 1 week, 30% after 2 weeks, and 0% after 3 weeks.[4] Relying on CT of the brain to make a diagnosis of SAH after 1 week is thus an uncertain affair. In the acute or hyperacute period, MRI of the brain with proton density or FLAIR sequences has equivalent sensitivity to CT for detecting SAH.[11,12]

If brain imaging does not show SAH, then CSF should be obtained to look for xanthochromia. Many clinicians measure the difference in red blood cell (RBC) counts between the first and last tube of CSF collected as a means to differentiate between SAH and a traumatic lumbar puncture. The belief is that a relatively unchanging RBC count in the thousands would support SAH. A large decrease in RBC counts would indicate a traumatic lumbar puncture. This belief is unreliable, however. Although such an RBC decrease occurs more frequently in traumatic lumbar puncture, it may also occur in SAH.[13] Conversely, many CSF samples from traumatic lumbar puncture show a stable RBC count between tubes.[13]

Examination of CSF for xanthochromia, breakdown products of hemoglobin, is a much more reliable method.[14,15] Many clinicians err by evaluating for xanthochromia only by visual inspection. After centrifugation, the tube with CSF is held to a white sheet of paper to look for the characteristic yellow-tinged fluid of xanthochromia. It is best to evaluate by spectrophotometry, however.[14] If CSF is obtained more than 12 hours and less than 1 week after onset of symptoms, the sensitivity of xanthochromia is 97% to 100%.[14,15]

Patients who have intracerebral hemorrhage develop focal neurologic signs that increase gradually over minutes, sometimes hours. After focal signs increase, headache, vomiting, and decrease in level of consciousness may develop if the ICH is large.[7] Patients usually have risk factors for hemorrhage, such as hypertension, use of amphetamine or cocaine, or an iatrogenic or intrinsic bleeding diathesis.[16] The most frequent cause of a bleeding diathesis is prescription anticoagulants (eg, warfarin). CT and MRI show a hematoma, a localized collection of blood, within the brain.

What if the Hemorrhage is Subarachnoid?

SAH is most often attributable to leakage of blood from an aneurysm. Less often, arteriovenous malformations that abut on pial surfaces can bleed. Amyloid angiopathy, severe hypertension, bleeding disorders, drugs, and occult trauma are less frequent causes. Evaluation centers on defining an aneurysm or other bleeding lesion. Vascular imaging, usually including cerebral dye contrast angiography, is needed. CT angiography (CTA) or magnetic resonance angiography (MRA) is used for preliminary screening but may not be definitive. Treatment of patients who have aneurysms is aimed at destroying the aneurysm's rebleeding potential either by direct surgical clipping or coating or by endovascular techniques that contain and thrombose the aneurysmal sac. Because subarachnoid blood often induces vasoconstriction that can cause secondary brain ischemia, another therapeutic aim is to use drugs, such as nimodipine, that decrease vasoconstriction and to maximize cerebral blood flow after the aneurysm is treated.

What if the Hemorrhage is Intracerebral?

The most frequent and important cause of ICH is uncontrolled hypertension.[17,18] Hypertensive hemorrhages most often are located in the lateral ganglionic region (putamen and internal capsule), subcortex, cerebellum, thalamus, and pons.[19] Some hypertensive hematomas are located in cerebral lobes. In isolated patients who have lobar hemorrhage, surgical intervention or activated factor VII infusion may be considered. Treatment includes control of hypertension without being overly aggressive and thereby reducing brain perfusion pressure. Hemorrhages caused by bleeding disorders or prescription medications are treated by reversing the bleeding diathesis. Surgical, radiosurgical, and endovascular control of vascular malformations are considered in appropriate patients.

What if the Problem is Ischemia? Is the Ischemia Due to Systemic Hypoperfusion, in Situ Vascular Occlusive Disease (Thrombosis), or Embolism?

There are three different mechanisms of brain ischemia: (1) diffusely diminished blood flow to the brain caused by a systemic process; (2) blockage, or thrombosis, of an artery supplying the brain related to in situ processes within that artery; and (3) embolic occlusion of arteries feeding the brain. Thrombosis and embolism are not mutually exclusive. A thrombus that forms in situ in an artery often embolizes to an intracranial distal artery, causing artery-to-artery brain embolism. Differentiating global hypoperfusion and thromboembolism is usually easy, but separation of thrombosis and embolism is difficult without extensive brain and vascular imaging.

Patients who have systemic hypoperfusion report lightheadedness, visual blurring, dampened and distant-sounding auditory stimuli, and difficulty thinking and concentrating. Patients feel faint, especially when standing. They have no premonitory TIAs. The blood pressure may be low and the pulse may be fast. Cardiac arrhythmia or arrest is a frequent cause of systemic hypoperfusion. Patients undergoing surgery, especially cardiac bypass surgery, are prone to hypoperfusion.[20] Pulmonary embolism, gastrointestinal bleeding, and hypovolemia from various causes can produce the same syndrome. There are usually no lateralized neurologic deficits. When present, signs are typically symmetric and emphasize visual, cognitive, and behavioral abnormalities. Brain imaging may be normal or show border-zone territory infarcts between major intracranial arteries.

Thromboembolism is characterized by the sudden or rapid onset of focal neurologic signs. Preceding TIAs may have occurred. Neurologic examination shows signs attributable to a brain region supplied by a single cerebral or posterior circulation artery. Usually a lesion can be placed in one of six general sites: (1) left cerebral hemisphere supplied by the internal carotid artery (ICA) and its anterior cerebral artery and middle cerebral artery (MCA) branches; (2) right cerebral hemisphere, anterior circulation; (3) brainstem or cerebellum, territory supplied by the vertebrobasilar arteries; (4) left posterior hemisphere in the territory of the left posterior cerebral artery (PCA); (5) right PCA territory; or (6) small deep hemisphere lesion (lacunar). Clinicians usually localize a lesion by using a pattern-matching strategy. The patient's findings are matched with prototypic findings for each of the above locations as shown in **Box 2**.[1]

The duration of neurologic signs has a direct correlation with the likelihood of stroke and of detecting lesions with brain imaging. If neurologic signs last less than an hour, the patient probably had a TIA. CT or MRI of the brain will most probably not show an infarct.[21] If signs persist longer than 1 hour, however, CT or MRI of the brain will frequently show an infarct.[21]

MRI of the brain is a much more sensitive test than CT for detecting acute infarcts. MRI diffusion-weighted sequences can detect an infarct within as few as 30 minutes of the first stroke symptoms.[22,23] In the acute period, CT of the brain can show subtle, early signs of infarct, such as loss of the insular ribbon, focal cortical swelling of the MCA, or loss of differentiation between gray and white matter. Hypodensities associated with infarct do not typically appear on CT imaging for several hours.[24,25] In stroke patients imaged 2 hours after their symptoms began, CT of the brain noncontrast had 77% sensitivity for early signs of stroke. MRI brain with diffusion-weighted imaging

---

Box 2
Frequent patterns of findings according to stroke location

Left anterior circulation (left ICA-MCA)–nonlacunar; right hemiparesis, hemisensory loss, hemianopia, aphasia

Right anterior circulation (right ICA-MCA)–nonlacunar; left hemiparesis, hemisensory loss, hemianopia; left neglect, decreased awareness of the deficit, abnormal drawing and copying, abnormal visuospatial abilities

Vertebrobasilar system (brainstem and cerebellum)—vertigo, diplopia, crossed motor or sensory signs (one side of the face and the contralateral body), ataxia; bilateral motor or sensory signs

Left PCA–right hemianopia, alexia without agraphia; right hemisensory symptoms

Right PCA–left hemianopia, left hemisensory symptoms, topographic disorientation

Lacunar infarction (four frequent syndromes): (a) ipsilateral weakness of face, arm, and leg, (b) ipsilateral sensory symptoms of face, arm, and leg, (c) hemiplegia and ipsilateral ataxia, (d) dysarthria and clumsiness of one hand

From Caplan LR, Hon FK. Clinical diagnosis of patients with cerebrovascular disease. Prim Care 2004;31(1):100; with permission.

---

had 100% sensitivity, however.[26] Rapid vascular imaging (CTA, MRA, or transcranial Doppler ultrasound) often shows occlusion of an intracranial artery.

What if the Cause of Ischemia is Systemic Hypoperfusion?

The aim is to correct the cause and to maximize brain blood flow quickly. Cardiac disease should be treated. Blood pressure should be restored. Intravenous fluids should be used first. If the blood pressure does not respond, then pressors should be used.

If the patient has significant anemia, then blood transfusion should be considered.

What if the Cause of Ischemia is Thromboembolism?

Thromboembolism is the most frequent cause of brain ischemia.[27] The initial evaluation should be rapid, efficient, and thorough. Neurologic signs should be characterized. Standard stroke scales, such as the National Institutes of Health stroke scale, should be used whenever possible to quantify neurologic deficits. Brain imaging (CT or MRI) should be performed quickly to determine the presence, location, and extent of brain infarction. Vascular imaging also should be performed quickly to identify an occlusive lesion. Is all of the brain territory supplied by the occluded artery already infarcted, normal, or "stunned" (nonfunctioning but not yet infarcted)? If there is considerable at-risk brain tissue, and the infarct is not too large, an effort should be made to recanalize the obstructed artery.

This recanalization is done most often using thrombolytic agents administered either intravenously or intra-arterially. Mechanical means (angioplasty, stenting, or mechanical removal or breakup of clot) and surgery sometimes are used to open or bypass the blockage. Intravenous tissue plasminogen activator (TPA) should be given within 3 hours of stroke onset, and intra-arterial TPA should be given within 6 hours whenever possible.[28,29] Endovascular treatments, using the MERCI clot retriever device for example, should be started within 8 hours.[30,31] These time windows are not set in stone, however. The decision to administer a thrombolytic or use an endovascular device should be guided not only by time windows but also by an understanding of whether there is important salvageable brain, the likelihood of opening an occluded artery and by which technique, and the potential risks of treatment.

Important aims are to prevent worsening and to prevent stroke recurrence after the acute period. Defining causative vascular lesions and any other cardiovascular-cerebrovascular-hematologic disorders that pose a threat for future brain injury is essential for choosing the correct prophylactic agent. Recognition and treatment of risk factors, such as hypertension, diabetes, smoking, obesity, inactivity, and hyperlipidemia, are essential. In most patients who have thromboembolism, prescription of agents that decrease the formation of platelet-fibrin "white thrombi" or erythrocyte-fibrin "red thrombi" is indicated. So-called "platelet antiaggregants" (aspirin, clopidogrel, modified-release dipyridamole alone or in combination with aspirin, and cilostazol) are used to prevent the formation of white thrombi.[32] Anticoagulants (heparin, warfarin, factor Xa inhibitors, and direct thrombin inhibitors) are used to prevent red thrombi. Correctable cardiac, aortic, and cervicocranial lesions are sought. Lesions that cause severe stenosis of cervicocranial arteries sometimes are treatable by surgical or endovascular techniques (stenting).

What is the Process of Diagnosis and Evaluation?

The history is crucial. Let the patient tell the story uninterrupted. This approach offers insight into the patient's intelligence, language skills, organizing skills, and concerns. As the story unfolds, aided by accompanying family or significant others, the clinician should generate "what" and "where" hypotheses and test them actively. The information used to make what diagnoses is listed in **Box 3**, and the information used to arrive at where diagnoses is listed in **Box 4**.[1]

The patient's age, sex, and past illnesses give the first clues. In an elderly hypertensive man who developed a slight left hemiplegia 4 days ago, hypertension raises the possibility of intracerebral hemorrhage. His age also favors some types of hemorrhage (eg, amyloid angiopathy or minor trauma). Alternatively, hypertension might have caused penetrating artery disease (the cause of lacunar infarcts) or accelerated the development of large artery extracranial and intracranial atherosclerosis. Already there are three hypotheses about stroke type. Then the clinician considers whether the account of the early symptoms and their subsequent course favors one of these

---

Box 3
Data from the clinical encounter used to make *what* (stroke mechanism) diagnoses

Demographic: age, race, sex

Past known medical conditions and family history (eg, hypertension, hyperlipidemia, diabetes, valvular disease, bleeding disorders)

Present medical conditions found on general and vascular examination (eg, elevated blood pressure, heart murmur, bruit)

TIAs—same or different vascular territories from present stroke/TIA

Activity at onset—noted after sleep, during vigorous activity

Course of the deficit (eg, sudden and maximal at onset, gradually progressing, fluctuating)

Accompanying symptoms and signs (eg, headache, vomiting, loss of consciousness, seizures, papilledema)

From Caplan LR, Hon FK. Clinical diagnosis of patients with cerebrovascular disease. Prim Care 2004;31(1):101; with permission.

> **Box 4**
> **Data used for the *where* diagnosis**
>
> Neurologic symptoms described by the patient
>
> Neurologic signs found on examination
>
> Matching of the symptoms and signs with known vascular syndromes
>
> Vascular examination
>
> Brain neuroimaging (CT and MRI)
>
> Vascular diagnostic tests (carotid and transcranial Doppler ultrasound, MRA, CTA, conventional angiography)
>
> *From* Caplan LR, Hon FK. Clinical diagnosis of patients with cerebrovascular disease. Prim Care 2004;31(1):102; with permission.

hypotheses or suggests a different possibility. This process of generating and testing what hypotheses should continue throughout the patient encounter.

At the same time, the physician should be considering the where diagnosis, the localization of the lesion in the nervous system and the arteries that supply these regions. The patient's description of what is or was wrong should generate anatomic hypotheses.

In most patients, the findings conform to one of six general patterns as listed in **Box 2**.[1] Full awareness of a left hemiparesis by the patient makes a subcortical or brainstem locus more likely than a frontal or parietal lobe cortical lesion. If a homonymous visual field defect is present, the lesion must be supratentorial and posteriorly located in the contralateral cerebral hemisphere, most often in the territory of the PCA. An arm monoparesis or a great discrepancy in the degree of weakness in the patient's face, arm, hand, and leg suggests a cortical, paracentral localization. As the history-taking proceeds, the physician should construct hypotheses of the brain lesion's location.

What are the Demographics of Cerebrovascular Disorders?

Age, sex, race, family history, and medical history strongly affect the probability of various stroke mechanisms. Some illnesses heavily favor only one mechanism. For instance, rheumatic mitral stenosis with atrial fibrillation strongly suggests cardiac origin embolism.[33,34] Others, such as hypertension, predispose to many possibilities. Race and sex affect the likelihood of particular vascular occlusive lesions. In general, white men have more extracranial occlusive disease of the ICA and vertebral artery origins in the neck; women, blacks, and Asians have more intracranial large artery occlusive disease.[35,36] Blacks and Asians have a higher frequency of ICH.[37] **Table 3** shows estimates of the relative weights attributable to the various risk factors.[1]

Risk factors also help clinicians assess the chances of future vascular disease — stroke, coronary artery disease, and peripheral vascular occlusive disease. These risk factors should be identified and discussed with the patient and family.

How do Past and Recent Cerebrovascular Events Inform the Process of Diagnosis?

A history of a stroke or TIA can yield important clues to the present cerebrovascular event. As arteries gradually occlude, there often are brief attacks related to intermittent reduced distal blood flow and embolization of white platelet-fibrin aggregates, red fibrin-dependent clots, and plaque material into the intracranial branches supplied by

Table 3
Weighting of ecologic factors

	Thrombosis	Lacune	Embolus	ICH	SAH
Hypertension	+ +	+ + +	—	+ +	+
Severe hypertension	—	+	—	+ + + +	+ +
Coronary disease	+ + +	—	+ +	—	—
Claudication	+ + +	—	+	—	—
Atrial fibrillation	—	—	+ + + +	—	—
Sick sinus syndrome	—	—	+ +	—	—
Valvular heart disease	—	—	+ + +	—	—
Diabetes	+ + +	+	+	—	—
Bleeding diathesis	—	—	—	+ + + +	+
Smoking	+ + +	—	+	—	+
Cancer	+ +	—	+ +	—	—
Old age	+ + +	+	+	+	—
Black or Asian origin	+	+	—	+ +	—

From Caplan LR, Hon FK. Clinical diagnosis of patients with cerebrovascular disease. Prim Care 2004;31(1):103; with permission.

that artery. In the Harvard Stroke Registry, about 50% of patients who had large artery occlusive lesions and 25% of patients who had penetrating artery disease had preceding TIAs in the same vascular territory as their subsequent stroke.[38] In patients who had large artery lesions (eg, the cervical ICA), TIAs are spread over a long interval and often are heterogeneous; thus, transient monocular blindness may occur in one attack, hand and face numbness in a second attack, and aphasia with hand weakness in a third attack. In patients who have penetrating artery disease, attacks usually occur during a shorter time span and closer to the time of the stroke. Attacks often are similar in their features and reflect the subcortical blood supply (eg, tingling on the left side of the body in each attack most often is due to disease of a thalamogeniculate branch artery supplying the lateral thalamus).

Patients whose present stroke is a small deep infarct caused by penetrating artery or branch atheromatous disease often have had past lacunar strokes in other locations. Similarly, patients who have emboli originating from the heart also often have had prior embolic strokes or unrecognized brain infarcts in other vascular territories. These past lacunes and embolic brain infarcts sometimes are evident only on CT and MRI. Patients who have lobar intracerebral hemorrhages may have had other smaller bleeds detectable by susceptibility-weighted (T2*) MRI.[39]

The nature of prior attacks or TIAs as shown by history, examination, or imaging provides insight to the present event. Most individuals are naive about the workings of their bodies, especially their nervous systems. A patient may attribute temporary hand numbness and weakness to a local lesion in the limb and may not think of reporting it. Similarly, most patients may not report having white flashes in their left visual field 10 days before the visit, thinking it a symptom for the eye doctor. To elicit the history of prior TIAs or strokes, the clinician must often ask repeatedly about specific symptoms, perhaps in different ways: Did your foot or leg ever become temporarily limp? Did your vision ever fade temporarily in one eye? Did your speech ever fail you or seem garbled, slurred, or wrong? Family members may remember spells that the patient does not recognize or recall. The patient may not recall symptoms the first time the questions are asked but may remember the events later. One patient who had transient monocular blindness when questioned about loss of vision on three occasions always gave a negative response. The day after he said no for the third time, he spontaneously said, "Doc, now I remember. About a week ago I was in line at the food store, and my left eye went gray for about a minute. The clerk said that I must have gotten a speck of dirt in the eye. Because it went away, I didn't make much of it."[40]

What is the Course of Development of Strokes?

Each stroke subtype has its usual common signature of development and evolution. Emboli most often (>80%) occur suddenly and create deficits that are maximal immediately.[36,38,41] For instance, patients might suddenly slump in their chair with a hemiplegia. In contrast, intracerebral hemorrhages grow gradually over minutes, and signs increase gradually. If the hematoma becomes large, headache, vomiting, and decreased consciousness ensue, after the initial signs of focal brain dysfunction. SAH also begins suddenly. Blood released into the cerebrospinal fluid under arterial pressure causes severe headache, vomiting, and transient interruption in posture or activities. In contrast to ICH, focal symptoms of brain dysfunction usually are not present at outset. In patients who have large artery occlusive disease, fluctuations of symptoms and signs are characteristic, with stepwise increases in deficits, temporary improvements or return to normal function, and gradual but erratic progression of symptoms and signs during a few days. These fluctuations and changes are presumed to be caused by changes in the systemic circulation affecting collateral blood flow and propagation and embolization of thrombi distally into distal branches. Transcranial Doppler monitoring has shown that microemboli are common in patients who have occlusive disease of large arteries. Decreased perfusion in these arteries impedes washout of these microemboli. **Table 4** compares the early course of deficits in patients who have embolism and in situ thrombosis derived from various stroke registries.[1]

Few patients can give an absolutely accurate account of the development of symptoms. Patients who have right-hemisphere frontal and parietal lobe strokes may not recognize any deficit. Family and friends can supply useful data. The clinician should have the patient walk through the events before and after the stroke began. A patient

Table 4
Early course of deficit in patients who had in situ thrombosis versus embolism in various stroke registries

	Thrombosis			Embolism		
Course	HSR	MRSR	LSR[a]	HSR	MRSR	LSR[a]
Maximal at onset	40%	45%	66%	79%	89%	82%
Stepwise/stuttering	34%	30%	—	11%	10%	—
Progressive	—	—	27%	—	—	13%
Gradual smooth	13%	14%	—	5%	1%	—
Fluctuating	13%	11%	7%	5%	—	5%

Abbreviations: HSR, Harvard Stroke Registry; MRSR, Michael Reese Stroke Registry; LSR, Lausanne Stroke Registry.
[a] In the LSR, gradual smooth and stepwise/stuttering are considered as progressive.
From Caplan LR, Hon FK. Clinical diagnosis of patients with cerebrovascular disease. Prim Care 2004;31(1):105; with permission.

reported that she gradually developed a left-sided paralysis that morning. When she described the events in more detail, she said, "At the breakfast table, my left hand and arm went weak and clumsy, and I dropped the coffee cup from my hand. I went upstairs to my bedroom, and I walked OK on the stairs. I rested for a half hour, and then when I came downstairs my hand was all right. I cleaned the room without trouble. An hour later, my hand and arm went weak again. This time I stumbled on the steps and had to limp with my left leg. When I called my daughter, my words were slurred. I lay down again, but this time, when I tried to get up, I couldn't use my left side at all."[40] This fluctuating pattern of development of the deficit is characteristic of a so-called "thrombotic stroke," in which the deficit is due to occlusion of a feeding artery with distal hypoperfusion. In this case, the symptoms fit the pattern of a pure motor hemiparesis most likely caused by penetrating artery or branch atheromatous disease.

Is There a Relationship Between a Patient's Activity and the Onset of a Stroke?

Most strokes and TIAs occur during activities of daily living. Emboli can be precipitated by a cough, sneeze, suddenly rising from bed during the night to go to the bathroom, or sexual intercourse (especially paradoxical emboli). SAH and ICH can be precipitated by intercourse or emotional stress. In patients who have large artery occlusive disease, standing or rising after bending can precipitate brief TIAs. Vigorous turning or stretching of the neck can cause extracranial arterial dissections. The physician always should inquire what the patient was doing before and during the attack. Was there any unusual or vigorous physical activity or emotional duress in the minutes, hours, or days before the attack?

What are Associated Symptoms of a Stroke?

Headache, loss of consciousness, vomiting, and seizures all provide clues to the cause of the stroke. Headaches, unusual for the patient before the stroke, may signify large artery occlusive disease or recent elevation in blood pressure. Headache at stroke onset is invariable in SAH and sometimes occurs in brain embolism. In ICH, headache usually follows the onset of other symptoms and signs. Vomiting is frequent near the onset of SAH and is common in large supratentorial and infratentorial ICH. Vomiting also is frequent in patients who have cerebellar and medullary infarcts. Seizures are slightly more common in patients who have embolic infarcts and lobar ICH than in patients who have other stroke subtypes. Loss of consciousness is frequent in patients who have SAH, large ICH, brainstem infarcts that affect the tegmentum bilaterally, or bilateral thalamic infarcts.

What General and Neurologic Examinations Should Be Performed on Stroke Patients?

The general and neurologic examinations should be planned ahead of time, after the history. What features could be found during the examination that would clarify the stroke mechanism and the anatomy? In a patient who has left hemiparesis, visual field testing, higher cortical function testing (eg, neglect, drawing and copying, and somatosensory testing) and careful cranial nerve examination should allow more precise localization. The neck should be auscultated with a stethoscope for carotid and vertebral artery bruits, and a careful cardiac and peripheral vascular examination is warranted. Are there any signs of systemic bleeding or head injury? At times, the examination uncovers findings completely unsuspected from the history. The patient who has left hemiparesis might have additional right-sided weakness and a bilateral Babinski sign or nystagmus suggesting brainstem (pontine) localization. An enlarged nodular liver may indicate metastatic disease. As the examination proceeds, the physician should continue to weigh what and where hypotheses and their probabilities.

Cardiac, ophthalmologic, vascular, and dermatologic examinations are important in all patients suspected of having cerebrovascular disease. Especially in young patients, the skin examination can yield the diagnosis. Fabry disease, Sneddon syndrome, Behçet disease, and Ehlers-Danlos type IV are all examples of disorders with dermatologic and cerebrovascular manifestations. Patients who have Fabry disease, an X-linked lysosomal disease, may have angiokeratomas, which are dark red or purple punctate telangiectasias. Angiokeratomas usually occur in clusters around the umbilicus, scrotum, hips, and thighs. These patients are at risk for ischemic infarcts.[42] Sneddon syndrome is a noninflammatory arteriopathy of small and medium-sized vessels that can result in multiple, often lacunar infarcts and occurs primarily in young people.[43,44] This disorder is suggested by a "fishnet pattern" of purple and blue discolorations, usually involving the legs.[44] Behçet disease, a multisystem inflammatory disorder that can lead to central nervous system infarcts, cerebral venous thrombosis, and encephalitis, can present with oral aphthous ulcers, genital ulcers, and erythema nodosum.[45] Ehlers-Danlos type IV (or vascular Ehlers-Danlos syndrome) causes susceptibility to dissections, aneurysms, thrombosis, and hemorrhage.[46] Manifestations include excessive bruising, joint hypermobility, and thin, translucent skin.[46] Skin laxity is less frequent compared with other types of Ehlers-Danlos. Given the link between dermatologic findings and uncommon stroke syndromes, stroke patients should be examined undressed.

Clinical localization of the brain lesion depends primarily on neurologic examination findings. The most vital and most frequently missed signs of brain dysfunction involve abnormalities of (1) higher cortical function, (2) level of alertness, (3) visual and oculomotor systems, and (4) gait. Evaluating visual fields is essential because it assesses the functioning of large segments of the parietal, temporal, and occipital lobes. If papilledema is observed during funduscopic evaluation it indicates increased intracranial pressure, which may be due to a host of causes, including large arterial stroke, tumor, hydrocephalus, and cerebral venous thrombosis. Also, walk the patient when possible, even in the emergency room setting. In sum, these are parts of the examination most often overlooked by non-neurologists, which provide clues to anatomic localization.

What are the Necessary Laboratory and Imaging Studies?

Often the patient already has had some investigations. It is best to obtain the history and examine the patient before reviewing such accompanying information. After the history and general and neurologic examinations, laboratory and imaging studies not already performed should be planned to test the existing hypotheses. Ordinarily a brain imaging test, either CT or MRI, is the first test in a patient who has had a stroke or has neurologic signs. The presence of a hemorrhage dictates a battery of tests that are different than if the process were ischemic. Most patients require some blood testing, including hemoglobin, hematocrit, white blood cell count, platelet count, prothrombin time, and activated partial thromboplastin time (aPTT). Vascular diagnostic tests and cardiac testing usually are planned optimally after the results of imaging and blood tests are known, but for convenience they often are done at the same time as brain imaging.

MANAGEMENT STRATEGIES ACCORDING TO TIMING OF EVENTS
What if the Patient Had an Acute Stroke?

In the case of acute stroke, hospital admission is nearly always in order. For both deep and cortical ischemic infarcts, usually a triad of tests should be ordered during admission, including: blood screening tests (complete blood count, platelet count, prothrombin time, aPTT, fibrinogen, hemoglobin A$_{1c}$, fasting glucose, fasting lipid panel), cardiac tests (electrocardiography and transthoracic echocardiography), and noninvasive vascular tests (extracranial and intracranial ultrasound, MRA, or CTA). No matter if the lesion is in the anterior or posterior circulation, MRA or CTA of the brain should be performed. Localization of the ischemia determines the main arteries to be studied, however. If the lesion is in the right cerebral hemisphere, a carotid duplex and color-flow Doppler scan of the ICA in the neck and transcranial Doppler of the anterior circulation arteries are indicated. Alternatively, MRA or CTA of the internal carotid artery could be performed. If the lesion is in the posterior circulation, head and neck MRA or CTA could be done with attention to the vertebrobasilar arteries. In addition, transcranial Doppler using a suboccipital window to insonate the intracranial vertebral arteries and basilar artery could be used.

What if the Patient Had a Remote (Non-Acute) Stroke?

If the patient has had a remote stroke (ie, a stroke >1 week old), a scan brought with the patient (or a reliable report of the films by a neuroradiologist) should suffice to inform whether the lesion was a hemorrhage or an infarct and its location. If it was a hemorrhage, the site, size, and pattern of spread should be evident. If the problem was ischemic, the scan might show the infarct or have only slight or nondiagnostic abnormalities. If the studies are old, inadequate, or nondiagnostic, a new scan (optimally MRI) should be ordered.

What if the Patient Had a Hemorrhage?

If the patient is hypertensive and the ICH is in a typical location for a hypertensive hematoma (putamen, caudate, thalamus, cerebellum, or pons), antihypertensive therapy is indicated without the need for other evaluation except blood screening. Ordinarily, all patients should have a platelet count, prothrombin time, and aPTT. Inquiry about the use of drugs (cocaine, diet pills, or methamphetamine) and medicines (especially warfarin derivatives) is important. The hemorrhage's location might suggest a contusion caused by trauma. An angioma or arteriovenous malformation may be evident from the films. If such a lesion is present and potentially treatable, angiography may be needed.

What if the Patient Had One or More Transient Ischemic Attacks in the Absence of a Stroke?

If the evaluation can be performed urgently (that day), outpatient preliminary testing is an option. If the nature or frequency of the attacks is worrisome, hospital admission is prudent. Usually, CT or MRI of the brain, MRA of the brain, and ultrasound or MRA of the neck are scheduled concurrently. Blood screening, as described previously, also is done. If the pattern of the clinical findings or the scan suggests large artery occlusive disease (TIAs in the same vascular territory), cardiac testing can be postponed until the results of carotid ultrasound or MRA of the neck are available. If there is only one attack, or there were attacks in many vascular territories, especially if there is clinical evidence of cardiac disease, cardiac testing is scheduled first or concurrently with noninvasive vascular testing. When the clinical localization is unclear, a review of the scan is necessary before deciding on the order and nature of the cardiac and vascular testing.

REFERENCES

1. Caplan LR, Hon FK. Clinical diagnosis of patients with cerebrovascular disease. Prim Care 2004;31(1):95–109.
2. Rosamond WD, Folsom AR, Chambless LE, et al. Stroke incidence and survival among middle-aged adults: 9-year follow-up of the Atherosclerosis Risk in Communities (ARIC) cohort. Stroke 1999;30(4):736–43.
3. Thom T, Haase N, Rosamond W, et al. Heart disease and stroke statistics—2006 update: a report from the American Heart Association statistics committee and stroke statistics subcommittee. Circulation 2006;113:e85–151.
4. Gijn JV, Dongen KJ. The time course of aneuysmal haemorrhage on computed tomograms. Neuroradiology 1982;23:153–6.
5. Leblanc R. The minor leak preceding subarachnoid hemorrhage. J Neurosurg 1987;66(1):35–9.
6. Ostergaard JR. Headache as a warning symptom of impending aneurismal subarachnoid haemorrhage. Cephalalgia 1991;11(1):53–5.
7. Gorelick PB, Hier DB, Caplan LR, et al. Headache in acute cerebrovascular disease. Neurology 1986;36:1445–50.
8. Kassell NF, Torner JC, Haley EC, et al. The international cooperative study on the timing of aneurysm surgery. Part 1: overall management results. J Neurosurg 1990;73:18–36.
9. Garfinkle AM, Danys IR, Nicolle DA, et al. Terson's syndrome: a reversible cause of blindness following subarachnoid hemorrhage. J Neurosurg 1992;76(5):766–71.
10. Adams HP, Kassell NF, Torner JC, et al. CT and clinical correlations in recent aneurismal subarachnoid hemorrhage: a preliminary report of the Cooperative Aneurysm Study. Neurology 1983;33:981–8.
11. Wiesmann M, Mayer TE, Medele R, et al. Diagnosis of acute subarachnoid hemorrhage at 1.5 Tesla using proton-density weighted FSE and MRI sequences. Radiologe 1999;39(10):860–5.
12. Wiesmann M, Mayer TE, Yousry I, et al. Detection of hyperacute subarachnoid hemorrhage of the brain by using magnetic resonance imaging. J Neurosurg 2002;96(4):684–9.
13. Buruma OJ, Janson HL, Den Bergh FA, et al. Blood-stained cerebrospinal fluid: traumatic puncture or haemorrhage? J Neurol Neurosurg Psychiatr 1981;44(2):144–7.
14. Soderstrom CE. Diagnostic significance of CSF spectrophotometry and computer tomography in cerebrovascular disease: a comparative study in 231 cases. Stroke 1977;8(5):606–12.
15. Vermeulen M, Hasan D, Blijenberg BG, et al. Xanthochromia after subarachnoid hemorrhage needs no revisitation. J Neurol Neurosurg Psychiatr 1989;52:826–8.
16. Kase CS, Caplan LR. Intracerebral hemorrhage. Boston: Butterworth-Heinemann; 1994.
17. Woo D, Haverbusch M, Sekar P, et al. Effect of untreated hypertension on hemorrhagic stroke. Stroke 2004;35:1703–8.
18. Feldmann E, Broderick JP, Kernan WN, et al. Major risk factors for intracerebral hemorrhage in the young are modifiable. Stroke 2005;36:1881–5.
19. Barnett HJ, Mohr JP, Stein BM, editors. Stroke pathophysiology diagnosis and management. Philadelphia: Churchill Livingstone; 1998. p. 673.
20. Selim M. Perioperative stroke. N Engl J Med 2007;356(7):706–13.

21. Kimura K, Minematsu K, Yasaka M, et al. The duration in symptoms in transient ischemic attack. Neurology 1999;52(5):976–80.
22. Brant-Zawadzi M, Pereira B, Weinstein P, et al. MR imaging of acute experimental ischemia in cats. AJNR Am J Neuroradiol 1986;7(1):7–11.
23. Kucharczyk J, Mintorovitch J, Asgari HS, et al. Diffusion/perfusion MR imaging of acute cerebral ischemia. Magn Reson Med 1991;19(2):311–5.
24. Gilman S. Imaging the brain. First of two parts. N Engl J Med 1998;338:812–20.
25. Bourquain H, Elsner E, Gerber J, et al. Prospektiver Wert der fruhen CT bei zerebraler Ischaemie. Klin Neuroradiol 1998;8:135–6.
26. Fieback J, Jansen O, Schellinger P, et al. Comparison of CT with diffusion-weighted MRI in patients with hyperacute stroke. Neuroradiology 2001;43:628–32.
27. Albers GW, Amarence P, Easton JD, et al. Antithrombotic and thrombolytic therapy for ischemic stroke. Chest 2001;119:300–20.
28. The National Institute of Neurological Disorders and Stroke rt-PA Stroke Study Group. Tissue plasminogen activator for acute ischemic stroke. N Engl J Med 1995;333:1581–7.
29. Furlan A, Higashida R, Wechsler L, et al. Intra-arterial prourokinase for acute ischemic stroke. The Proact II study: a randomized controlled trial. Prolyse in acute cerebral thromboembolism. JAMA 1999;282(21):2003–11.
30. Smith WS, Sung G, Starkman S, et al. Safety and efficacy of mechanical embolectomy in acute ischemic stroke: results of the MERCI Trial. Stroke 2005;36:1432–40.
31. Smith WS, Sung G, Saver J, et al. Mechanical thrombectomy for acute ischemic stroke: final results of the Multi MERCI Trial. Stroke 2008;39:1205–12.
32. Sacco RL, Adams R, Albers G, et al. Guidelines for prevention of stroke in patients with ischemic stroke or transient heart attack. Circulation 2006;113:e409–49.
33. Carter AB. Prognosis of cerebral embolism. Lancet 1965;2:514–9.
34. Levine HJ. Which atrial fibrillation patients should be on chronic anticoagulation? J Cardiovasc Med 1981;6:483–7.
35. Caplan LR, Gorelick PB, Hier DB. Race, sex, and occlusive cerebrovascular disease: a review. Stroke 1986;17:648–55.
36. Caplan LR, Wityk RJ, Glass TA, et al. The New England Medical Center Posterior Circulation Registry. Ann Neurol 2004;56:389–98.
37. Broderick JP, Brott T, Tomsick T, et al. The risk of subarachnoid and intracerebral hemorrhage in blacks as opposed to whites. N Engl J Med 1992;326:733–6.
38. Mohr JP, Caplan LR, Melski JW, et al. The Harvard Cooperative Stroke Registry: a prospective registry. Neurology 1978;28:754–62.
39. Nighoghossian N, Hermier M, Adeleine P, et al. Old microbleeds are a potential risk factor for cerebral bleeding after ischemic stroke: a gradient-echo T2*-weighted brain MRI study. Stroke 2002;33:735–42.
40. Caplan LR. Caplan's stroke: a clinical approach. 3rd edition. Boston: Butterworth-Heinemann; 2000.
41. Caplan LR, Hier DB, D'Cruz L. Cerebral embolism in the Michael Reese stroke registry. Stroke 1983;14:530–6.
42. Mehta A, Ricci R, Widmer U, et al. Fabry disease defined: baseline clinical manifestations of patients in the 366 patients in the Fabry outcome survey. Eur J Clin Invest 2004;34:236–42.

43. Fetoni V, Grisoli M, Salmaggi A, et al. Clinical and neuroradiological aspects of Sneddon's syndrome and primary antiphospholipid antibody syndrome. a follow up study. Neurol Sci 2000;21:157–64.
44. Aladdin Y, Hamadeh M, Butcher K. The Sneddon syndrome. Arch Neurol 2008; 65(6):834–5.
45. Akman-Demir G, Serdaroglu P, Banu Tasci. The neuro-Behçet study group. Clinical patterns of neurological involvement in Behçet's disease: evaluation of 200 patients. Brain 1999;122:2171–81.
46. Zilocchi M, Macedo TA, Oderich GS, et al. Vascular Ehlers-Danlos syndrome: imaging findings. Am J Roentgenol 2007;189:712–9.

Movement Disorders

Meghan K. Harris, MD, Natalya Shneyder, MD, Aimee Borazanci, MD, Elena Korniychuk, MD, Roger E. Kelley, MD, Alireza Minagar, MD*

KEYWORDS

- Tremor • Parkinson disease • Restless leg syndrome
- Wilson's disease • Huntington's disease
- Involuntary movements • Drug-induced tremor

PARKINSON DISEASE

How is Parkinson Disease Defined?

Idiopathic Parkinson disease is a progressive disabling neurodegenerative disease that manifests with the following neurologic symptoms: resting tremor, flexed posture, loss of postural reflexes, bradykinesia, and rigidity.

What are the Clinical Features of Parkinson Disease?

The salient clinical features of Parkinson disease consist of resting tremor, bradykinesia or akinesia, cogwheel rigidity, and loss of corrective postural reflexes. Less specific features include dementia; dystonia; psychiatric disorders, such as hallucinations, delusions, and depression; sleep disorders, such as restless legs syndrome, parasomnias, and REM behavior disorders; and autonomic dysfunction. Sensory symptoms are usually less recognized but extremely common symptoms of Parkinson disease. These include olfactory dysfunction and pain secondary to rigidity and dystonias. Resting tremor is present in most patients and usually begins unilaterally; it is almost always prominent in the distal part of the extremity. As disease worsens, the tremor becomes bilateral. Parkinson disease tremor frequency is in the 4- to 6-Hz range and is described as supination-pronation ("pill-rolling") type. This clinical feature assists clinicians to differentiate it from essential tremor, which usually has a higher frequency and is a flexion-extension form of movement.[1] Bradykinesia, or slowness of movements, is the most characteristic and disabling motor feature in Parkinson disease, causing difficulties in performing daily activities, such as writing and personal hygiene. Other manifestations of bradykinesia are "mask face," reduced arm swing during gait, and loss of spontaneous movements. Rigidity, which occurs in neck, shoulders, wrist, and ankles, leads to the characteristic stooped posture, anteroflexed head, and flexed knees and elbows of patients who have Parkinson disease. Postural instability usually presents later in the course of the disease. The pull test, during which the patient is quickly pulled backward or forward by the shoulders, is used to assess

Department of Neurology, Louisiana State University Health Sciences Center, 1501 Kings Highway, Shreveport, LA 71130, USA
* Corresponding author.
E-mail address: aminag@lsuhsc.edu (A. Minagar).

Med Clin N Am 93 (2009) 371–388
doi:10.1016/j.mcna.2008.09.002
0025-7125/08/$ – see front matter © 2009 Elsevier Inc. All rights reserved.

retropulsion or propulsion. Taking more than two steps indicates an abnormal postural response. There are several debilitating nonmotor symptoms that can occur in patients who have Parkinson disease. Dementia eventually develops in approximately 35% to 40% of patients who have Parkinson disease. Hallucinations and psychotic behavior resulting from drug treatment are common. Depression and fatigue occur in almost 50% of patients. Autonomic and sleep disturbances are also common features of the disease.

What is the Epidemiology of Parkinson Disease?

The prevalence of Parkinson disease is 1% to 2% in the population 65 years of age or older, and up to 4% in individuals older than 85 years. The usual age of onset is the seventh decade, although up to 10% of those affected are younger than 50 years of age. In the United States, there are currently up to 1 million patients who have diagnosed Parkinson disease.[1] About 40,000 cases of Parkinson disease are diagnosed annually. Lifetime risk for Parkinson disease is 2.0% in males and 1.3% in females. Incidence of Parkinson disease is lower in African Americans than whites.

What is the Cause and Pathogenesis of Parkinson Disease?

The cause of Parkinson disease remains unknown; however, it seems that interactions between genetic background and environmental factors play significant roles in its development. The role of genetic factors in the pathogenesis of Parkinson disease has been discussed for many years. Currently, 13 chromosome loci have been identified and linked to familial forms of Parkinson disease. Mapping of *PARK* genes (**Table 1**) that are associated with development of Parkinson disease supports the role of genetic factors in pathogenesis of Parkinson disease.[2]

One hypothesis on pathogenesis of Parkinson disease links mitochondrial abnormalities and environmental agents to its development. Impaired protein degradation is likely to follow mitochondrial dysfunction and oxidative damage. The folding process of proteins is impaired resulting in an increase of misfolded proteins. The ubiquitin-proteasome system and autophagy-lysosomal pathway are two major degradation systems that are involved in the pathogenesis of nigral neuronal death and the neurodegenerative process in Parkinson disease.

Table 1 Genes responsible for parkinsonism		
Type/Gene	**Locus**	**Pattern of Inheritance**
PARK 1/α-Synuclein	4q21-23	Autosomal dominant
PARK 2/Parkin	6q25.2-27	Autosomal recessive
PARK5/UCH-L1	4p14	Autosomal dominant
PARK3/unknown	2p13	Autosomal dominant
PARK4/SNCA	4p21-23	Autosomal dominant
PARK6/PINK1	1p35-35	Autosomal recessive
PARK7/ DJ-1	1p36	Autosomal recessive
PARK8/LPRK2	12p11.2-q13.1	Autosomal dominant
PARK9/ATP13A2	1p36	Autosomal recessive
PARK10/unknown	1p32	Sporadic
PARK11/unknown	2q36-37	Autosomal dominant
PARK12/unknown	Xq21-25	Sporadic
PARK13/Omi/HtrA2	2p13	Autosomal dominant?

What Neuropathologic Features does Parkinson Disease have?

Characteristic neuropathologic features of Parkinson disease consist of degeneration and loss of the pigmented neurons of the pars compacta of the substantia nigra and the presence of Lewy bodies. A Lewy body is an eosinophilic intracytoplasmic inclusion that occurs in the locus coeruleus, raphe nucleus, olfactory bulb, and other locations in patients who have Parkinson disease. These intracytoplasmic inclusions consist of dense accumulation of α-synuclein, ubiquitin, and torsinA. These lesions may be responsible for motor and nonmotor symptoms of Parkinson disease.

How do We Diagnose Parkinson Disease?

Parkinson disease remains a clinical diagnosis. Brain imaging may be only supportive. Possible Parkinson disease requires at least two of the following four features: resting tremor, bradykinesia, rigidity, and asymmetry of onset. Clinical response to levodopa or a dopamine agonist also lends further support to the diagnosis. There should be absence of features that would support a so-called "Parkinson-plus" disorder, such as progressive supranuclear palsy, corticobasal ganglionic degeneration, or multisystem atrophy. These features include postural instability in the first 3 years, freezing in the first 3 years, hallucinations not related to levodopa in the first 3 years, dementia preceding motor symptoms, autonomic dysfunction, or supranuclear gaze palsy.[3]

What is the Differential Diagnosis of Parkinson Disease?

Differential diagnosis of Parkinson disease includes essential tremor and other parkinsonism syndromes, such as progressive supranuclear palsy, multiple system atrophy (parkinsonism-type and cerebellar-type), corticobasal ganglionic degeneration, diffuse Lewy body disease, and drug-induced parkinsonism.[1,4]

How is Parkinson Disease Managed?

There is no cure for Parkinson disease and its treatment is mainly symptomatic management of motor and nonmotor features. Available therapeutic approaches include pharmacologic, nonpharmacologic, and surgical procedures. It is important to educate patients about the disease to address safety issues and the role of occupational therapy and regular exercise. Pharmacologic treatment of Parkinson disease includes carbidopa/levodopa, dopamine agonists, amantadine, catechol-O-methyltransferase (COMT) inhibitors, and combination of levodopa and COMT and anticholinergics (**Table 2**). Carbidopa/levodopa remains the most effective agent for treatment of motor symptoms of Parkinson disease. Carbidopa/levodopa decreases rigidity, tremor, and bradykinesia, but has its limitations in controlling motor fluctuations. It may contribute to dyskinesia and neuropsychiatric complications, such as hallucinations. Nausea is the most common side effect, but may be reduced by taking medication following meals. Carbidopa/levodopa is usually administered orally in three or four divided doses. COMT inhibitors in combination with levodopa are used to extend levodopa half-life and decrease the end-of-dose wear-off effect. Dopamine agonists (bromocriptine, pergolide, pramipexole, and ropinirole) are used as monotherapy in early Parkinson disease. Adverse effects of dopamine agonists include nausea and vomiting, orthostatic hypotension, sedation, cardiac arrhythmia, and psychosis. Sleep attacks are an uncommon side effect of dopamine agonists, along with compulsive gambling and sexual activity, about which patients should be warned.

Amantadine possibly acts by direct stimulation of dopamine receptors and inhibiting dopamine reuptake. It has been shown to help with rigidity and akinesia, but it has

Table 2 Anti-Parkinson medications	
Medication	Daily Dose (mg)
Anticholinergic agents	
• Trihexyphenidyl	6–10 div tid
• Benztropine	1–2 q hs
• Amantadine	200 div bid
Dopamine agonists	
• Bromocriptine	7.5–60 div tid
• Pramipexole	1.5–4.5 div tid
• Ropinirole	9–24 div tid
• Carbidopa/Levodopa (10/100; 25/250; 25/100)	200/2000 div tid, qid
• Selegiline	10 div bid
• COMT inhibitors	200 with each levodopa dose

Abbreviations: COMT, catechol-O-methyltransferase; div, divided.

minimal effects on tremor. Livedo reticularis, blurred vision, constipation, urinary retention, cognitive deterioration, and hallucinations are adverse effects.

Anticholinergics (benztropine, biperiden, trihexyphenidyl, and procyclidine) are used for reducing tremor in patients who have Parkinson disease, but they have no effect on rigidity or bradykinesia. It is believed that anticholinergics exert their effects by decreasing the amount of acetylcholine that occurs as a result of dopamine deficiency. These agents should be used cautiously in the elderly because of their adverse effects, which include blurred vision, memory impairment, confusion, delirium, urinary retention, and constipation.

What are the Surgical Interventions for Parkinson Disease?

Currently deep brain stimulation is regarded as standard of care for medication-refractory symptoms of Parkinson disease. The subthalamic nucleus and globus pallidus interna are the preferred brain targets of this surgical procedure, which may improve bradykinesia, postural instability, rigidity, and gait dysfunction. Deep brain stimulation (DBS) of the ventral intermediate nucleus of the thalamus is used for treatment of tremor. This treatment does not improve rigidity, bradykinesia, or gait impairment, however. DBS of the internal segment of the globus pallidus suppresses bradykinesia and rigidity and reduces dyskinesia.[5,6]

ESSENTIAL TREMOR
How is Essential Tremor Defined?

Essential tremor is characterized by involuntary shaking most often in the hands or forearms with no other neurologic signs or posturing. The tremor is described as postural (occurring with voluntary maintenance of a position against gravity) or kinetic (occurring during voluntary movement). It may involve the cranial musculature in about 30% of cases with the head being most frequently involved followed by voice.[7] Mild asymmetry is not uncommon. The frequency of essential tremor is 4 to 12 Hz, with older patients exhibiting frequencies in the lower range and younger patients exhibiting frequencies in the higher range.[8] Essential tremor can be disabling for many patients, with up to 85% of affected individuals reporting significant changes in their livelihood and socializing.[9]

What is the Epidemiology of Essential Tremor?

Essential tremor is one of the most common movement disorders. The prevalence ranges widely between epidemiologic studies with data suggesting estimates from 0.4% to 4.8%.[10] Incidence has been assessed in a retrospective 45-year study showing an age-adjusted incidence of 17.5/100,000/y with the incidence of essential tremor rising sharply after age 49.[11] It can be seen in people of any age but its prevalence tends to increase in those aged 65 and older.[8] Patients who have a positive family history of essential tremor have been observed to have a younger age of onset.

What Genetic Factors are Involved in the Development of Essential Tremor?

Essential tremor is frequently described as familial, with a positive family history in 17% to 100% of patients. It is usually inherited as an autosomal dominant trait but may have variable penetrance.[12] A few susceptibility loci have been found. The first was found in a study of 75 members of 16 Icelandic families. A link was identified in the FET1 (also known as ETM1) gene located on chromosome 3q13.[12] Another gene, designated ETM2, mapped to chromosome 2p22–25 in a large American family of Czech descent who had many members affected by ET.[13] In the same family, an ancestral haplotype on chromosome 2p24.1 was also found.

What is the Pathophysiology of Essential Tremor?

The cause of essential tremor remains unknown. Suggestions that essential tremor originates from an abnormal oscillation within thalamocortical and cerebello-olivary loops can be supported by reports that have noted that essential tremor is reduced in lesions of the cerebellum and thalamus. Positron emission tomography (PET) studies of patients who have essential tremor have demonstrated an increase in cerebellar blood flow during the tremor and at rest, which can be observed to decrease with the consumption of alcohol.[14,15] Other areas of increased blood flow revealed by functional MRI imaging include the dentate nucleus, red nucleus and contralaterally in the thalamus, globus pallidus, and primary sensorimotor cortex. A reduced N-acetyl-L-aspartate to creatine ratio in the cerebellar cortex, which is consistent with neuronal loss, has been shown on magnetic resonance spectroscopy.[16]

What is the Differential Diagnosis of Essential Tremor?

The differential diagnosis includes Parkinson disease tremor, dystonic tremor, cerebellar tremor, rubral tremor, psychogenic tremor, and asterixis. Tremor may be observed alone or in the context of other neurologic diseases, such as idiopathic Parkinson disease, Parkinson-plus syndromes, multiple sclerosis, Wilson disease, Huntington chorea, and cerebellar degenerative diseases. Drugs, toxins, and systemic illnesses may also precipitate tremor.

How can the Diagnosis for Essential Tremor be Made?

Essential tremor is a clinical diagnosis and the proposed diagnostic guidelines consist of the following core criteria:

Bilateral action (postural or kinetic) tremor of the hands and forearms (but not rest tremor)
Isolated head tremor with no signs of dystonia
Absence of other neurologic signs with the exception of the cogwheel phenomenon

Secondary criteria consist of long duration (>3 years), positive family history, and beneficial effect of alcohol.[17]

What is the Treatment of Essential Tremor?

Reassuring the patient that he or she does not have a progressive neurologic disease, such as Parkinson disease, is an important first step. No medication is necessary if the tremor does not cause functional impairment or embarrassment to the patient. If medical treatment is required, the two medications that are considered first-line therapies in suppressing tremor are propranolol and primidone. Propranolol is a nonselective beta-adrenergic antagonist that has been shown to be more effective than drugs with selective B1-adrenergic activity.[18] An average dose of 120 mg/d of propranolol has been shown to significantly reduce tremor in these patients. One study showed that long-acting propranolol was as effective as conventional propranolol, and compliance with the long-acting formulation is significantly better.[19] Propranolol is usually well tolerated; however, relative contraindications include asthma, congestive heart failure, insulin-dependent diabetes mellitus, and atrioventricular block. Primidone is an anticonvulsant medication that is metabolized to phenylethylmalonamide and phenobarbitone. It is usually started at 25 mg/d or less to avoid acute adverse effects, including somnolence, flulike symptoms, vertigo, nausea, and ataxia. The primidone dosage may be increased by 25-mg or 50-mg increments until efficacy or a dose of 250 mg/d is achieved. It has been shown that low-dose therapy (<250 mg/d) is just as effective as high-dose therapy (750 mg/d).[20]

Second-line medications, which include alprazolam, gabapentin, topiramate, nimodipine, clozapine, clonidine, and theophylline, may be tried if propranolol and primidone fail to improve tremor. Botulinum toxin A seems to suppress tremor amplitude when injected into intrinsic hand muscles but no significant recovery of function is noted because it is associated with a dose-dependent, reversible weakness.[20] The injections may have more clinical impact when used to treat voice tremor and possibly head tremor; adverse reactions, such as breathiness, hoarseness, and swallowing difficulties, may occur after treatment of voice tremor.[19]

Thalamotomy and thalamic DBS are surgical procedures that have been shown to effectively reduce limb tremor; however, both carry risk for certain complications, such as hemorrhage, infection, or dysarthria.[20] There is currently insufficient evidence to support use of these procedures to reduce head or voice tremor.

RESTLESS LEGS SYNDROME
What is Restless Legs Syndrome?

Restless legs syndrome is characterized by an irresistible urge to move, usually the legs, to stop an uncomfortable or strange sensation. The movement relieves the sensation temporarily. The symptoms are most often worse at night than during the day. It can be idiopathic, which usually starts at a younger age, and can progressively get worse over the years, or it can be secondary, usually starting more suddenly and associated with a medical condition or drugs.

What is the Epidemiology of Restless Legs Syndrome?

Restless legs syndrome is often an under-diagnosed condition that exists in about 10% of the adult population. It can be mild in most cases, but it seriously affects the quality of life in 2.5% of the population. Patients seeking treatment represent only a small portion of those affected. The ratio of women to men is 2:1.[21]

How is Restless Legs Syndrome Diagnosed?

The National Institute of Health established the following criteria to aid in the diagnosis of restless legs syndrome: (1) an urge to move the limbs with or without sensations, (2) improvement with activity, (3) worsening at rest, and (4) worsening in the evening or night.

Supportive clinical features[22] of restless legs syndrome include: (1) history of restless legs syndrome–like symptoms in other family members, (2) relief with dopamine agonist therapy, (3) periodic limb movements in sleep and during wakefulness, and (4) ferritin level less than 50 μg/L.

What is the Cause and Pathophysiology of Restless Legs Syndrome?

The exact cause of restless legs syndrome remains unknown; however, many conditions associated with dopamine production and metabolism have been linked to restless legs syndrome along with genetic factors. Genetic factors play a role in the development of restless legs syndrome; about 60% of cases have been reported as familial with an autosomal dominant pattern with variable penetrance.[23] Restless legs syndrome may be associated with peripheral neuropathy. Several factors support the involvement of dopamine metabolism in the pathogenesis of restless legs syndrome. Medications that increase dopamine activity are effective in relieving symptoms of primary and secondary restless legs syndrome, but dopamine antagonists can exacerbate symptoms. Aggravation of symptoms at night is also indirect confirmation of dopamine metabolism involvement. The level of dopamine activity is influenced by the circadian rhythm with an increase in the level of activity in the morning and decrease of the level at night.[24] Iron is another factor that is involved in pathogenesis of restless legs syndrome because iron is a necessary element in dopamine production pathway. In patients who have restless legs syndrome low iron levels have been identified in the substantia nigra.[25,26] In addition, restless legs syndrome can be associated with low serum iron levels; during diagnostic work-up, serum iron and ferritin levels should be assessed.

Folate deficiency has also been associated with restless legs syndrome. Folate is also involved in the dopamine pathway in the central nervous system as a cofactor of tyrosine hydroxylase production, which is a catalyst in the production of levodopa, which is subsequently decarboxylated into dopamine.[25]

What are the Clinical Manifestations of Restless Legs Syndrome?

The primary and most recognizable feature of restless legs syndrome is the need to move the legs. Sometimes patients describe the need to move other parts of the body also. Patients describe the sensation in their legs as itching, burning, creeping, tingling, and even pain. Sometimes they are unable to describe the sensation, but describe feeling the need to move the legs. Any relaxing activity during the day or night may precipitate the symptoms but they are usually worse at night. Patients who take naps during the day also report symptoms, which may indicate a circadian rhythm involvement. The urge to move is relieved partially or totally by movement; however, this relief is only temporary and the sensation or urge to move can return as soon as the movement subsides. Often, there is a disturbance of sleep secondary to the symptoms. The neurologic examination is usually normal in idiopathic cases; however, patients may have signs of peripheral neuropathy or other signs that may point to a secondary cause of restless legs syndrome.

What is the Differential Diagnosis of Restless Legs Syndrome?

The differential diagnosis of restless legs syndrome includes peripheral neuropathy, positional discomfort, neuroleptic- or other medication–induced akathisia, dyskinesia, peripheral vascular disease, and moving toes. Peripheral neuropathy can be confirmed or ruled out by electrophysiologic studies and its clinical manifestations generally do not improve with movements. Positional discomfort is relieved by specific movements and changing a position of one body part. In neuroleptic-induced akathisia, the patient improves with dopamine blockers and symptoms do not worsen at night. Painful legs with moving toes is a rare disorder with almost continuous movements of the toes as opposed to the whole body stretching and walking, which is seen in restless legs syndrome.[22]

How is Restless Legs Syndrome Treated?

The primary treatment of restless legs syndrome is dopaminergic drugs, such as levodopa, non-ergot dopamine agonists (ropinirole, pramipexole), and ergot derivatives (bromocriptine, pergolide, cabergoline). Non-ergot preparations are preferred to ergot secondary to a more favorable side effect profile. The main potential problem with dopaminergic drugs in the treatment of restless legs syndrome is augmentation, which is a switch of symptoms to an earlier time of day and increase in severity and frequency. Augmentation may be overcome by adding an earlier dose of drug to the regimen, but if symptoms progress to an earlier time, the drug should be tapered off and an alternative medication, such as carbidopa/levodopa or gabapentin, or a benzodiazepine, such as clonazepam, should be considered. Severe intolerable symptoms may require a chronic opioid treatment approach with an agent such as methadone. Iron therapy is promising but cannot be used as monotherapy because it takes a moderate amount of time to raise the serum ferritin level.[26]

HUNTINGTON DISEASE
What is the Definition of Huntington Disease?

Huntington disease is an autosomal dominant, progressive neurodegenerative disorder typically affecting middle-aged adults. It is characterized by a distinct phenotype that includes chorea and dystonia, incoordination, cognitive decline, and various psychiatric and behavioral disorders that generally evolve into dementia.[27]

What is the Epidemiology?

Worldwide prevalence of Huntington disease shows a stable but striking regional variation. The prevalence of Huntington disease has many variations ranging from 0.5/100,000 in Finland to 10/100,000 in parts of the United Kingdom. In Japan, the prevalence of the disease is 0.5/100,000 and the rate is much lower in most of Asia.[27] African populations show a similarly reduced prevalence. In the United States, 5 to 7 whites per 100,000 are affected with Huntington disease. Asymptomatic individuals account for two to four times as many cases as symptomatic individuals. The higher incidence of Huntington disease in the white population compared with African or Asian people relates to the higher frequency of huntingtin alleles with 28 to 35 CAG repeats in whites.[27] The Australian Aboriginal population has shown similar prevalence to that of European origin. Because of the lack of European genetic influence, cases of Huntington disease are not documented in native North or South Americans. The Lake Maracaibo region in Venezuela and the Tasmanian region are two of several regions of the world where the high prevalence of Huntington disease has been shown to have originated from a single gene carrier migrating to that region.

What is the Genetic Basis of Huntington Disease?

In 1983, two years after the US-Venezuela Huntington Disease Collaborative Research Project began, a genetic marker was recognized on the short arm of chromosome 4.[28] It was not until 10 years later that the mutant Huntington disease gene was finally identified. Pathogenesis of Huntington disease involves the mutation of the huntingtin protein. Huntingtin protein (htt) is a 3144-amino acid antiapoptotic protein of unknown function that is expressed in all human and mammalian cells. The highest concentrations can be found in the brain and testes.[27] The *IT-15* gene, which is a 210-kb gene located near the tip of the short arm of chromosome 4 (4p16.3), encodes for the huntingtin protein. Patients with Huntington disease have an expanded and unstable trinucleotide CAG (cytosine-adenine-guanine) repeat in the *IT-15* gene within exon 1.[29] Huntington disease is therefore considered one of the trinucleotide repeat disorders. The huntingtin protein becomes toxic when the CAG repeat, which codes for a polyglutamine stretch at the amino terminus, becomes expanded.[30] This expanded polyglutamine segment is considered the mutant form of the huntingtin protein and leads to cellular dysfunction and neuronal death. The American College of Medical Genetics and the American Society of Human Genetics suggested that laboratories use the following standards when reporting results of patients tested for Huntington disease: fewer than 27 CAG repeats, normal individual; 27 to 35 repeats, normal but repeats may expand in future generations; 36 to 39 repeats, abnormal but may show variable or reduced penetrance; 40 or more repeats, abnormal.[31]

The number of CAG repeats has significant implications for age at onset, disease severity, and stability of the gene between generations. There is a robust inverse correlation between the number of polyglutamine repeats and the age at disease onset so that longer repeat lengths are associated with earlier onset of Huntington disease.[32] This correlation accounts for about 60% of the variation in age of onset. The number of CAG repeats is not an absolute prediction of disease onset. The causes of such a wide variation are not clear; however, rare genetic modifiers, such as GluR6 and ApoE, may contribute, along with environmental factors. The CAG repeat length accounts for about 50% of the disease variance. The effect of trinucleotide length on the rate of progression of Huntington disease is not well defined.

What are the Neuropathologic Features of Huntington Disease?

The most prominent neuropathologic features of Huntington disease consist of neuronal loss and gliosis in the cortex and striatum, particularly the caudate nucleus.[33] Initially, neuronal injury occurs in the caudate tail, in the medial paraventricular caudate, and in the dorsal part of the putamen. As the neurodegenerative process progresses, further neuronal loss and an increase in astrocytes can be observed in widespread cortical and subcortical regions. Pathologic observation of affected striatum shows loss of GABAergic spiny projection neurons with preservation of the aspiny interneurons and large aspiny acetylcholinesterase-positive neurons. There is a decrease of important neurotransmitters and neuropeptides, such as γ-aminobutyric acid (GABA), calbindin, enkephalin, and substance P, as a result of selective loss of the medium spiny neurons.

How is Huntington Disease Diagnosed?

A confirmed family history of Huntington disease combined with clinical manifestations in a patient is sufficient for a diagnosis of the disease. Neuroimaging (MRI and CT) typically reveals severe atrophy of the caudate nucleus in patients who have moderate disability but may also be relatively normal in patients in the early stages of

Huntington disease. This atrophy can be detected in a presymptomatic state by the finding of head of caudate hypometabolism by PET scan. In some cases, caudate nucleus atrophy may be detected anatomically before the onset of symptoms. There is an inverse correlation between the area of the head of the caudate nucleus and the duration of the disease. The degree of cortical atrophy may be more conspicuous than caudate atrophy in elderly patients who have Huntington disease. A patient who has a questionable clinical syndrome of Huntington disease can undergo DNA testing to confirm the diagnosis. The patient's cognitive decline can be evaluated and monitored by neuropsychologic examination.

What is the Differential Diagnosis of Huntington Disease?

Clinical manifestations of Huntington disease, such as chorea, dystonia, and dementia, can present with other diseases. The most likely disorder to be confused with Huntington disease is choreoacanthocytosis, which causes dementia, involuntary movements, and caudate atrophy. Patients who have choreoacanthocytosis display abnormal red blood cell morphology, neuropathy, seizures, myopathy, elevated creatine phosphokinase, self-mutilation, and an unusual eating dystonia. These manifestations are not seen in patients who have Huntington disease. Chorea can have numerous causes and can manifest in disorders such as Sydenham chorea, chorea gravidarum hyperthyroidism, systemic lupus erythematosus, polycythemia vera, neurosyphilis, external pallidal atrophy, dentatorubropallidal atrophy, Wilson disease, Pick disease, Creutzfeldt-Jakob disease, neuronal ceroid lipofuscinosis, multiple system atrophy, glutaric aciduria, Lesch-Nyhan disease, benign familial chorea, and drug-induced chorea. Many drugs, such as estrogens, carbamazepine, phenytoin, anticholinergics, amphetamines, and drugs that cause tardive dyskinesia, can have chorea as an adverse effect.

How is Huntington Disease Treated?

Huntington disease has no definitive cure and presently our therapeutic options are limited. Medical, social work, and physical therapy teams should provide a coordinated effort to develop treatment strategies for patients who have Huntington disease. Therapy of Huntington disease is tailored to the individual. Common symptoms of Huntington disease include depression, mania, delusions, paranoia, and chorea. Selective serotonin reuptake inhibitors are effective in treating depression symptoms, along with other aspects related to depression, such as rumination, perseveration, and obsessive-compulsive disorder. Suicide remains a major concern. For patients who have Huntington disease with symptoms of bipolar disorder, mood stabilizers, such as valproate, carbamazepine, lamotrigine, or lithium, may be effective. Side effects of valproate and carbamazepine include blood dyscrasias and hepatic abnormalities, which require periodic monitoring of complete blood count and liver function test. For those who have delusions and paranoia symptoms neuroleptics are effective; they are also effective in treating chorea. Low doses of neuroleptics are well tolerated but high doses of neuroleptics may impair a patient's motor and cognitive functions. For those patients who have psychosis, the atypical antipsychotics, such as risperidone, clozapine, olanzapine, and quetiapine, provide sufficient control of psychotic symptoms with a lower risk for extrapyramidal adverse effects and tardive dyskinesia. Nutrition is another concern regarding management in patients who have Huntington disease because their caloric requirements may be increased. As the disease progresses, patients may become bedridden, mute, and rigid, with dysphagia and aspiration eventually occurring. The individual patient's plan in palliative care must be addressed in managing the latter stage of the disease.

DRUG-INDUCED MOVEMENT DISORDERS
What is the Definition of Drug-Induced Movement Disorders?

Drug-induced movement disorders (DIMDs) involve a group of disorders that include acute dystonia, akathisia, neuroleptic malignant syndrome, tardive dyskinesia, neuroleptic-induced parkinsonism, asterixis, chorea, and serotonin syndrome. Acute DIMDs, such as akathisia and acute dystonic reaction, can manifest within minutes of drug ingestion. Akathisia is a feeling of inner restlessness and a constant urge to move. Neuroleptic malignant syndrome is a rare complication in patients treated with neuroleptics and can be life threatening. Symptoms of NMS include autonomic dysfunction, altered mental status, hyperthermia, and muscle rigidity.[34] Patients who have been on neuroleptic treatment for 3 months or longer are susceptible to acquiring tardive dyskinesia, which is defined as involuntary repetitive movements. Asterixis is a motor disturbance marked by arrhythmic, intermittent lapses of an assumed posture attributable to interruptions of sustained muscle contraction, resulting in a "flapping" of the outstretched pronated hands. Serotonin syndrome presents as a life-threatening adverse drug reaction that can manifest within minutes of exposure to the offending medication. Clinical findings of serotonin syndrome include tachycardia, myoclonus, rigidity, tremor, ataxia, hyperreflexia, hyperthermia, confusion, and coma.[35]

What are the Epidemiology and Risk Factors?

Because various medications can induce movement disorders the incidence of DIMDs is difficult to quantify. Dopamine receptor blockers, however, account for most cases of DIMDs. The risk for development of DIMDs with atypical antipsychotics is much less than with conventional drugs. DIMDs also occur more frequently with parenteral drugs than with oral drugs.[36]

What is the Pathogenesis?

The exact pathogenesis of DIMDs remains unknown. There are two diverging hypotheses to explain the pathogenesis of DIMD causing acute dystonias regarding either a hypodopaminergic or a hyperdopaminergic state associated with dopaminergic receptor blockade in the caudate, putamen, or globus pallidus. The delay between receptor blockade and the onset of symptoms of acute dystonia suggests involvement of other mechanisms, such as secondary dopamine-receptor hypersensitivity. Hypotheses about the underlying cause of akathisia include dopamine blockade in the mesocortical dopamine pathway and involvement of central serotonergic and adrenergic neurotransmitter systems. In serotonin syndrome, no single receptor seems to be completely responsible; however, agonism of 5HT2A and 5HT1A receptors located in the brainstem seems to contribute substantially.

How are Drug-Induced Movement Disorders Diagnosed?

DIMDs do not usually require further testing for diagnosis. They are differentiated from non–drug-induced dystonic reactions, such as torticollis, by their acute onset, presence of precipitating factors, and cessation when the precipitating factor is removed. Focal seizures and hypocalcemia are included in the differential diagnosis of DIMDs; if the diagnosis is unclear in any way, an EEG and calcium level can be obtained to help aid in the diagnosis.

How are Drug-Induced Movement Disorders Treated?

Most treatments are aimed at reducing or stopping the offending agent. Dystonia is treated by this method, which may briefly worsen the dystonia initially. If discontinuing the offending agent is not possible, switching to a less potent drug is the next step. Intramuscular or intravenous benztropine, diphenhydramine, or diazepam may be used to treat acute dystonia.

Akathisia usually has a favorable prognosis. Reducing the dose of the insulting drug is the first step in treatment; however, if this is not possible then switching to a less potent antipsychotic treatment is the next step. If symptoms still persist, evidence-based treatment is strongest for beta-blockers, such as propranolol, although benzodiazepines may also be beneficial. Other choices for management include anti-cholinergics (especially if parkinsonian features are present) and amantadine.

Neuroleptic malignant syndrome treatment involves not only withdrawing the insulting drug but also supportive measures, such as fluid and electrolyte correction, lowering the temperature of the patient, and management of cardiopulmonary and renal complications. Dantrolene, bromocriptine, lisuride, benzodiazepines, and N-methyl-D-aspartate receptor blockers (ie, amantadine and memantine) have been used in the treatment of neuroleptic malignant syndrome.

Treatment of tardive dyskinesia involves stopping the offending drug, or at least lowering the dose. If withdrawing the antipsychotic drug is not possible, switching to an antipsychotic with a low propensity to cause the disorder (quetiapine or clozapine) would be the next step. Other medications that have shown to be effective include propranolol, clonidine, GABA agonists (valproate and clonazepam), anticholinergics (trihexyphenidyl), and vitamin E. The dopamine-depleting agent, tetrabenazine, is the only licensed treatment of tardive dyskinesia in the United Kingdom (not yet available in the United States), but can produce symptoms of depression.

Serotonin syndrome is serious and severe cases should be monitored in an ICU. Removal of the causative agent is the initial treatment. In most cases, symptoms resolve within 24 hours of cessation of the causative agent. Symptoms of agitation can be managed by benzodiazepines. Other drug treatments that have been used include propranolol, diphenhydramine, chlorpromazine, diazepam, methysergide, and cyproheptadine.

WILSON DISEASE
What is Wilson Disease?

Wilson disease, also known as progressive hepatolenticular degeneration,[37] is an autosomal recessive systemic disorder of copper metabolism. It is characterized by impaired incorporation of copper into ceruloplasmin and its reduced biliary excretion, which leads to decreased serum concentration of ceruloplasmin and excessive deposition of copper initially in the liver and later into the brain and other organs. The defective gene is located on the long arm of chromosome 13q14.3, which codes for a P-type adenosine triphosphatase protein (ATP7B).[38] ATP7B binds copper and transports it across cellular membranes for exocytosis from hepatocytes.

What are the Neurologic Manifestations Caused by Wilson Disease?

About half of all patients who have Wilson disease have a neurologic or psychiatric problem. Postural and intention tremors are the most common neurologic manifestation of Wilson disease. Other common symptoms include ataxia, titubation, dysarthria, chorea, akinetic-rigid syndrome, postural and gait abnormalities, and generalized dystonia. Cognitive and psychiatric problems can include inappropriate and uncontrolled grinning, drooling, cognitive impairment with below-average memory function, depression, anxiety, psychosis, and organic mood disorders.[39]

What is the Epidemiology of Wilson Disease?

The best estimate for the prevalence of Wilson disease is about 1 in 30,000 to 1 in 40,000 live births in most populations. The carrier frequency of the abnormal ATP7B gene is about 1 in 100.

How do you Diagnose Wilson Disease?

Wilson disease can be suspected when a patient presents with liver or neurologic manifestations. Mild to moderate elevations in alanine transaminase (ALT), aspartate transaminase (AST), and bilirubin can be seen, with AST usually greater than ALT. Uric acid may be decreased from associated renal tubular acidosis. The most common specific screening test for Wilson disease is a measurement of serum ceruloplasmin level. Serum ceruloplasmin is usually low (<20 mg/dL); however, in 10% of patients, serum ceruloplasmin level may be close to normal. Elevated 24-hour urine copper concentration is also characteristic with more then 40 μg (600 nmol) considered abnormal. Kayser-Fleischer rings may be seen with a slit-lamp ocular examination. Abnormal hyperintense signals in the bilateral lentiform and caudate nuclei, thalamus, brainstem, and white matter are characteristic MRI findings in the brain.[40–42] The liver biopsy with quantification of hepatic copper is the most specific test to provide a definitive diagnosis of Wilson disease. Genetic testing is possible but not very useful because of a high variety of disease-specific mutations.

What is the Differential Diagnosis?

Wilson disease must be differentiated from other genetic extrapyramidal disorders, including Huntington disease, juvenile parkinsonism, dopa-responsive dystonia, neurodegeneration with brain iron accumulation, idiopathic torsion dystonia, chorea-acanthocytosis, and benign familial chorea. The combination of neurologic or psychiatric features with the presence of a Kayser-Fleischer ring or hepatic disease is a diagnostic clue. Early schizophrenia, drug abuse, or a personality disorder can obscure the diagnosis, especially if the initial manifestations are psychiatric.

How is Wilson Disease Treated?

Once diagnosed, Wilson disease requires aggressive treatment, which prevents severe neurologic and psychiatric manifestations and can even reverse them to some extent.[40] Avoidance of foods rich in copper, especially liver and shellfish, is recommended. The mainstay of treatment is focused on the inhibition of copper absorption or an increase of copper elimination. Currently available pharmacologic agents include penicillamine, zinc acetate, trientine, and ammonium tetrathiomolybdate. Zinc acetate blocks copper absorption. The typical dose is 50 mg three times a day. Side effects include abdominal discomfort. Penicillamine and trientine have a similar mechanism of action. Both chelate and allow for urinary excretion of copper. The standard doses are penicillamine 250 to 500 mg four times a day and trientine 600 mg three times a day. They have similar side effects, including acute hypersensitivity, bone marrow suppression, Goodpasture syndrome, and chronic effects on collagen and the immune system. Trientine is known for its lower frequency of side effects as compared with penicillamine. Ammonium tetrathiomolybdate promotes copper/protein complex formation to prevent copper absorption and to promote detoxification of circulating copper but it can cause copper deficiency anemia. It is slowly titrated from 20 mg three times a day up to 60 mg with the option of possibly adding an additional three doses of 20 to 60 mg. Albumin dialysis is provided along with chelating therapy. Liver transplantation is indicated for fulminant liver failure in patients who fail to respond to medication. It has been shown to result in reduction of neurologic and psychiatric symptoms.[43]

TOURETTE SYNDROME
What is Tourette Syndrome?

Tourette syndrome is a hyperkinetic disorder characterized by combination of multiple motor and vocal tics that typically starts in childhood. It is frequently associated with psychiatric comorbidities, such as obsessive-compulsive disorder, impulse control disorder, and attention deficit hyperactivity disorder.

What is the Epidemiology of Tourette Syndrome?

The disease can be seen in all ethnic and racial groups with a strong predisposition for males over females by a ratio of 4:1. The peak incidence falls into early preadolescence with further resolution of symptoms in adult life in 50% of the cases.[11] There are mixed prevalence rates recorded in various studies that make an accurate prevalence rate difficult to establish. Some studies estimate the prevalence of Tourette syndrome as 0.1% to 1% of the general population.[44] One observational study recorded a prevalence of tics in 18.7% of 13- to 14-year-old students and Tourette syndrome in 1.85% of the same population.[45]

What is the Cause and Pathophysiology of Tourette Syndrome?

Multiple mechanisms have been proposed as the cause of Tourette syndrome; however, the exact cause is still unknown. Genetic, autoimmune, and environmental factors seem to be involved. There is a complex mechanism of inheritance that can be different in different families. Several different theories connect Tourette syndrome with the centromeric region of chromosome 5[46] and an autosomal dominant mechanism of inheritance with incomplete penetrance, but none of them has been solidly proved. There is strong evidence that the first-degree relatives of a proband have an increased risk for Tourette syndrome or multiple chronic tics. Several large families have been described with multiple family members having a spectrum of involvement in tic expression from mild transient tics, to chronic tic syndrome, to actual Tourette syndrome. Genetics do not explain the entire clinical picture, however, and environmental (including intrauterine) factors and autoimmune mechanisms[47] have been postulated to influence the clinical expression of the disorder. Antineuronal or antinuclear antibodies obtained from some patients who have Tourette syndrome have been shown to increase oral stereotypies in rats that have been infused with the sera.[48]

The imbalance of dopamine and serotonin metabolism has been studied as a potential pathophysiologic mechanism of the disease. By PET studies, a significant increase in dopamine release has been shown in the ventral striatum with predisposition to the left. Additional PET studies show that glucose reuptake and regional cerebral blood flow are decreased in the same area. Serotonin transporter binding protein is increased in the midbrain and striatum.[49] An impaired limbic-motor interaction has been implicated from PET studies of regional cerebral metabolic rates showing positive functional coupling between motor and lateral orbitofrontal circuits, which is a reversal of the normal interrelationship.[50] The volume of the left lenticular nucleus is reduced, which has been demonstrated by volumetric MRI studies.[51]

How can the Diagnosis of Tourette Syndrome be Made?

The DSM-IV[52] criteria for the diagnosis of Tourette syndrome include the following:

History or finding of multiple motor tics
History or finding of one or more vocal tics
Onset before 18 years of age

Duration of more than 1 year
Tics cause marked distress or significant impairment in daily functioning

Tics are involuntary or semivoluntary sudden, rapid, stereotyped motor movements or sounds. They can easily be confused with chorea or other hyperkinetic disorders. Tics can be divided into simple tics (abrupt, purposeless, and isolated movements) or complex tics (coordinated, sequenced movements resembling normal motor acts or gestures that are inappropriately intense and timed). Simple motor tics include shoulder shrugs, eye blinking, and head jerks. In 80% of cases, tics initially started in the face and neck area. Complex motor tics include touching, throwing, hitting, and jumping. Other examples of complex motor tics are grabbing or exposing one's genitalia (copropraxia), imitating gestures (echopraxia), or imitating sounds (echolalia). Phonic tics can involve vocal cords or can be generated by mouth, throat, and nose, and present as clearing the throat, coughing, and nose blowing. Simple phonic tics are inarticulate noises, whereas complex phonic tics include words, word fragments, or musical elements. Up to 20% of patients express coprolalia, which is the obsessive use of obscene language. Tics can be stopped voluntary for a while but usually produce an uncomfortable feeling, which eventually must be relieved by executing the tic behavior.

What is the Treatment of Tourette Syndrome?

Because of the complexity of the disease, a multidisciplinary approach with a team consisting of a neurologist, psychiatrist, psychologist, and other appropriate specialists is required. The goal is to access the maximum control with the smallest number of side effects possible. The general principles are to start medication in the lowest possible dose and slowly titrate until the lowest effective dose is obtained or intolerable adverse effects become a problem.

For tics, the standard treatment may be typical and atypical neuroleptics, if clearly believed to be clinically indicated. The older drugs include fluphenazine, pimozide, haloperidol, thiothixene, trifluoperazine, and molindone. Their use is restricted by severe and in 50% of patients permanent side effects of drug-induced movement disorders, from acute dystonic reactions to tardive syndromes. Fluphenazine is effective and least sedating. Pimozide is effective but it can cause prolongation of the Q-T interval and requires frequent EKG follow up. Haloperidol, the first and oldest of this group of medications, has the greatest number frequent side effects, including sedation, depression, weight gain, and school phobia. Newer neuroleptics, such as risperidone, olanzapine, quetiapine, and ziprasidone, tend to have fewer side effects than the typical antipsychotics and can be just as effective at reducing tics. Clonidine, an alpha blocker, (0.05–0.5 mg/d) also has tic-suppressant effects and can be used in children who have associated attention deficit hyperactivity disorder for whom antipsychotics are contraindicated. Presynaptic catecholamine depletors, such as reserpine and tetrabenazine, have been shown to suppress tics. The side effects of reserpine (0.1–1 mg three times daily) include postural hypotension, parkinsonism, and depression. Tetrabenazine is not currently available in the United States.

The treatment of concomitant obsessive-compulsive disorder includes the use of antidepressants, tryptophan, monoamine oxidase inhibitors, mianserin (a selective serotonin antagonist), and benzodiazepines. In mild to moderate cases, selective serotonin reuptake inhibitors have replaced older antidepressants. They are recommended in treatment of Tourette syndrome associated with obsessive-compulsive disorder and other behavioral changes. These include fluoxetine (20–60 mg/d), sertraline (50–200 mg/d), paroxetine (20–60 mg/d), and fluvoxamine ($\geq$ 50 mg/d). They may improve obsessive-compulsive disorder symptoms without affecting tic severity. The effectiveness of these drugs is dose dependent, so doses higher than standard antidepressant doses are often required. Clomipramine (initiated at 25 mg/d) is equally effective but its side effects (anticholinergic, cardiotoxic, and seizure-potentiating) make it less commonly used. Clonazepam (0.5–5 mg/d) may be used as once-daily medication because it may relax the patient and ameliorate concomitant emotional and behavioral abnormalities.

Botulinum toxin can be used in the area of tics. It is especially effective when tics involve strong, forced movements of the neck that can cause physical trauma. Botulinum therapy can stop the involuntary movements and premonitory sensory component associated with the tics. The effects can last 3 to 4 months and repetitive injections are required. Botulinum injections are usually free from serious complications, but caution should be used when injecting into the neck area because of potential dysphasia.

Behavioral techniques and support groups have been used for treatment of tics. Vagus nerve stimulation and deep nerve stimulation have been tried as surgical procedures. Thalamic area, globus pallidus interna and externa, and the anterior limb of the internal capsule/nucleus accumbens have been tried as targets.[53]

Education of the patients and their families is important. Parents need to understand their child's limited ability to suppress the tics, which become most prominent when the child feels nervous or under stress. Parents should inform the child's teachers of the diagnosis and of any medications for this disorder. In severe cases home education can be recommended as temporary measure.

REFERENCES

1. Alvarez MV, Evidente VG, Driver-Dunckley ED. Differentiating Parkinson's disease from other parkinsonian disorders. Semin Neurol 2007;27(4):356–62.
2. Dekker MCJ, Bonifati V, van Duijn CM. Parkinson's disease: piecing together a genetic jigsaw. Brain 2003;126:1–12.
3. Jankovick J. Parkinson's disease: clinical features and diagnosis. J Neurol Neurosurg Psychiatr 2008;79:368–76.
4. Esper CD, Factor SA. Current and future treatments in multiple system atrophy. Curr Treat Options Neurol 2007;9(3):210–23.
5. Zesiewicz T, Hauser R. Medical treatment of motor and nonmotor features of Parkinson's disease. Minneapolis (MN): American Academy of Neurology; 2007. p. 12–38.
6. Siddiqui M, Okun M. Deep brain stimulation in Parkinson's disease. Minneapolis (MN): American Academy of Neurology; 2007. p. 39–57.
7. Deuschl G, Bain P, Brin M. Consensus statement of the Movement Disorder Society on tremor. Ad Hoc Scientific Committee. Mov Disord 1998;13(Suppl 3):2–23.
8. Elble RJ. Diagnostic criteria for essential tremor and differential diagnosis. Neurology 2000;54(11 Suppl. 4):S2–6.
9. Bain PG, Findley LJ, Thompson PD, et al. A study of hereditary essential tremor. Brain 1994;117:805–24.
10. Lorenz D, Deuschl G. Update on pathogenesis and treatment of essential tremor. Curr Opin Neurol 2007;20(4):447–52.
11. Rajput AH, Offord KP, Beard CM, et al. Essential tremor in Rochester, Minnosota: a 45 year study. J Neurol Neurosurg Psychiatr 1984;47:466–70.
12. Glucher JR, Jonsson P, Kong A, et al. Mapping of a familial essential tremor gene, FET1, to chromosome 3q13. Nat Genet 1997;17:84–7.

13. Higgins JJ, Pho LT, Nee LE. A gene (ETM) for essential tremor maps to chromosome 2p22-p25. Mov Disord 1997;12:859–64.
14. Jenkins JH, Bain PG, Colebatch JG, et al. A positron emission tomography study of essential tremor; evidence for overactivity in cerebellar connections. Ann Neurol 1993;34:82–90.
15. Boecker H, Wills AJ, Ceballos-Baumann A, et al. The effect of ethanol on alcohol-responsive essential tremor: a positron emission tomography study. Ann Neurol 1996;39:650–8.
16. Louis ED, Shungu DC, Chan S, et al. Metabolic abnormality in the cerebellum in patients with essential tremor: a proton magnetic resonance spectroscopic imaging study. Neurosci Lett 2002;333:17–20.
17. Bain P, Brin M, Deuschl G, et al. Criteria for the diagnosis of essential tremor. Neurology 2000;54(Suppl 4):S7.
18. Jefferson D, Jenner P, Marsden CD. Adrenoreceptor antagonists in essential tremor. J Neurol Neurosurg Psychiatr 1979;42:904–9.
19. Cleeves L, Findley LJ. Propranolol and propranolol-LA in essential tremor: a double blind comparative study. J Neurol Neurosurg Psychiatr 1988;51:379–84.
20. Zesiewicz TA, Elble R, Louis ED, et al. Practice parameter: therapies for essential tremor: report of the quality standards subcommittee of the American academy of neurology. Neurology 2005;64:2008–20.
21. Thomas K, Watson CB. Restless legs syndrome in women: a review. J Womens Health 2008;17(5):859–68.
22. Walters AS. Restless legs syndrome and periodic limb movements. Minneapolis (MN): American Academy of Neurology; 2007. p. 115–38.
23. Lavigne GJ, Montplaisir JY. Restless legs syndrome and sleep bruxism: prevalence and association among Canadians. Sleep 1994;17(8):739–43.
24. Satija P, Ondo WG. Restless legs syndrome: pathophysiology, diagnosis and treatment. CNS drugs 2008;22(6):497–518.
25. Patrick L. Restless legs syndrome: pathophysiology and the role of iron and folate. Altern Med Rev 2007;12:101–12.
26. Earley CJ, Horska A, Mohamed MA, et al. A randomized, double-blind, placebo-controlled trial of intravenous iron sucrose in restless legs syndrome. Sleep Med 2008, in press.
27. Walker, Francis O. Huntington's disease. The Lancet 2007;369:218–28.
28. Gusella JF, Wexler NS, Conneally M, et al. A polymorphic DNA marker genetically linked to Huntington's disease. Nature 1983;306:234–8.
29. Greenamyre J, Timothy. Huntington's disease—making connections. N Engl J Med 2007;356:518–20.
30. Sandrine AL, Saudou F, Sandrine H. Phosphorylation of huntingtin by cyclin-dependent kinase 5 is induced by DNA damage and regulates wild-type and mutant huntingtin toxicity in neurons. J Neurosci 2007;27:7318–28.
31. Quarrell OW, Rigby AS, Barron L, et al. Reduced penetrance alleles for Huntington's disease: a multi-centre direct observational study. J Med Genet 2007;44:68–72.
32. Shelbourne PF, Keller-McGandy C, Bi LW, et al. Triplet repeat mutation length gains correlate with cell-type specific vulnerability in Huntington disease brain. Hum Mol Genet 2007;16:1133–42.
33. Roth J, Klempis J, Jech R, et al. Caudate nucleus atrophy in Huntington's disease and its relationship with clinical and genetic parameters. Funct Neurol 2005;20:127–30.
34. Jackson N, Doherty J, Coulter S. Neuropsychiatric complications of commonly used palliative care drugs. Postgrad Med J 2008;84:121–6.

35. Haddad PM, Dusun SM. Neurological complications of psychiatric drugs: clinical features and management. Human Psychopharmocol 2008;23:15–26.
36. Dressler D, Benecke R. Diagnosis and management of acute movement disorders. J Neurol 2005;252:1299–306.
37. Roberts EA, Schilsky M. AASLD guideline: a practice guideline on Wilson disease. Hepatology 2003;37:1475–92.
38. Davies LP, Macinture G, Cox DW. New mutations in the Wilson disease gene, ATP7B: implications for molecular testing. Genetic testing 2008;12(1):139–45.
39. Ala A, Walker AP, Ashkan K, et al. Wilson's disease. Lancet 2007;369:397–408.
40. Sinha S, Taly AB, Prashanth LK, et al. Sequential MRI changes in Wilson's disease with de-coppering therapy: a study of 50 patients. Br J Radiol 2007;80(957):744–9.
41. Das M, Misra UK, Kalita J. A study of clinical, MRI and multimodality evoked potentials in neurologic Wilson disease. Eur J Neurol 2007;14(5):498–504.
42. Huang CC, Chu NS, Yen TC, et al. Dopamine transporter binding in Wilson's disease. Can J Neurol Sci 2003;30:163–7.
43. Sevmis S, Karakayali H, Aliosmanoglu I, et al. Liver transplantation for Wilson's disease. Transplant Proc 2008;40(1):228–30.
44. Houeto JL, Gire P. Tics and Tourette syndrome: diagnosis, course and treatment principles. Presse Med 2008;37(2Pt 2):263–70.
45. Hornsey H, Banerjee S. The prevalence of Tourette's syndrome in 13–14 year olds in mainstream schools. J Child Psychol Psychiatry 2001;42:1035–9.
46. Laurin N, Wigg KG, Feng Y, et al. Chromosome 5 and Gilles de la Tourette syndrome: linkage in a large pedigree and association study of six candidates in region. Am J Med Genet 2008 [Pubmed publication ahead of print].
47. Hoekstra PJ, Kallenberg CG, Korf J, et al. Is Tourette's syndrome an autoimmune disease? Mol Psychiatry 2002;7:437–45.
48. Taylor JR, Morshed SA, Parveen S, et al. An animal model of Tourette's syndrome. Am J Psychiatry 2002;159:657–60.
49. Wong DF, Brasic JR, Singer HS, et al. Mechanisms of dopaminergic and serotonergic neurotransmission in Tourette syndrome: clues from an in vivo neurochemistry study with PET. Neuropsychopharmacology 2008;33:1239–51.
50. Jeffries KJ, Schooler C, Schoenbach C, et al. The functional neuroanatomy of Tourette's syndrome: an FDG PET study: functional coupling of regional cerebral metabolic rates. Neuropsychopharmacology 2002;27:92–104.
51. Peterson BS, Thomas P, Kane MJ, et al. Basal ganglia volumes in patients with Gilles de la Tourette syndrome. Arch Gen Psychiatry 2003;60:415–24.
52. American Psychiatric Association. Diagnostic and statistical manual of mental disorders. 4th edition. Washington: American Psychiatric Association; 1994.
53. Ackermans L, Temel Y, Visser-Vandewalle V. Deep brain stimulation in the Tourette's syndrome. Neurotherapeutics 2008;5(2):339–44.

Memory Complaints and Dementia

Roger E. Kelley, MD*, Alireza Minagar, MD

KEYWORDS

- Dementia • Memory complaints • Alzheimer's disease
- Normal pressure hydrocephalus • Dementia with Lewy bodies
- Multi-infarct dementia • Congophilic angiopathy

WHAT IS THE DEFINITION OF DEMENTIA AND WHAT ARE THE POSSIBLE CAUSES?

Dementia is a progressive loss of cognitive function on a chronic basis for which several possible causes exist. The most common forms of dementia are outlined in **Box 1**. Alzheimer's disease (AD) remains the most common form of dementia, but there seems to be considerable overlap in terms of neurodegenerative disease in general. In other words, it is felt that vascular dementia in combination with AD may be the second most common form of dementia, and vascular dementia alone may be the third most common form of dementia. On the other hand, dementia with Lewy bodies (DLB), characterized by cognitive impairment with features of parkinsonism and visual hallucinations, may be the second or third most common form of dementia in the elderly, according to some studies.[1] It may be difficult to sort out if the combination of dementia with parkinsonism may be primary Parkinson's disease in association with dementia or the combination of Parkinson's disease with AD rather than DLB.

It has been practical to differentiate treatable forms of dementia from untreatable. AD can be listed as a "treatable" form of dementia because cholinesterase inhibitors are available, but it is well recognized that the response to treatment is generally less than dramatic. Treatable forms of dementia include hypothyroidism, vitamin B_{12} deficiency, nonconvulsive status epilepticus, general paresis from tertiary syphilis, normal pressure hydrocephalus, chronic subdural hematoma, benign brain tumor, and cryptococcal meningitis. Infectious causes may respond to treatment that arrests the process, but that does not necessarily improve cognitive function. This is the case for general paresis and HIV-related dementia, including AIDS dementia complex. On the other hand, prion disease, the process responsible for Creutzfeldt-Jakob disease, remains completely untreatable. Herpes simplex encephalitis has a predilection for the temporal lobes and can leave afflicted individuals with severe memory impairment, if they survive. The sooner the agent acyclovir is initiated for this viral central nervous system infection, however, the better the overall outcome.

Department of Neurology, LSU Health Sciences Center, 1501 Kings Highway, Shreveport, LA 71103, USA
* Corresponding author.
E-mail address: rkelly@lsuhsc.edu (R.E. Kelley).

Med Clin N Am 93 (2009) 389–406
doi:10.1016/j.mcna.2008.09.008
0025-7125/08/$ – see front matter © 2009 Elsevier Inc. All rights reserved.

medical.theclinics.com

Box 1
Differential diagnosis of dementia

Neurodegenerative

   AD

   Frontotemporal dementia

   Parkinson's disease

   Progressive supranuclear palsy

   Huntington's disease

   Dementia with Lewy bodies

Metabolic/deficiency state

   Vitamin B_{12} deficiency

   Thyroid disease

   Alcohol-related

Vascular

   Multi-infarct

   Cerebral autosomal dominant arteriopathy with subcortical infarcts and leukoencephalopathy

   Congophilic angiopathy

   Chronic subdural hematoma

   Postsubarachnoid hemorrhage

Infectious

   Neurosyphilis

   HIV-related

   Cryptococcal meningitis

   Herpes simplex encephalitis

   Postencephalitic

Structural

   Brain tumor

   Normal pressure hydrocephalus

Epileptiform

   Partial complex status epilepticus

   Absence status

Other

   Pseudodementia from depression

   Posttraumatic Creutzfeldt-Jakob disease

   Multiple sclerosis

   Limbic encephalitis

   Morvan's syndrome

WHAT ARE THE SUBCATEGORIES OF DEMENTIA RELATED TO NEURODEGENERATIVE DISEASE?

There is considerable overlap for neurodegenerative disease in terms of cognitive involvement.[2] Under this broad category, one includes the dementia of AD, DLB, dementia associated with Parkinson's disease, dementia associated with progressive supranuclear palsy, dementia associated with Huntington's disease, frontal-temporal lobe dementia, Pick's disease, multisystemic atrophy, corticobasal ganglionic degeneration, striatonigral degeneration, and probably primary progressive aphasia. The presence of significant dementia in any of these neurodegenerative processes can significantly impact the prognosis and potential response to therapy. Typically, one differentiates cortical from subcortical dementia in terms of selective involvement of specific cognitive capacities related to the localization of the pathology. Cortical dementia with AD as the hallmark disease process is characterized by memory disturbance (recent more so than remote) along with possible aphasic disturbance, loss of executive function, inattention, motor impersistence, agnosia, and apraxia. Subcortical dementia, such as that seen with progressive supranuclear palsy, is characterized by slowing of thought processes, impairment of task-specific activities, and impaired communication ability other than typical aphasia. Response to visual input also tends to be impaired significantly in persons affected by subcortical dementia.

WHAT ARE SOME OTHER EXPLANATIONS FOR DEMENTIA?

Other disease processes are not uncommonly associated with dementia. For example, it is not at all uncommon to see cognitive impairment in patients who have multiple sclerosis, which can be devastating and impede any potential for employability. Chronic alcoholism is well recognized as a cause of dementia. The dementia associated with alcoholism can be related to a direct neurotoxic effect from chronic excessive alcohol consumption. An individual who has alcoholism is also more susceptible to falls, with secondary head trauma, and predisposition to subdural hematoma. Specific cognitive complaints, such as profound memory loss, can be seen with development of Wernicke-Korsakoff syndrome.

The term "pseudo-dementia" is used to denote cognitive complaints related to clinically significant depression. It can mimic dementia, especially if the patient is so distracted that it creates a barrier to registration of new information. Typically, however, such patients are readily aware of their deficit and are able to seek out evaluation on their own.

WHAT IS THE PROPER APPROACH FOR EVALUATION OF THE PATIENT WITH MEMORY COMPLAINTS?

Typical patients with significant dementia are brought to the doctor's office by a significant other or family members. Patients tend to be oblivious to the proceedings and often have a bemused or quizzical expression on their face. Occasionally, they are defensive or irritable. It is important for the clinician to gauge the situation in an appropriate fashion. A gentle approach is best, and one often must intercede with family members who are trying their best to emphasize the gravity of the situation while patients try to downplay their input. Experienced clinicians all have their favorite way to assess cognitive function. The Mini-Mental State Examination has become a popular initial choice for screening purposes.[3] An abnormal test result supports the presence of dementia and should lead to further evaluation of causes of dementia. A normal or equivocal test result does not exclude the diagnosis of a dementing illness, however.

The addition of clock-drawing, in which patients are asked to fill in the numbers of a clock and provide a specified time, can be a useful adjunctive test.

Mild cognitive impairment (MCI) is becoming an increasingly used term for patients who have mild cognitive disturbance.[4] Application of the Clinical Dementia Rating Scale can be useful in the detection of early cognitive impairment, which might progress to AD over time.[5] Such detection becomes increasingly important as newer preventive therapies for persons at risk for developing AD become available. The Clinical Dementia Rating Scale is a structured assessment of the subject and person familiar with the subject. This scale is set up as follows: 0 is for asymptomatic individuals, 0.5 is for mild or questionable cognitive impairment, 1 is for mild dementia, 2 is for moderate dementia, and 3 is for severe dementia.

WHAT ADDITIONAL DIAGNOSTIC TESTING IS INDICATED IN THE EVALUATION OF COGNITIVE IMPAIRMENT?

Formal neuropsychological testing can be useful for assessing patients with atypical presentations.[6] Such testing has the potential to differentiate AD from vascular dementia in patients who have prominent, but not necessarily specific, white matter changes on their MRI brain scan. Once it has been decided that dementia is present, certain diagnostic testing is fairly standard (**Box 2**). It is important to obtain a complete blood count to assess for a systemic process affecting bone marrow production.

Box 2
Diagnostic testing in dementia

Standard tests

    Noncontrast CT brain scan

    Metabolic panel

    Complete blood count

    Serum B_{12} level

    Thyroid profile

    Depression screening

Tests in selected circumstances

    MRI brain scan

    EEG

    Syphilis serology

    HIV testing

    Lumbar puncture

    Cerebral positron emission tomographic scan

    Cerebral single-photon emission computed tomographic scan

    Cerebral functional MRI scan

    Apolipoprotein E4 allele

    Cerebrospinal fluid biomarkers for AD

    Genetic testing for DLB or Creutzfeldt-Jakob disease

    Genetic testing for frontotemporal dementia

An erythrocyte sedimentation rate test should be considered if an inflammatory, infectious, or neoplastic process is under consideration. A metabolic profile helps to eliminate a possible encephalopathy that could result from a low or high serum calcium level, a low serum glucose level, a low serum sodium level, a low serum phosphate level, or a low serum magnesium level. A thyroid profile is necessary to exclude cognitive impairment related to hypothyroidism. A serum B_{12} level is performed in recognition that B_{12} deficiency can lead to myriad neurologic deficits, including dementia. Syphilis serology and HIV testing is also important in susceptible populations.

It is generally accepted that a brain scan is indicated in all patients with dementia to evaluate for a possible structural process, such as brain tumor or subdural hematoma, find evidence of cerebrovascular disease, or find evidence of communicating hydrocephalus, which would raise the possibility of normal pressure hydrocephalus as an explanation for the dementia. The noncontrast CT brain scan is probably adequate when there is clear clinical evidence to support AD or DLB as the most likely explanation for the dementia.[7] One expects to see some degree of cortical atrophy and possibly some secondary enlargement of the ventricular system on either CT or MRI brain scan (**Fig. 1**) when these entities are the most likely explanation for the dementia. A contrast-enhanced study is indicated when there is clinical suspicion of a mass lesion. The contrast-enhanced study is safer as the gadolinium used in the MRI brain scan is not iodine based and is not associated with a significant risk of allergic reaction or renal toxicity. The MRI is more sensitive for microvascular changes, and such findings may help to support vascular dementia related to small vessel occlusive disease (ie, multiple lacunar-type infarcts).[8] The MRI brain scan is also clearly superior to the CT brain scan for the evaluation of demyelinating disease, such as multiple sclerosis.

Cerebrospinal fluid (CSF) examination can help to confirm neurosyphilis and is mandatory for the evaluation of cryptococcal meningitis. CSF evaluation for tau protein and other pathogenetic markers of AD, such as beta-amyloid (Aβ), remains primarily

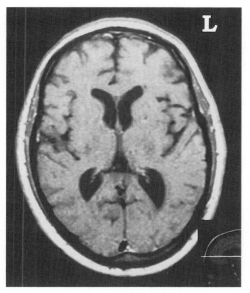

Fig. 1. T1-weighted MRI brain scan demonstrates diffuse cortical atrophy with secondary ventricular dilatation in a patient with dementia.

in the research realm. In a recent study by Ringman and colleagues,[9] however, the authors found that the CSF Aβ $Aβ_{42}$ to $Aβ_{40}$ ratio was reduced in familial AD nondemented mutation carriers, whereas CSF tau and p-tau$_{181}$ levels were elevated in presymptomatic carriers. They also reported that $Aβ_{42}$ was elevated in the plasma of carriers and may decrease as dementia develops. The EEG can help to determine a subclinical status epilepticus as an explanation for the cognitive disturbance. This is especially relevant if the patient has a fluctuating course of mental impairment or has manifestations of partial complex epilepsy, such as staring spells or stereotypic behavior. The EEG also can show a characteristic pattern with Creutzfeldt-Jakob disease, in which one can see slow wave discharges in a burst-suppression pattern. Periodic lateralized epileptiform discharges, which are most prominent in the temporal lobe region, are supportive of herpes simplex encephalitis.

Functional neuroimaging is currently being recognized as potentially helpful in the evaluation of dementia.[10] It has been reported that cerebral positron emission tomography can reveal a characteristic pattern of biparietal hypometabolism (**Fig. 2**) in early stages of AD and might be particularly useful in identifying people at risk for developing AD.[11] Similar information may be provided by the less expensive single-photon emission computed tomographic brain scan. Diffusion-weighted and fluid-attenuated inversion recovery MRI can be more sensitive for certain ischemic and demyelinating processes.[12] Magnetic resonance angiography and spiral CT angiography are noninvasive means of assessing the cerebral vasculature in suspected cases of large vessel occlusive disease and vasculitic processes. Routine cerebral angiography remains more accurate and should be considered if there is the potential for the results to impact on therapeutic intervention. A summary of potential diagnostic testing in the evaluation of memory complaints, including dementia, is provided in **Box 2**.

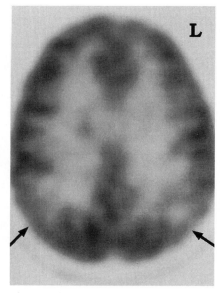

Fig. 2. 18-FDG cerebral positron emission tomographic scan reveals bi-parietal hypometabolism (*arrows*) in a patient with early AD.

WHAT IS MEANT BY THE TERM "MILD COGNITIVE IMPAIRMENT"?

MCI refers to subtle cognitive impairment, especially in elderly persons, that is readily recognized by the patient and companions but does not qualify, in degree, as actual dementia.[13] It is often viewed as a precursor to true dementia, and memory impairment is the most common manifestation. MCI becomes clinically relevant when cognitive impairment impacts on quality of life, such as making poor financial decisions or disrupting personal interactions. The same type of neuropsychiatric symptoms not uncommonly seen with dementia can be part of MCI.[14]

The detection of mild cognitive deficit that is evolving into clinically significant dementia is becoming increasingly important. It is estimated that approximately 10% of the population older than age 65 have dementia and that at least 25% of the population older than age 85 have dementia. Researchers recognize a continuum of progressive cognitive deficits that has serious implications for functional independence and quality of life for older individuals. For example, one of our greatest sources of independence in this country is the ability to drive a motor vehicle. Clinicians frequently must address this issue in patients who are showing cognitive decline, however. There is a slowing of reaction time, some loss in judgment ability, and forgetfulness as to where one is going and how to get there in this population. Screening tests for such deficit, even when the Mini-Mental State Examination score is normal, are becoming increasingly pertinent. For example, a recently introduced Memory Impairment Screen[15] is reported to be a reliable alternative test for the detection of early dementia.

HOW DOES ONE DEFINE AND DIAGNOSE ALZHEIMER'S DISEASE?

AD remains the most common form of dementia, and there is a virtual epidemic of this disorder as people live longer. There is an increasing prevalence with increasing age. The disease can present at a relatively young age, however, and has been referred to as "presenile dementia" of the Alzheimer's type when it afflicts individuals who are younger than age 60. The female to male ratio is roughly 2:1, which might reflect, at least in part, on the greater longevity of women. The diagnosis of AD is based on well-established criteria.[16] Characteristic features of AD are provided in **Box 3**. A definite diagnosis of AD requires the presence of clinical characteristics of AD, including dementia, and pathologic confirmation by either brain biopsy or autopsy. The pathologic hallmark of AD is an excessive number of amyloid plaques within certain areas of the brain, such as the hippocampus. The finding of neurofibrillary tangles also supports the diagnosis, but these silver-staining, cytoplasmic filaments can be found in several other neurologic conditions.

Probable AD requires the presence of dementia with memory loss, generally recent much more impaired than remote, along with at least one other realm of cognitive disturbance and in the absence of delirium.[17] Specific cognitive functions that can be involved, other than memory, include language disturbance, apraxia, agnosia, and impaired activities of daily living. Additional supportive features can include impaired judgment, behavioral disturbance (eg, personality change with increasing irritability, disinhibition, and other psychiatric manifestations), weight loss, family history of a similar disorder, especially if confirmed pathologically, and supportive diagnostic testing. In more advanced disease, once can see prominent cortical release signs, long tract signs, myoclonus, gait instability, and seizures.[17]

Possible AD represents a fairly typical clinical picture in terms of the features of dementia of the Alzheimer's type but with atypical features. These atypical features can include fairly sudden onset, more rapid progression than generally seen, a fluctuating

---

Box 3
Characteristic features of Alzheimer's disease

Clinical features

    Impairment of memory, especially short-term

    Change in personality

    Impairment of judgment

    Loss of language skills

    Loss of executive function

    Social withdrawal

    Apathy with loss of initiative

    Loss of orientation

    Loss of abstract ideation

    Tendency toward irritability and depression

Pathologic features

    Presence of amyloid (neuritic) plaques

    Presence of neurofibrillary tangles

    Presence of granulovacuolar degeneration

    Loss of cortical neurons

    Presence of congophilic angiopathy in up to 40% of patients

---

course, associated neurologic deficits not usually seen with AD, or coexistent disease that may impact on the neurologic picture.

WHAT DIAGNOSTIC STUDIES ARE INDICATED IN THE EVALUATION OF POSSIBLE ALZHEIMER'S DISEASE?

Diagnostic studies in AD are generally useful for excluding other possible causes. For example, it can be difficult to differentiate AD from vascular dementia on the basis of neuropsychological testing alone.[18] The MRI or CT brain scan typically shows some degree of cortical atrophy but no evidence of significant cerebrovascular disease, a tumor, subdural hematoma, or hydrocephalus. A noncontrast CT brain scan is usually the most cost-effective and practical neuroimaging study unless there are atypical features. The EEG, if performed, either is normal or shows nonspecific slowing. The CSF examination results, if clinically indicated, should be normal, although a nonspecific elevation of the protein may be seen. The evaluation for tau and neuronal thread protein[19,20] is more in the research realm, as is Apolipoprotein E (APOE) genotyping.[21] Certain individuals may have an atypical course, and the presence of supportive evidence can be reassuring. It also can be reassuring if the family is reluctant to accept the diagnosis without further testing. For example, the presence of an apolipoprotein E4 allele, especially if homozygous, can support a diagnosis of AD in a patient with otherwise unexplained dementia. The cerebral positron emission tomographic scan or single-photon emission CT scan as a less expensive but less precise alternative can support the clinical suspicion of AD if one observes the characteristic pattern of biparietal hypometabolism (**Fig. 2**) or hypoperfusion. Functional MRI, such as magnetization transfer imaging, may allow differentiation between normal aging from MCI and AD.[22] Fleisher and colleagues[23] reported on four cognitive measures that can help in the prediction of progression of amnestic MCI to AD, including the Symbol Digit Modalities Test, Delayed 10-Word List Recall, New York University Paragraph Recall Test (Delayed), and the ADAS-cog total score. There seemed to be some enhancement with Apolipoprotein E4 (APOE4) status, and the estimated predictive accuracy over 36 months was 80%.

WHAT TREATMENT IS CURRENTLY AVAILABLE FOR ALZHEIMER'S DISEASE?

The treatment for AD remains limited. Researchers have reported some potential neuroprotective benefit of vitamin E at a dose of 2000 IU per day,[24] but this was not observed in a more recent study of MCI,[25] in which donepezil was observed to lower the rate of progression to AD during the first 12 months of treatment. Donepezil is in a class of cholinesterase-inhibiting drugs that also includes rivastigmine, galantamine, and tacrine.[26] Tacrine is no longer commonly used because of its potential for liver toxicity. Donepezil remains attractive because of the once-a-day dosing and the ease of building up to the maintenance dose of 10 mg/d after an initial dose of 5 mg/d for 28 days. Rivastigmine requires much more cautious titration of the dose because of potential gastrointestinal toxicity. The initial dose is often 1.5 mg/d or no more than 1.5 mg twice a day with a potential maintenance dose of 6 to 12 mg/d in a twice-a-day regimen. Rivastigmine is also available as a once-a-day patch that is reported to significantly enhance its tolerability. Galantamine, the latest cholinesterase inhibitor to be released for use in the United States, is started with an initial dose of 4 mg with meals twice a day. After 4 weeks, the dose can be increased to 8 mg with meals twice a day. This dose tends to be the most effective and best tolerated maintenance dose, but one can go up to 12 mg twice a day after another 4 weeks. Some patients respond better to one cholinesterase inhibitor than another, which is the main reason for keeping an open mind about which is the best agent for a particular patient.

The cholinesterase inhibitors produce an increased level of acetylcholine in the brain, which seems to be their primary mechanism of action. There is a deficiency of this neurotransmitter in AD, and the improvement in acetylcholine levels can translate into a modest benefit on cognitive skills in patients with mild to moderate AD. Recent studies suggested that cholinesterase inhibitors have a neuroprotective effect in AD.[27] These agents can promote bradycardia, and bradycardia and asthma are relative contraindications to these agents. Donepezil also can promote a hypersensitivity reaction in patients who are sensitive to piperidine derivatives.

It is not uncommon to see depression as a clinically significant feature of AD. Selective serotonin reuptake inhibitors and other newer antidepressants, which do not have a significant risk of cardiac toxicity in older individuals, can be helpful for certain patients who have AD. Sleep disturbance can play a deleterious role in patients with AD. It is generally best to avoid sedative-hypnotics, if at all possible, because they can contribute to the confusion. On the other hand, innocuous agents such as melatonin at a dose of up to 10 mg at bedtime or diphenhydramine can achieve a desirable effect on insomnia. Antipsychotic medications are indicated when there is severe behavioral disturbance in an effort to protect the patient and caregivers. The newer atypical antipsychotic agents, such as olanzapine, quetiapine, and risperdone, are considered to be superior to the older typical antipsychotics, such as haloperidol, in light of a better side-effect profile. These newer agents are considerably more expensive, however.

Several agents may hold promise for AD, but the results of limited clinical trials, to date, have been contradictory. These agents include estrogen supplement in women, nonsteroidal anti-inflammatory agents, statin drugs, and the herb Gingko biloba. The agent memantine, an N-methyl-D-aspartate antagonist, has been reported to be of some benefit for moderate to severe AD.[28] This agent may be available for use in the United States in the near future. In an effort to protect against plaque deposition in AD, innovative ways to protect against accumulation of Aβ proteins in brain parenchyma have led to the development of a monoclonal antibody, bupanizeumab. This is given intravenously and is currently in phase III clinical trial.[29]

WHAT ARE SOME POSSIBLE PREVENTIVE MEASURES FOR ALZHEIMER'S DISEASE?

Preventive measures also may hold promise. It is possible that agents that interfere with the deposition of Aβ proteins and tau proteins have a neuroprotective effect. Anti-inflammatory agents may have potential in this regard; one study reported a reduced incidence of AD with chronic use of nonsteroidal anti-inflammatory drugs but not H2 receptor antagonists.[30] This result was not found to be beneficial in a study of celecoxib and naproxen, however.[31] High dietary intake of vitamins E and C reportedly may lower the risk of AD.[32] The potential benefit of estrogen therapy for protection against AD remains controversial.[33] It is being increasingly recognized that the so-called "enriched environment" can be helpful. This belief is based on the concept that mental activity with efforts to promote intellectual stimulation can potentially slow the progression of AD.

WHAT IS THE CONTRIBUTION OF CEREBROVASCULAR DISEASE TO DEMENTIA?

Vascular dementia along with AD accounts for approximately 80% of all cases of dementia.[34] Vascular dementia is also known as multi-infarct dementia, and it becomes increasingly important as a contributing mechanism to cognitive decline as people age.[35] The risk of vascular dementia correlates with risk factors for stroke.[36] Two important mechanisms that have been cited include (1) volume and location of tissue loss by a large artery distribution infarction and (2) subtle but progressive cognitive decline secondary to evolution of small vessel arterial occlusive disease, which is usually in a subcortical pattern.[37] It has been estimated that the prevalence of poststroke dementia is on the order of 13.6% to 32%,[38] and it is usually evident within the first 6 months of ictus. The incidence rates of dementia after stroke are on the order of 24% to 33.4% at 3 to 5 years, however, which probably reflects a contribution from changes related to AD in at least some of these patients.[39]

WHAT IS THE MECHANISM OF SMALL VESSEL OCCLUSIVE CEREBROVASCULAR DISEASE IN DEMENTIA?

Small vessel occlusive disease is most commonly associated with longstanding hypertension that results in lipohyalinosis of small penetrating arteries of the brain. Contributing factors include age, diabetes mellitus, hyperlipidemia, and genetic predisposition. The subcortical dementia associated with small vessel disease may correlate with subcortical white matter changes seen on MRI brain scan, which is termed "leukoaraiosis."[39] Diagnoses such as Binswanger's disease have been given to patients with neurologic deficits, including impaired cognition, who have such white matter changes (**Fig. 3**). Such changes can be seen with cerebral autosomal dominant arteriopathy with subcortical infarcts and leukoencephalopathy, which is a genetically transmitted disorder, familial amyloid angiopathy, and various coagulopathies.[40]

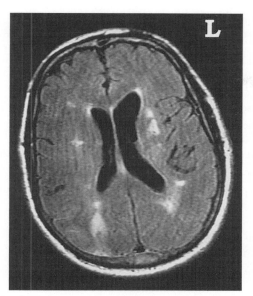

Fig. 3. Fluid-attenuation inversion recovery MRI brain scan demonstrates increased signal intensity changes in the subcortical region in a patient with recurrent small vessel stroke and secondary cognitive impairment.

WHAT IS THE IMPORTANCE OF RECOGNIZING PATIENTS AT SIGNIFICANT RISK FOR VASCULAR DEMENTIA? WHAT CAN BE DONE ABOUT IT?

Prestroke cognitive decline is a recognized precursor of dementia for AD and vascular dementia with or without a component of AD.[40] Clinical features that may help to distinguish primary vascular dementia from AD are listed in **Box 4**. In reference to the contribution of cerebral ischemia to dementia, a recent study reported the increased risk of dementia in elderly subjects who had clinically silent infarcts on brain MRI.[41] From a cerebrovascular standpoint, higher risk patients can be identified and measures taken to prevent ongoing cerebral ischemia.[42] These measures can include antiplatelet agents in patients with cerebral atherosclerosis, lipid-lowering agents, especially the statins, optimal blood pressure control, improved diabetic control, carotid endarterectomy and other vascular procedures in appropriate candidates, and anticoagulant therapy when there is either a higher risk cardiogenic source of embolus or a prothrombotic state. In terms of glucose control in type 2 diabetes mellitus, the Action to Control Cardiovascular Risk in Diabetes Study Group (ACCORD) found an actual deleterious effect of intensive blood sugar control in higher risk patients, which may cause us to rethink this aspect of vascular protection.[43] Cholinesterase inhibition also seems to be beneficial in treating vascular dementia.[44]

WHAT IS THE SIGNIFICANCE OF DEMENTIA WITH LEWY BODIES?

Lewy bodies are abnormal intracytoplasmic (eosinophilic) neuronal inclusions. They stain with monoclonal antibodies to ubiquitin, which is a polypeptide associated with breakdown of protein. Commonly associated with the neuropathology of Parkinson's disease, Lewy bodies are commonly found in brainstem nuclei, such as the locus ceruleus and substantia nigra, in this disorder. More recently recognized was the

---

Box 4
Features that may help to distinguish Alzheimer's disease from vascular dementia

Alzheimer's disease

Slowly progressive course over 5–10 years

Can be familial

Onset usually after age 60 in most subjects

Insidious onset of short-term memory loss accompanied by loss of other realms of cognition over time

Cortical atrophy and secondary ventricular dilatation appears on CT or MRI brain scan

Nonspecific subcortical low density changes shown on CT brain scan

Increased signal intensity changes shown on T2-weighted or fluid-attenuated inversion recovery MRI brain scan

Vascular dementia

Abrupt onset or step-wise decline

Close association with risk factors for stroke

Onset often in 70s or 80s

Deficit reflective of vascular territory involved

Improvement possible after an event

Vascular territory involvement or extensive subcortical leukoaraiosis seen on brain scan

---

presence of Lewy bodies in a specific form of cortical dementia termed DLB, which is believed to be the second most common type of neurodegenerative-mediated dementia,[45] with up to 15% to 25% of elderly demented subjects having this pathologic finding at autopsy.

WHAT CLINICAL FEATURES SUPPORT THE DIAGNOSIS OF DEMENTIA WITH LEWY BODIES?

The characteristic features of DLB are outlined in **Box 5**. The most common manifestations outside of dementia are features of parkinsonism, visual hallucinations, and delusions. Psychiatric features are common[46] and can help to distinguish DLB from AD. It can be difficult to distinguish Parkinson's disease associated with dementia from AD with coexistent Parkinson's disease from the so-called "pure" form of DLB, however.[47,48]

WHAT THERAPEUTIC INTERVENTIONS ARE CURRENTLY AVAILABLE TO POSSIBLY HELP PATIENTS WHO HAVE DEMENTIA WITH LEWY BODIES?

The major therapeutic initiative is to control the neurobehavioral disturbance with psychotropic medications. It is imperative to avoid medications that are commonly associated with extrapyramidal side effects because they may exacerbate the parkinsonian features. It is worthwhile to try carbidopa/levodopa in patients who have functional compromise related to their parkinsonian component; however, dopamine agonists should be avoided because of their potential for adverse behavioral effects. Cholinesterase inhibitors have not clearly demonstrated benefit for treatment of cognitive deficits of DLB, but they are often tried in an effort to offer patients and family

---

Box 5
Characteristic features of dementia with Lewy bodies

Clinical features

    Clinically significant cognitive impairment

    Fluctuating level of alertness

    Recurrent visual hallucinations that are often vivid and well formed

    Parkinsonism

    Loss of postural stability with secondary falls

    Transient loss of consciousness

    Sensitivity to neuroleptics

Pathologic features

    Presence of brainstem or cortical Lewy bodies

    Associated—but not essential—pathologic features

    Lewy-related neurites

    Plaques of all morphologic types

    Cell loss, especially the brainstem, with predilection for the substantia nigra, locus coeruleus, and nucleus basalis of Meynert

    Spongiform changes

---

something in terms of specific treatment for the dementia. Antidepressants may be helpful, because depression commonly accompanies the disease.

WHAT ARE THE IMPLICATIONS OF DEMENTIA IN ASSOCIATION WITH PARKINSON'S DISEASE?

The association of dementia with Parkinson's disease carries a significantly worse prognosis in terms of functional disability. This clinical picture is viewed as the greatest therapeutic challenge in this disorder.[48] In a recent 8-year prospective study of dementia in Parkinson's disease that was performed in Norway,[49] 78.2% of 224 patients with Parkinson's disease developed dementia over the 8-year prospective study period. Unfortunately, there is no specific treatment for the dementia component, although as with DLB, cholinesterase inhibitor therapy is often tried.

HOW DOES ONE SORT OUT THE POSSIBLE CLINICAL FEATURES TO SUPPORT THE DIAGNOSIS OF FRONTOTEMPORAL DEMENTIA?

This neurodegenerative disease tends to overlap with AD, but certain features can potentially distinguish one from the other. It is estimated that this disorder may account for up to 10% of all dementias compared with 50% to 60% for AD.[50] This dementia category can include Pick's disease, nonspecific frontal degeneration, and frontal degeneration with anterior spinal neuron loss[51] and primary progressive aphasia.[52] Pick's disease can affect any lobe of the brain in a selective fashion (ie, lobar atrophy); the pathologic hallmark is intracytoplasmic silver-staining inclusion bodies, which are termed "Pick's bodies." Characteristics of frontotemporal dementias include onset usually before age 65, predilection for men, positive family history in up to 50% of patients, and initial deficits that can consist of impaired language function, behavioral changes, cortical release signs, and extrapyramidal features. As with many of the neurodegenerative disorders associated with dementia, there is little to offer in terms of specific therapy. The cholinesterase inhibitors are not likely to have a beneficial effect because choline acetyltransferase levels are not reduced compared with controls.

HOW DOES ONE ARRIVE AT A DIAGNOSIS OF PROGRESSIVE SUPRANUCLEAR PALSY?

Progressive supranuclear palsy is characterized by subcortical dementia in association with extrapyramidal features, loss of ocular motility on a supranuclear basis, and axial dystonia. The age of onset is usually in the 60s, and men seem to be affected more commonly than women. There is progressive loss of functional ability, with a prominent tendency toward sudden falls related to postural instability. As with most neurodegenerative disorders, severe functional incapacity or death occurs within 5 to 10 years of onset of symptoms. No specific treatment is available, although some patients respond to medications prescribed for Parkinson's disease. Behavioral changes can be prominent and may respond to psychotropic medication.[53]

WHAT CHARACTERIZES NORMAL PRESSURE HYDROCEPHALUS?

Normal pressure hydrocephalus is characterized by the triad of dementia, urinary incontinence, and gait apraxia.[54] The diagnosis is supported by the finding of a communicating hydrocephalus on either CT or MRI brain scan (**Fig. 4**). There has been a great deal of debate about the response of normal pressure hydrocephalus to shunting.[55] From a clinical standpoint, patients with a known cause of their communicating hydrocephalus (eg, prior subarachnoid or intracerebral hemorrhage with secondary ventriculitis or central nervous system infection) and patients with fairly abrupt onset tend to be more responsive to shunting procedure than patients with an indolent course without an identifiable explanation.[56] Detection of the hydrocephalus when gait problems

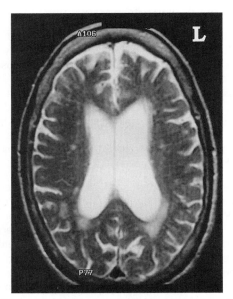

Fig. 4. T2-weighted MRI brain scan shows diffusely enlarged ventricles in a 72-year-old woman with MCI, progressive gait instability, and loss of bladder control. This patient improved with ventriculoperitoneal shunting for presumed normal pressure hydrocephalus.

are the primary manifestation—especially before the development of significant dementia—also tends to be associated with a more favorable response to shunting.[57]

WHAT HELPS TO SUPPORT THE DIAGNOSIS OF NORMAL PRESSURE HYDROCEPHALUS?

The patient illustrated in **Fig. 4** represents the not uncommon dilemma of significantly enlarged ventricles in an elderly patient who also has some degree of cortical atrophy. This patient presented with significant gait instability with secondary falls, MCI, and some subtle loss of bladder control. The results of her isotope cisternogram were equivocal. The neurosurgeon did not initially feel that a ventriculoperitoneal shunt was indicated in light of the cisternogram results. She then underwent a cine phase contrast MR study, which suggested hyperdynamic CSF flow in the region of the aqueduct of Sylvius, manifested as increased CSF flow void.[58] This finding led to a lumbar puncture with the removal of 30 cc of CSF, which was associated with a significant improvement in her ability to ambulate within several hours. The improvement persisted for several days according to the patient and her family. She has had a persistent benefit from the ventriculoperitoneal shunt over the past year with no further falls and some subtle improvement in her cognitive capacity.

WHAT ARE SOME OTHER CAUSES OF DEMENTIA?

Dementia is generally an integral part of the Huntington's disease triad of dementia, chorea, and autosomal dominant inheritance. The disease has been attributed to trinucleotide-repeat expansion with loss of striatal neurons that contain gamma-butyric acid. Genetic testing for susceptibility to the disease is available and can impact on genetic counseling of family members. Antidepressant therapy can be beneficial in patients who have Huntington's disease because of the high incidence of depression. Drugs that inhibit dopaminergic transmission can help to alleviate the chorea. Studies have demonstrated that N-methyl-D-aspartate receptor sensitivity may contribute to the pathogenesis of the disorder. In an effort to promote a neuroprotective effect against this hypersensitivity, a study of amantadine, a noncompetitive N-methyl-D-aspartate antagonist, was conducted, which demonstrated some benefit.[59]

JUST HOW TREATABLE (OR UNTREATABLE) ARE CERTAIN CAUSES OF DEMENTIA?

It is always exciting when one can detect a truly treatable cause of the dementia. Unfortunately, such instances are not that common. Evaluation for vitamin B_{12} deficiency and thyroid disease is part of the routine screen. Neurosyphilis, which is currently uncommon, is treatable, but the patient often has residual manifestations, especially if the disease has evolved to general paresis with dementia. Cryptococcal meningitis can be treated with antifungal therapy with generally good results if the disease is caught early. The same is true for herpes simplex encephalitis. HIV-related dementia tends to persist despite antiviral agents currently available. The abnormal accumulation of prion protein[60] is at least part of the pathogenesis of Creutzfeldt-Jakob disease. which is a devastating disorder with no treatment currently available. It is generally a sporadic disorder characterized by subacute progressive dementia and is often accompanied by myoclonus. It can be heralded by personality change and sleep disturbance. The clinical course can be acute. An EEG can be helpful in the diagnosis if it shows a fairly characteristic pattern of bursts of high-voltage slow and sharp wave activity superimposed on a low-voltage background. This periodic pattern has been termed "burst suppression." Pathologically, one sees spongiform changes; hence, the alternative designation of subacute spongiform encephalopathy.

There is increasing interest in voltage-gated channelopathies, which can be seen on an autoimmune basis and are part of a paraneoplastic process.[61] Limibic encephalitis and Morvan's syndrome have been reported to be associated with a dementing illness that can be responsive to immunosuppressive therapy.

REFERENCES

1. Ince PG, Irving D, McArthur F. Quantitative neuropathological study of Alzheimer-type pathology in the hippocampus: comparison of senile dementia of Alzheimer type, senile dementia of Lewy body type, Parkinson's disease, and non-demented elderly control patients. J Neurol Sci 1991;106:142–52.
2. Hardy J. Pathways to primary neurodegenerative disease. Mayo Clin Proc 1999; 74:835–7.
3. Folstein MF, Folstein SE, McHugh PR. Mini-mental state: a practical method for grading the cognitive state of patients for the clinician. J Psychiatr Res 1975; 12:189–98.
4. Peterson RC, Doody R, Kurz A, et al. Current concepts in mild cognitive impairment. Arch Neurol 2001;58:1985–92.
5. Morris JC. Clinical dementia rating: a reliable and valid diagnostic and staging measure for dementia of the Alzheimer's type. Int Psychogeriatr 1997;9(Suppl 1):173–6.
6. O'Connor DW, Blessed G, Cooper B, et al. Cross-national interrater reliability of dementia diagnosis in the elderly and factors associated with disagreement. Neurology 1996;47:1194–9.
7. Katzman R. Should a major imaging procedure (CT or MRI) be required in the workup of dementia? An affirmative view. J Fam Pract 1990;31:401–5.
8. de Groot JC, de Leeuw F-E, Oudkerk M, et al. Periventricular cerebral white matter lesions predict rate of cognitive decline. Ann Neurol 2002;52:335–41.
9. Ringman JM, Younkin SG, Pratico D, et al. Biochemical markers in persons with preclinical familial Alzheimer disease. Neurology 2008;71:85–92.
10. Bookheimer SY, Strojwas MH, Cohen MS, et al. Patterns of brain activation in people at risk for Alzheimer's disease. N Engl J Med 2000;343:450–6.
11. de Leon MJ, Convit A, Wolf OT, et al. Prediction of cognitive decline in normal elderly subjects with 2-[18-F]fluoro-2-D-glucose/positron-emission tomography (FDG/PET). Proc Natl Acad Sci U S A 2001;98:10966–71.
12. Bakshi R, Ariyaratana S, Benedict RH, et al. Fluid-attenuated inversion recovery magnetic resonance imaging detects cortical and juxtacortical multiple sclerosis lesions. Arch Neurol 2001;58:742–8.
13. Bennet DA, Wilson RS, Schneider JA, et al. Natural history of mild cognitive impairment in older persons. Neurology 2002;59:198–205.
14. Lyketsos CG, Lopez O, Jones B, et al. Prevalence of neuropsychiatric symptoms in dementia and mild cognitive impairment. Results from the cardiovascular health study. JAMA 2002;288:1475–83.
15. Buschke H, Kuslansky G, Katz M, et al. Screening for dementia in the memory impairment screen. Neurology 1999;52:231–8.
16. Small GW, Rabins PV, Barry PP, et al. Diagnosis and treatment of Alzheimer disease and related disorders: consensus statement of the American Association for Geriatric Psychiatry, the Alzheimer's Association, and the American Geriatrics Society. JAMA 1997;278:1363–71.
17. Cummings JL, Vinters HV, Cole GM, et al. Alzheimer's disease: etiologies, pathophysiology, cognitive reserve, and treatment opportunities. Neurology 1998;51(Suppl 1):S2–17.

18. Looi JCL, Sachdev PS. Differentiation of vascular dementia from AD on neuropsychological tests. Neurology 1999;53:670–8.
19. Kahle PJ, Jakowec M, Teipel SJ, et al. Combine assessment of tau and neuronal thread protein in Alzheimer's disease CSF. Neurology 2000;54:1498–504.
20. Growden JH. Biomarkers of Alzheimer disease. Arch Neurol 1999;56:281–3.
21. Mayeux R, Saunders AM, Shea S, et al. for the Alzheimer's Disease Centers Consortium on Apolipoprotein E and Alzheimer's Disease. Utility of the apolipoprotein E genotype in the diagnosis of Alzheimer's disease. N Engl J Med 1998;338:506–11.
22. van der Flier WM, van den Heuvel MJ, Weverling-Rijnsburger AWE, et al. Magnetization transfer imaging in normal aging, mild cognitive impairment, and Alzheimer's disease. Ann Neurol 2002;52:62–7.
23. Fleisher AS, Sowell BB, Taylor C, et al. for the Alzheimer's Disease Cooperative Study. Clinical predictors of progression to Alzheimer disease in amnestic mild cognitive impairment. Neurology 2007;68:1588–95.
24. Sano M, Ernesto C, Thomas RG, et al. A controlled trial of selegiline, alpha-tocopherol, or both as treatment for Alzheimer's disease. N Engl J Med 1997;336:1216–22.
25. Peterson RC, Thomas RG, Grundman M, et al. for the Alzheimer's Disease Cooperative Study Group. Vitamin E and donepezil for the treatment of mild cognitive impairment. N Engl J Med 2005;353:2379–88.
26. Mayeux R, Sano M. Treatment of Alzheimer's disease. N Engl J Med 1999;341:1670–9.
27. Mohs RC, Doody RS, Morris JC, et al. for the "312" Study Group. A 1-year, placebo-controlled preservation of function survival study of donepezil in AD patients. Neurology 2001;57:481–8.
28. Reisberg B, Doody R, Stoffler A, et al. for the Memantine Study Group. Memantine in moderate-to-severe Alzheimer's disease. N Engl J Med 2003;348:1333–41.
29. Nitsch RM, Hock C. Targeting beta-amyloid pathology in Alzheimer's disease with Abeta immunotherapy. Neurotherapeutics 2008;5:415–20.
30. Zandi PP, Anthony JC, Hayden KM, et al. for the Cache County Study Investigators. Reduced incidence of AD with NSAID but not H2 receptor antagonists: the Cache County Study. Neurology 2002;59:880–6.
31. ADAPT Research Group, Martin BK, Szekely C, et al. Cognitive function over time in the Alzheimer's Disease Anti-inflammatory Prevention Trial (ADAPT): results of a randomized, controlled trial of naproxen and celecoxib. Arch Neurol 2008;65:896–905.
32. Engelhart MJ, Geerlings MI, Ruitenberg A, et al. Dietary intake of antioxidants and risk of Alzheimer disease. JAMA 2002;287:3223–9.
33. Zandi PP, Carlson MC, Plassman BL, et al. for the Cache County Memory Study. Hormone replacement therapy and incidence of Alzheimer disease in older women: the Cache County Study. JAMA 2002;288:2123–9.
34. Meyer JS, Xu G, Thornby J, et al. Is mild cognitive impairment prodromal for vascular dementia like Alzheimer's disease? Stroke 2002;33:1981–5.
35. Desmond DW, Moroney JT, Sano M, et al. Incidence of dementia after ischemic stroke: results of a longitudinal study. Stroke 2002;33:2254–62.
36. Schmidt R, Schmidt H, Fazekas F. Vascular risk factors for dementia. J Neurol 2000;247:81–7.
37. Erkinjuntti T. Types of multi-infarct dementia. Acta Neurol Scand 1987;75:391–9.
38. Henson H, Durieu I, Guerouaou D, et al. Poststroke dementia: incidence and relationship to prestroke cognitive decline. Neurology 2001;57:1216–22.

39. O'Sullivan M, Lythgoe DJ, Pereira AC, et al. Patterns of cerebral blood flow reduction in patients with ischemic leukoaraiosis. Neurology 2002;59:321–6.

40. Tatemichi TK. How acute brain failure becomes chronic: a view of the mechanisms of dementia related to stroke. Neurology 1990;40:1652–9.

41. Vermeer SE, Prins ND, den Heijer T, et al. Silent brain infarcts and the risk of dementia and cognitive decline. N Engl J Med 2003;348:1215–22.

42. Straus SE, Majumdar SR, McAlister FA. New evidence for stroke prevention: scientific review. JAMA 2002;288:1388–95.

43. The Action to Control Cardiovascular Risk in Diabetes Study Group. Effects of glucose lowering in type 2 diabetes. N Engl J Med 2008;358:2545–59.

44. Malouf R, Birks J. Donepezil for vascular cognitive impairment. Cochrane Database Syst Rev 2004;1:CD004395.

45. McKeith IG, Galasko D, Kosaka K, et al. for the Consortium on Dementia with Lewy Bodies. Consensus guidelines for the clinical and pathological diagnosis of dementia with Lewy bodies (DLB): report of the consortium on DLB international workshop. Neurology 1996;47:1113–24.

46. Klatka LA, Louis ED, Schiffer RB. Psychiatric features in diffuse Lewy body disease: a clinicopathologic study using Alzheimer's disease and Parkinson's disease comparison groups. Neurology 1996;47:1148–52.

47. Minoshim S, Foster NL, Sima AAF, et al. Alzheimer's disease versus dementia with Lewy bodies: cerebral metabolic distinction with autopsy confirmation. Ann Neurol 2001;50:358–65.

48. Lang AE, Lozano AM. Parkinson's disease: second of two parts. N Engl J Med 1998;339:1130–43.

49. Aarsland D, Andersen K, Larsen JP, et al. Prevalence and characteristics of dementia in Parkinson disease. Arch Neurol 2003;60:387–92.

50. Mendez MF, Cherrier M, Perryman KM, et al. Frontotemporal dementia versus Alzheimer's disease: differential cognitive features. Neurology 1996;47:1189–94.

51. Armstrong RA, Lantos PL, Cairns NJ. Overlap between neurodegenerative disorders. Neuropathology 2005;25:111–24.

52. Mesulam M-M. Primary progressive aphasia. Ann Neurol 2001;49:425–32.

53. Litvan I, Mega MS, Cummings JL, et al. Neuropsychiatric aspects of progressive supranuclear palsy. Neurology 1996;47:1184–9.

54. Vanneste JAL. Diagnosis and management of normal-pressure hydrocephalus. J Neurol 2000;247:5–14.

55. Vanneste J, Augustijn P, Dirven C, et al. Shunting normal-pressure hydrocephalus: do the benefits outweigh the risks? A multicenter study and literature review. Neurology 1992;42:54–9.

56. Thomsen AM, Borgesen SE, Bruhn P, et al. Prognosis of dementia in normal-pressure hydrocephalus after a shunt operation. Ann Neurol 1986;20:304–10.

57. Graff-Radford NR, Godersky JC. Normal-pressure hydrocephalus: onset of gait abnormality before dementia predicts good surgical outcome. Arch Neurol 1986;43:940–2.

58. Dixon GR, Friedman JA, Luetmer PH, et al. Use of cerebrospinal fluid flow rates measured by phase-contrast MR to predict outcome of ventriculoperitoneal shunting for idiopathic normal-pressure hydrocephalus. Mayo Clin Proc 2002;77:509–14.

59. Metman LV, Morris MJ, Farmer C, et al. Huntington's disease: a randomized, controlled trial using NMDA-antagonist amatadine. Neurology 2002;59:694–9.

60. Prusiner SB. Shattuck lecture: neurodegenerative disease and prions. N Engl J Med 2001;344:1516–26.

61. Vernino S. Autoimmune and paraneoplastic channelopathies. Neurotherapeutics 2007;4:305–14.

Review of Sleep Disorders

Lori A. Panossian, MD[a], Alon Y. Avidan, MD, MPH[b],*

KEYWORDS

- Insomnia • Parasomnia • Sleep apnea • Circadian rhythm
- Classification • Management

EPIDEMIOLOGY AND CLASSIFICATION
How Prevalent are Sleep Disorders and What are their Potential Consequences?

Sleep disorders are extremely common in the general population and can lead to significant morbidity. Sleep disturbances lasting at least several nights per month have been reported by 30% of the population.[1] Sleep disorders may cause or exacerbate preexisting medical and psychiatric conditions and are associated with high rates of depression, anxiety, and impaired daytime functioning.[2] They may also lead to poor occupational performance, motor vehicle accidents, cardiovascular and endocrine disorders, or heightened pain perception.[1,3,4]

How are Sleep Disorders Categorized?

The International Classification of Sleep Disorders, second edition (ICSD-2) was published by the American Academy of Sleep Medicine with the goal of standardizing definitions and creating a systematic approach to diagnosis (**Box 1**).[5] The ICSD-2 subdivides sleep disorders into eight major categories: insomnia, sleep-related breathing disorders, hypersomnias of central origin, circadian rhythm disorders, parasomnias, and sleep-related movement disorders.[5]

CLINICAL APPROACH TO THE PATIENT WHO HAS SLEEP DISTURBANCES
When Should a Patient be Referred for a Sleep Study?

Although many sleep disorders can be diagnosed clinically, some require further evaluation in a sleep laboratory. In suspected sleep-related breathing disorders, a full-night polysomnogram (PSG) is recommended followed by continuous positive airway pressure (CPAP) titration. PSG is also indicated in severe forms of parasomnias, such as rapid eye movement (REM) sleep behavior disorder (RBD). Patients

[a] UCLA Department of Neurology, UCLA Medical Center, 710 Westwood Plaza 1241 RNRC, Los Angeles, CA 90095-1767, USA
[b] UCLA Department of Neurology, UCLA Neurology Clinic, UCLA Sleep Disorders Center, 710 Westwood Boulevard, Room 1-169 RNRC, Los Angeles, CA 90095-6975, USA
* Corresponding author.
E-mail address: avidan@mednet.ucla.edu (A.Y. Avidan).

Med Clin N Am 93 (2009) 407–425
doi:10.1016/j.mcna.2008.09.001
0025-7125/08/$ – see front matter. Published by Elsevier Inc.

Box 1
Major categories of sleep disorders

International Classification of Sleep Disorders, second edition, categories of sleep disorders

Insomnias

Sleep-related breathing disorders

Hypersomnias of central origin (not due to a circadian rhythm sleep disorder, sleep-related breathing disorder, or other causes of disturbed nocturnal sleep)

Circadian rhythm sleep disorders

Parasomnias

Sleep-related movement disorders

Isolated symptoms, apparently normal variants, and unresolved issues

Other sleep disorders

Data from American Academy of Sleep Medicine. The international classification of sleep disorders, 2nd edition: Diagnostic and coding manual. Sateia M, editor. Westchester (IL): American Academy of Sleep Medicine; 2005. p. xiii.

---

who have possible narcolepsy should be evaluated with a daytime nap study, the multiple sleep latency test (MSLT), for objective quantification of hypersomnia, and PSG performed the night before to document total sleep time and evaluate for other comorbid sleep disturbances. Alternatively, insomnia and restless legs syndrome (RLS) do not routinely require PSG because diagnosis is mainly clinically derived.[6] In some circumstances, a PSG may be helpful for some who present with insomnia that is refractory to traditional therapy and in whom other sleep disorders (ie, sleep apnea, motor disorders of sleep) are also suspected.

What are Some Important Components of a Sleep History?

The sleep history should include bedtime habits, timing of sleep onset and waking, daytime sleepiness, snoring, abnormal nocturnal leg kicking, nocturia, mood complaints, and cataplexy. Details about comorbid medical or psychiatric diagnoses, substance abuse, stressors, and family history should also be elicited.[7] Information-gathering tools include daily sleep logs that patients keep for several weeks; these provide a thorough overview of their home routines and may identify environmental or behavioral contributors.[7] The Epworth Sleepiness Scale (ESS) is a self-administered and validated questionnaire that quantifies the severity of daytime sleepiness; a score greater than 10 signifies significant sleepiness (**Table 1**).[7,8]

What are the Components of a Sleep Disorders–Specific Physical Examination?

An evaluation for obstructive sleep apnea (OSA) should include measurements of neck circumference and posterior airway size. Neck circumferences greater than 43 cm in men or 41 cm in women are associated with increased OSA risk. The Mallampati classification assigns a score to grade the severity of airway crowding, and a higher score together with nasal obstruction are risk factors for OSA (**Fig. 1**).[7] RLS may be associated with peripheral neuropathy, and in these patients a careful sensory examination of the lower extremities is indicated. Similarly, RBD may be a harbinger for alpha synucleinopathies, such as Parkinson disease, which may be become apparent on clinical evaluation and associated with nocturnal agitation and dream enactment.[7,9,10]

Table 1
Epworth Sleepiness Scale

How likely are you to fall asleep in the following situations, in contrast to feeling just tired? This refers to your usual way of life in recent times. Even if you have not done some of these things recently try to work out how they would have affected you. Use the following scale to choose the most appropriate number for each situation.

0 = no chance of dozing

1 = slight chance of dozing

2 = moderate chance of dozing

3 = high chance of dozing

Situation	Chance of Dozing
Sitting and reading	
Watching TV	
Sitting inactive in a public place (eg, a theater or meeting)	
As a passenger in a car for an hour without a break	
Lying down to rest in the afternoon when circumstances permit	
Sitting and talking to someone	
Sitting quietly after a lunch without alcohol	
In a car, while stopped for a few minutes in traffic	
Total Score =	

The ESS is an eight-point questionnaire that assesses the severity of daytime sleepiness in various situations.

Adapted from Johns MW. A new method for measuring daytime sleepiness: the Epworth Sleepiness Scale. Sleep 1991;14(6):540–5; with permission.

What Objective Tests can be Used to Measure Sleep?

The PSG is the mainstay of sleep laboratory testing. It consists of electrographic recordings of multiple physiologic parameters during drowsiness and sleep. Measurements may include electroencephalography (EEG) for sleep staging, electrooculogram (EOG) channels to measure eye movements, electromyography (EMG) measured superficially on the skin to assess for movement or atonia during REM sleep, airflow monitors, EKG leads, pulse oximetry, chest and abdominal excursion monitors to assess respiratory effort, auditory recordings of snoring, and video recording of movements in sleep.[7] An example of a PSG is provided in **Fig. 2** recorded during the night in a patient presenting with abnormal nocturnal behaviors and dream enactment. The clinical history was suggestive of RBD and was confirmed by the diagnostic PSG using expanded electromyographic leads documenting abnormal augmentation of the EMG tone during REM sleep and confirming RBD.

Patients who have suspected narcolepsy can undergo further evaluation with the MSLT on the morning after the PSG.[7,11,12] The MSLT uses electrographic recordings to assess a series of four to five naps taken the morning after the nocturnal PSG. Patients who have excessive sleepiness fall asleep faster and have abnormal sleep latencies of less than 8 minutes. Patients who have narcolepsy are more likely to have abnormal rapid onset of REM sleep intrusion during the daytime. The PSG criteria for narcolepsy include two or more sleep-onset REM periods during the MSLT and a mean sleep latency of less than 8 minutes.[11,12]

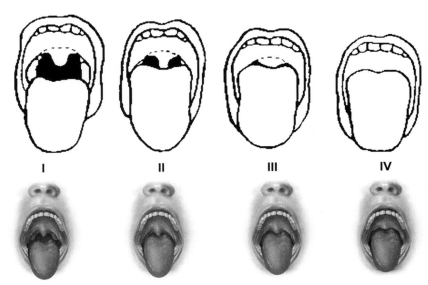

Fig. 1. Mallampati classification. The classification is determined by assessing the anatomy of the oral cavity and describes tongue size relative to oropharyngeal size. The test is conducted with the patient seated, the head held in a neutral position and the mouth wide open and relaxed. The subsequent classification is assigned based on the pharyngeal structures that are visible. Scoring is as follows: Class I: Full visibility of tonsils, uvula, and soft palate. Class II: Visibility of hard and soft palate, upper portion of tonsils, and uvula. Class III: Soft and hard palate and base of the uvula are visible. Class IV: Only hard palate visible. (*Data from* Mallampati SR, Gatt SP, Gugino LD, et al. A clinical sign to predict difficult tracheal intubation: a prospective study. Can Anaesth Soc J 1985;32:429–34.)

INSOMNIA
Diagnosis and Epidemiology

When does insomnia meet criteria for a sleep disorder?

Patients may complain of difficulty falling asleep (sleep-onset insomnia) or difficulty remaining asleep (sleep-maintenance insomnia) with frequent nocturnal awakenings or early morning awakenings associated with nonrestorative sleep.[7,9,10,13–15] According to a recent National Institutes of Health consensus, insomnia is defined as a disorder when occurring despite the patient's having adequate opportunity and circumstances to sleep, and must be associated with impairment of daytime functioning or mood symptoms.[5,14,15] Daytime impairment may manifest as inattention, impaired memory and concentration, poor performance in vocational or social settings, increased errors at work or while driving, tension headaches, gastrointestinal symptoms, or fatigue. Mood symptoms include decreased energy and motivation, irritability, restlessness, and anxiety.[14]

How common is insomnia?

Approximately 9% to 15% of the general United States population has reported symptoms of chronic insomnia with associated daytime consequences.[16] Similarly, the European population has an insomnia prevalence of 16.8%, with 64.5% of those also suffering from comorbid sleep or psychiatric disorders.[17] The risk for insomnia increases in women.[16] More than one third of the population older than 65 years of

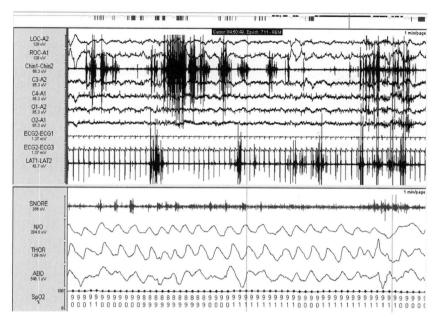

Fig. 2. Example of a 60-second epoch from a diagnostic PSG. Channels are as follows: EOG (left, LOC-A2; right, ROC-A1), chin EMG, EEG (left central, right central, left occipital, right occipital), two EKG channels, limb EMG (LAT), snore channel, nasal-oral airflow, respiratory effort (thoracic, abdominal) and oxygen saturation (SpO2). The patient was a 77-year-old man who was referred to the sleep disorders clinic for evaluation of recurrent violent nighttime awakenings. (*Data from* Avidan AY, Zee P, editors. Handbook of sleep medicine. Philadelphia: Lippincott Williams & Wilkins; 2006. p. 187–201.)

age has symptoms of insomnia. This finding seems to be related to physical inactivity, dissatisfaction with social life, and comorbid medical problems in older adults. When controlling for these factors, age alone is not a significant contributor.[18]

How serious a problem is insomnia?
Chronic insomnia can have a deleterious effect on patients' comorbid medical and psychiatric illnesses. For example, insomnia can heighten the perception of pain[19,20] and is associated with the development of endocrine disturbances.[4,21] Insomnia may also have an association with increased risk for hypertension or cardiovascular disease.[22] Insufficient sleep can lead to public health hazards, such as increased risk for motor vehicle accidents, occupational errors, and poor multitasking.[3,23]

Classification

What are some of the main causes of primary insomnia?
Insomnia can be primary or comorbid along with another medical or psychiatric condition. Primary insomnia can be divided into three categories: idiopathic insomnia, psychophysiologic insomnia, and paradoxical insomnia (also known as sleep state misperception).[15,24] Patients who have idiopathic insomnia suffer from pervasive sleep disturbance throughout their lives, beginning in early childhood, and are at risk for developing major depression and overuse of pharmacologic sleep aids or

alcohol because of distress or daytime impairment from the sleep deficit. The estimated prevalence is 0.7% to 1.0% among adolescents and young adults.[5]

Psychophysiologic insomnia develops as a result of maladaptive thought patterns and hyperarousal, including somatic tension, inability to relax at bedtime, racing thoughts, hypervigilance, or anxiety.[5] There is also believed to be an underlying physical state of heightened arousal, with increased catecholamine levels, elevated basal metabolic rate and body temperature, heart rate changes, and increased central nervous system metabolism.[25,26] Symptoms typically last one month or longer.[5]

Paradoxical insomnia is characterized by the complaint of severe insomnia and daytime sleepiness, but without any objective evidence of sleep disturbance. These patients typically have normal sleep patterns on PSG. Paradoxical insomnia is a rare condition with poorly understood pathophysiology.[5]

What comorbid disorders are associated with insomnia?

Insomnia can be comorbid with a psychiatric illness, such as depression, anxiety, or somatoform disorder; it can also occur in conjunction with medication use or substance abuse, including stimulants, corticosteroids, caffeine, alcohol, and many prescription drugs. Many medical conditions are associated with insomnia, including chronic pain, RLS, pulmonary disorders (such as chronic obstructive pulmonary disease and asthma), menopause, nocturia, and neurologic disorders.[5,13]

What is adjustment insomnia (acute insomnia)?

Adjustment insomnia is a short-lived sleep disturbance precipitated by anxiety from an identifiable stressor. The sleep disturbance is expected to resolve once the stressor has dissipated or the patient has adjusted. If symptoms last for more than a few months, acute insomnia may become chronic, particularly if maladaptive sleep behaviors develop, such as suboptimal stress management or poor sleep hygiene.[5,27]

What is sleep hygiene and how is it related to insomnia?

Sleep hygiene consists of optimizing routines and behaviors associated with sleep. Some patients develop habits that prevent the onset of relaxation and sleepiness at the appropriate time, resulting in insomnia due to inadequate sleep hygiene. Some problematic behaviors include maintaining erratic sleep and wake times, lying in bed awake for prolonged periods of time, addressing stressful or worrisome issues near bedtime, exposure to bright lights, such as TV or computer screens, around bedtime, late night eating or caffeine, nicotine or alcohol use, or prolonged daytime naps.[28]

Treatment

What are some nonpharmacologic treatment options for insomnia?

Cognitive-behavioral therapy (CBT) has demonstrated efficacy in treating chronic insomnia.[29–31] It is recommended as the first-line therapy for primary insomnia[30,32] and is also beneficial for many types of comorbid insomnia, including patient who have chronic pain, cancer, and depression. Although pharmacologic therapy may work more quickly, CBT provides better long-term sleep benefits as compared with pharmacologic therapy alone; CBT alone is also more effective than CBT combined with medication.[33] A potential limitation of CBT is that resources or trained providers may not be available to administer the recommended biweekly CBT sessions.[13,34]

What are the current pharmacologic treatment recommendations for insomnia in adults?

Hypnotic medications are shown in **Table 2** classified according to their mechanism of action and indication. Options include benzodiazepines, such as triazolam, estazolam,

	Duration	Recommended		
Table 2				
Food and Drug Administration–approved pharmacologic treatments of insomnia				
Generic Name	**of Action**	**Dose in Adults**	**Class**	**Indication**
Triazolam	Short	0.125–0.25 mg	Benzodiazepine	Sleep-onset insomnia
Temazepam	Intermediate	7.5–30 mg	Benzodiazepine	Sleep-maintenance insomnia
Estazolam	Intermediate	0.5–2 mg	Benzodiazepine	Sleep-maintenance insomnia
Zaleplon	Ultrashort	5–20 mg	Nonbenzodiazepine hypnotic	Sleep-onset and sleep-maintenance insomnia
Zolpidem	Short	5–10 mg	Nonbenzodiazepine hypnotic	Sleep-onset insomnia
Eszopiclone	Intermediate	1–3 mg	Nonbenzodiazepine hypnotic	Sleep-maintenance insomnia
Zolpidem extended-release	Long	6.25–12.5 mg	Nonbenzodiazepine hypnotic	Sleep-onset and sleep-maintenance insomnia
Ramelteon	Short	8 mg	Melatonin receptor agonist	Sleep-onset insomnia

Data from Silber MH. Chronic insomnia. N Engl J Med 2005;353:803–10.

and temazepam, and nonbenzodiazepine hypnotics, including zolpidem, zolpidem tartrate, zaleplon, and eszipiclone.[14,35] Zolpidem and zaleplon have a short duration of action and are useful in sleep-onset insomnia, whereas longer-acting agents, such as eszopiclone, zolpidem extended-release, or temazepam, are effective for sleep-maintenance insomnia.[13] The nonbenzodiazepine hypnotics have less potential for abuse, tolerance, or withdrawal,[35] but may be associated with increased propensity for rebound insomnia and amnestic reactions in higher doses.[14]

Melatonin receptor agonists, such as ramelteon, are a newer class of Food and Drug Administration (FDA)–approved agents for sleep-onset insomnia.[35,36] Rozerem is currently the only FDA-approved medication for the treatment of insomnia that is not schedule IV and has no abuse potential. Over-the-counter melatonin is also available but is not FDA regulated, and randomized controlled trials have shown no clear benefit unless insomnia is related to a circadian rhythm disorder.[37,38] Other over-the-counter sleep aids include antihistamines, such as diphenhydramine, which may reduce sleep latency but can cause side effects, such as daytime sedation and cognitive impairment.[14] Antihistamines are not approved for use as sleep aids and their long-term efficacy has not been proven.

Although not FDA approved for the indication, low-dose antidepressants are commonly prescribed for insomnia. In the short term, trazodone has been shown to improve sleep in primary insomnia and in patients who have comorbid depression, but its safety and efficacy have not been studied for long-term use.[14,35] Tricyclic antidepressants, such as amitriptyline and doxepin, can improve sleep efficiency but have the potential for adverse anticholinergic effects, daytime sedation, and suppression of REM sleep, resulting in REM sleep rebound with disturbing dreams; thus they are not indicated for short-term use in insomnia.

OBSTRUCTIVE SLEEP APNEA
Diagnosis and Epidemiology

How is obstructive sleep apnea diagnosed?
OSA is a form of sleep-disordered breathing, consisting of episodic upper airway obstruction with reduced blood oxygenation and brief arousals from sleep. An episode of complete airway obstruction despite ongoing respiratory effort is called an apnea, and partial obstruction with persistent effort is termed hypopnea. The events typically last 10 to 30 seconds, but can last for 1 minute or longer (**Fig. 3**). Blood oxygenation returns to baseline immediately after the event.[5] The severity of OSA is based in part on the apnea-hypopnea index (AHI), the ratio of apneas or hypopneas per hour of sleep measured during PSG.[6,39–41] OSA is generally diagnosed when the sleep study demonstrates an AHI of 5 or greater and there are associated symptoms of excessive daytime sleepiness (ie, as measured by the ESS), nonrefreshing sleep, or witnessed pauses in breathing during sleep.[5,42] The physical examination should include measurements of the body mass index, neck circumference, and Mallampati classification of tongue size to oropharyngeal size, all of which can confer a higher risk for OSA if elevated.[43]

How prevalent is obstructive sleep apnea in the population?
OSA is common and can affect children and adults. Prevalence is estimated at 2% of women and 4% of men aged 30 to 60 years.[44] Risk factors include increased age,

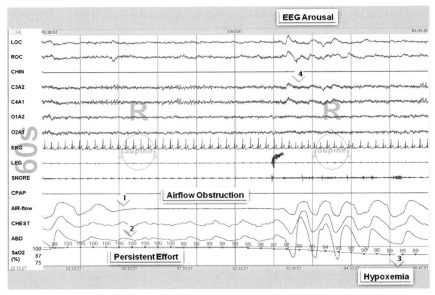

Fig. 3. A 60-second epoch (recorded during stage Rapid Eye Movement (REM) sleep) from a diagnostic polysomnogram of a older man with a history of pauses in his breathing, snoring and excessive daytime somnolence previously admitted to the stroke unit with left hemiparesis and right middle cerebral artery infarction. Obstructive sleep apnea characterized by nasal oral (N/O) breathing cessation (1) in the presence of persistent respiratory effort (2) and hypoxemia (3). An EEG arousal (4) signifies a change to a higher EEG frequency. Channels are as follows: Electrooculogram (left: LOC-A2, right: ROC-A1), chin EMG, EEG (left central, right central, left occipital, right occipital), electrocardiogram, limb EMG, snoring, nasal-oral airflow, respiratory effort (thoracic, abdominal), nasal pressure, and oxygen desaturation. The CPAP cahnnel is inactive.

male gender, obesity, and high cholesterol.[45] Snoring is also associated with an increased OSA risk, possibly related to snoring-induced pharyngeal edema and inflammation.[46] Sleep-disordered breathing is increased among older adults (mean age of 76 years old), with an estimated prevalence of 24% to 26%.[47] Among older adults, OSA with daytime sleepiness can cause significant cognitive difficulties, particularly in tests of attention.[48] Treatment with CPAP is effective in treating the cognitive and cardiovascular sequelae of OSA in the older population.[49]

Management

What are some behavioral interventions for obstructive sleep apnea?
Strategies aimed at minimizing airway obstruction may be beneficial in treating milder OSA, including sleeping with the head and trunk slightly elevated, avoiding the supine position at night, refraining from use of alcohol or sedatives, and weight loss.[42] Patients who have craniofacial structural problems may be candidates for oral appliances, such as mandibular advancement devices.[42]

What is the success rate of continuous positive air pressure?
Nightly use of nasal CPAP or bi-level positive airway pressure (BiPAP) is the mainstay of treatment of OSA. When used regularly, it is effective in reducing apneas and hypopneas and improving oxygenation and sleep, with associated improvements in daytime sleepiness and cognitive performance.[50] The cardiovascular complications of OSA may also diminish.[50] There is evidence that OSA is associated with systemic inflammation, with endothelial dysfunction and activated leukocytes, and that inflammation is reduced with use of CPAP.[51] Unfortunately, there are many barriers to the regular use of CPAP for at least 4 hours nightly, with a nonadherence rate of as high as 29% to 83%.[52] The reasons for this are multifactorial and may include physical side effects, such as nasal stuffiness, and psychologic obstacles.[52] The physical side effects can be ameliorated somewhat by use of heated humidification, nasal sprays, and correctly fitting the mask.[42]

What interventions are available for patients who have failed continuous positive air pressure?
In patients who have severe disease or cannot tolerate CPAP, surgical treatment of OSA may be an option. Strategies may include uvulopalatopharyngoplasty to reduce oropharyngeal soft tissue bulk, or tracheostomy in severe refractory cases associated with significant cardiovascular morbidity.[42,53–55] Although pharmacologic treatments have not been successful as OSA monotherapy, modafinil, a nonsympathomimetic wake-promoting agent, may be used during the day in conjunction with nightly CPAP to reduce symptoms of excessive daytime sleepiness (provided that patients are compliant with CPAP, are not sleep deprived, and have documented evidence of sleepiness based on such measures as the ESS). Patients who are adequately compliant with CPAP use and continue to have excessive daytime somnolence may have other underlying sleep disorder (ie, narcolepsy) or need adjustments to their CPAP settings and should be evaluated with a repeat PSG.

NARCOLEPSY
Diagnosis and Epidemiology

How is narcolepsy diagnosed?
Diagnostic criteria include symptoms of severe excessive daytime sleepiness occurring almost daily for at least 3 months that interfere with functioning, REM intrusion phenomena (ie, cataplexy, hypnagogic hallucinations, sleep paralysis), and

electrographic evidence of an abnormal MSLT, with a sleep latency of 8 minutes or less and at least two sleep-onset REM periods following a PSG.[5,56–58] Narcolepsy may occur with or without cataplexy. Cataplexy is defined as sudden self-limited episodes of loss of waking muscle tone, usually triggered by laughter or other strong emotions. The presence of cataplexy may be sufficient by itself to establish the diagnosis of narcolepsy and cataplexy, although sleep studies are often advised to quantitatively assess the level of sleepiness.[59] Patients may also have episodes of sleep paralysis, hypnagogic hallucinations, and fragmented sleep with frequent nocturnal arousals. Sleep paralysis occurs as patients transition from sleep to waking, and consists of episodes up to several minutes in duration of inability to move and occasionally feeling unable to breathe despite being awake. Hypnagogic hallucinations are vivid and often frightening perceptual hallucinatory experiences, which occur during the transition between waking and sleep. Sleep paralysis and hypnagogic hallucinations may rarely occur in normal individuals also. Fragmented nocturnal sleep and automatic behaviors may also occur when patients go about their daily activities in a mechanical fashion with no memory or conscious awareness of their actions.[5,58]

What is the population prevalence of narcolepsy?

Narcolepsy with cataplexy is rare, affecting approximately 0.02% to 0.18% of the general population in the United States and Europe.[5] The prevalence ranges from as low as 0.002% in Israel to 0.15% in Japan.[5,58] The disease may present at any age but is typically diagnosed before age 25. Men are slightly more likely to be affected than women.[5]

Pathophysiology

What causes narcolepsy?

Narcolepsy arises because of interplay between genetic and environmental factors. It is hypothesized that an autoimmune process results in loss of hypothalamic neurons responsible for producing the neuropeptide hypocretin. Hypocretin normally modulates an increase in muscle tone during wakefulness. Ninety percent of patients who have narcolepsy with cataplexy and 10% of those without cataplexy demonstrate reduced levels of cerebrospinal fluid hypocretin-1. Most of these patients are also positive for the major histocompatibility class II allele HLA DQ1B*0602.[5,56] Specific autoantibody markers for narcolepsy have not yet been found, however.[60]

Narcolepsy Management

What are the treatment options for narcolepsy?

Pharmacologic therapies for excessive daytime sleepiness include stimulants and other wakefulness-promoting agents (**Table 3**). Although traditionally stimulants, such as methylphenidate and dextroamphetamine, were used, first-line therapy now consists of the nonstimulant medication modafinil. Modafinil has a low potential for abuse, is well tolerated, and was effective in promoting wakefulness in clinical trials.[61,62] Sodium oxybate, the sodium salt of g-hydroxybutyrate, is also useful in the treatment of narcolepsy. It is a short-acting sedative hypnotic that is administered at night to help consolidate REM sleep and increase slow-wave sleep. It significantly reduces daytime sleepiness and also improves cataplexy and associated daytime symptoms of narcolepsy.[56] Other treatment options include selegiline, a monoamine oxidase B inhibitor that can improve alertness and also treats cataplexy symptoms; however, its use in high doses is limited by the need to maintain a low-tyramine diet.[56] Although sodium oxybate is the only approved medication for cataplexy in the United States, tricyclic antidepressants (TCAs), such as clomipramine, have

Table 3
Treatment options for narcolepsy and cataplexy

Generic Name	Usual Dose in Adults	Class	Indication
Dextroamphetamine	5–50 mg/d	Stimulant	EDS
Methylphenidate	10–40 mg/d	Stimulant	EDS
Modafinil	100–400 mg/d	Non-sympathomimetic wake-promoting agent	EDS
Selegiline	5–10 mg/d	Monoamine oxidase B inhibitor	EDS
Sodium oxybate	4.5–9.0 g/d	Gamma-hydroxybutyrate	Cataplexy and EDS
Clomipramine	10–200 mg/d	Heterocyclic antidepressant	Cataplexy
Fluoxetine	10–80 mg/d	Serotonin reuptake inhibitor	Cataplexy
Venlafaxine	75–375 mg/d	Norepinephrine reuptake inhibitor	Cataplexy

Abbreviation: EDS, excessive daytime sleepiness.

Data from Wise MS, Arand DL, Auger RR, et al. Treatment of narcolepsy and other hypersomnias of central origin. Sleep 2007;30(12):1712–27.

been used to treat cataplexy successfully for decades. TCAs may cause more severe rebound cataplexy if abruptly discontinued, however.[56,57] More recently serotonin and norepinephrine reuptake inhibitors have also been used for cataplexy, including fluoxetine and venlafaxine.[57,63] Nonpharmacologic therapy using regular bedtimes and strategically timed power naps may also improve alertness.[58,64]

CIRCADIAN RHYTHM SLEEP DISORDERS
Diagnosis and Epidemiology

What are some common types of circadian rhythm disorders?
Circadian rhythm refers to the body's internal timing system, which synchronizes its rhythmic cycles to external stimuli to follow a 24-hour day. Circadian rhythms affect sleep and wake cycles, cortisol release, body temperature, melatonin levels, and other physiologic variables. Patients who have circadian rhythm disorders have chronic or recurring sleep disturbances (insomnia or hypersomnia) because of misalignment between their endogenous circadian timing and external influences.[5,65–67]

The most common disorder is delayed sleep phase–type, characterized by sleep and wake times that are later than desired, often resulting in daytime sleepiness when conventional waking times are enforced. Individuals typically prefer to sleep from 2 to 6 AM until 10 AM to 1 PM. Although the general population prevalence is estimated at 0.17%, it occurs in approximately 7% of adolescents and is more common in men.[66] Advanced sleep phase–type is less common, and is characterized by earlier than desired sleep and awakening. In situations in which a conventional later bedtime is required, patients continue to awaken early and develop chronic sleep deprivation.[66] Jet lag is another form of circadian rhythm disturbance, attributable to rapid change in time zones altering the timing of exogenous light stimuli. This alteration results in transient symptoms of difficulty falling asleep at the appropriate time and daytime sleepiness. Jet lag is often more severe among older adults whose circadian rhythms take longer to adjust.[66]

How can a diagnosis be made?
Diagnosis of circadian rhythm disorders is based primarily on history and a sleep diary. Actigraphy, based on a wrist-mounted motion detector worn as an outpatient for at least 7 days, can help quantify time spent asleep. PSG is indicated only if another underlying sleep disorder is suspected.[66,68]

How are circadian rhythm disorders treated?
Delayed or advanced sleep phase–type disorders can be difficult to treat, and trials of various treatment modalities may be necessary. Management strategies include bright light therapy, chronotherapy, or melatonin. Light therapy, defined as exposure to bright light around 2500 lux for 2 to 3 hours in the mornings, has some benefit in retraining circadian rhythm to conform to conventional sleep times, especially when combined with avoiding light in the evening.[66,68] Chronotherapy in delayed sleep phase disorders consists of the patient delaying sleep time by 3 hours every 2 days until he or she adjusts to a conventional earlier bedtime and wake time. Although effective in some patients, compliance and maintenance after treatment completion are difficult, and it has not been demonstrated to consistently work in advanced sleep phase disorders.[66,68] Melatonin given in the afternoon or evening can also benefit patients who have delayed sleep phase.[66,68]

How is jet lag disorder best managed?
Options to minimize jet lag include behavioral strategies, such as good sleep hygiene, shifting sleep and wake times gradually before travel to conform to the destination's time zone, and avoiding bright light exposure before bedtime.[66,68] Melatonin administered before bedtime in the new time zone has also been shown to be effective, particularly immediate-release doses of 0.5 to 5 mg.[68] Nonbenzodiazepine hypnotics, such as zolpidem 10 mg at bedtime, may be used for short-term treatment of insomnia due to jet lag; however, hypnotics may have a higher risk for adverse effects. Caffeine improves daytime sleepiness from jet lag but may interfere with sleep architecture.[68]

PARASOMNIAS
Diagnosis and Epidemiology

What are parasomnias?
Parasomnias consist of undesirable experiences or behaviors that occur during transitions between sleep and waking. They represent central nervous system activation and intrusion of wakefulness into REM or non-REM sleep, producing nonvolitional motor, emotional, or autonomic activity. Non-REM sleep parasomnias include confusional arousals and sleep terrors, whereas REM sleep–associated parasomnias include nightmares and RBD.[69–76]

What are sleep terrors, and how do they differ from nightmares?
Sleep terrors occur in approximately 3% of children aged 4 to 12 years and may also commonly present around age 20 to 30 years. They are dramatic sudden arousals from non-REM sleep with associated screaming, fear, and increased autonomic activity. Patients may be disoriented, unresponsive to the environment, and typically do not remember the event afterward. By contrast, nightmares typically occur during REM sleep toward the end of the night and are not associated with autonomic activity or amnesia.[69,71,72,75,77] Treatment of night terrors is usually not indicated and the condition resolves over time, but severe cases may be treated with low-dose benzodiazepines at bedtime.[69]

How is rapid eye movement sleep behavior disorder diagnosed?
RBD consists of abnormal loss of muscle tone inhibition during REM sleep, permitting vigorous movements while dreaming. Sleep behaviors can include screaming, punching, and kicking for up to several minutes, sometimes resulting in injury to the patient or bed partner.[78] RBD may be associated with unusually vivid and often violent dreams. RBD is more common in men older than 50 years of age, and approximately 40% of cases are associated with an underlying neurodegenerative condition, such as Parkinson disease or multiple system atrophy.[78] There is also a high incidence of RBD among narcoleptics.[69] RBD may be mistaken for nocturnal seizures, but unlike epilepsy, RBD movements are not stereotyped.[70] Diagnosis is made based on clinical history and PSG, which demonstrates anomalous increases in muscle tone on EMG during REM sleep.[70]

Management

What are some management strategies for rapid eye movement sleep behavior disorder?
The goal of treatment is to minimize potentially injurious behaviors. Nonpharmacologic approaches include avoiding substances that may exacerbate RBD, such as antidepressants (selective serotonin reuptake inhibitors, monoamine oxidase inhibitors), caffeine, or alcohol, which can trigger RBD episodes,[79–81] and removing dangerous objects from the sleep environment to improve safety. Medications include clonazepam 0.25 to 1 mg at bedtime, tricyclic antidepressants, dopamine agonists or levodopa (particularly in patients who have underlying Parkinson disease), anticonvulsants such as carbamazepine, and melatonin at high doses.[69,70,78,82–85]

RESTLESS LEGS SYNDROME AND PERIODIC LIMB MOVEMENT DISORDER
Diagnosis and Epidemiology

How is restless legs syndrome diagnosed?
RLS is described clinically as an overwhelming urge to move the legs or sometimes the arms, particularly worse in the evening.[86,87] Succinctly, RLS can be defined as a "movement-responsive quiescegenic nocturnal focal akathisia usually with dysesthesias."[88] Symptoms are usually worse later in the day and may disrupt sleep initiation. RLS is diagnosed clinically based on the following four criteria: an urge to move the legs usually accompanied by an uncomfortable sensation; rest or inactivity exacerbating the urge to move the legs; physical activity temporarily relieving the urge to move the legs; and evening or nighttime predominance of the symptoms.[5,89]

What are some predisposing factors for restless legs syndrome?
Although the population prevalence of RLS in North America ranges from 5% to 10%, only 2.5% of patients have symptoms severe enough to necessitate clinical attention.[5,90] There is a higher prevalence of RLS among older adults and women. RLS may be primary or idiopathic, and 50% of these patients also have a positive family history.[5] RLS may also be secondary to other medical conditions, including pregnancy, end-stage renal disease, iron or folate deficiency, peripheral neuropathy, radiculopathy, rheumatoid arthritis, or fibromyalgia.[86,90] Medications, such as antihistamines, dopamine receptor antagonists, and antidepressants (with the exception of bupropion) may exacerbate RLS.[5]

What are periodic limb movements in sleep?
Periodic limb movements in sleep occur in 80% to 90% of patients who have RLS and may also commonly occur in older adults who do not have RLS.[5,86] Symptoms include

Table 4
Treatment of restless legs syndrome

Drug	Dose	Risks
Iron		
Ferrous sulfate	325 mg bid to tid Recommended for serum ferritin <50 μg	GI side effects: constipation. Role in treatment under current investigation
Dopamine agonists		
Pramipexole	0.125–0.5 mg, 2–3 h before bedtime. Start low and increase slowly[a]	Severe sleepiness, nausea, vomiting, sleep attacks, rare compulsive gambling, hallucinations, orthostatic hypotension
Ropinirole	0.25–2 mg 1–2 h before bedtime[a]	Severe sleepiness, nausea, vomiting, sleep attacks, rare compulsive gambling, hallucinations, orthostatic hypotension
Dopaminergic agents		
Levodopa/carbidopa	25/200 mg: 1/2 tab to 3 tabs 30 min before bedtime.	Nausea, sleepiness, augmentation of daytime symptoms, insomnia, sleepiness, gastrointestinal disturbances
Anticonvulsants		
Gabapentin	300–2700 mg/d divided tid	Daytime sleepiness, nausea
Benzodiazepines		
Clonazepam	0.125–0.5 mg half hour before bedtime	Nausea, sedation, dizziness
Clonidine		
Catapres	0.1 mg bidMay be helpful in patients who have hypertension	Dry mouth, drowsiness, constipation, sedation, weakness, depression (1%), hypotension
Opioids		
Propoxyphene and acetaminophen	300 mg/d	Nausea, vomiting, restlessness, constipation. Addiction, tolerance may be possible
Propoxyphene	65–135 mg at bedtime	
Codeine	30 mg	

[a] Only FDA-approved drugs for RLS as of August, 2008.
Data from Avidan AY, Zee P, editors. Handbook of sleep medicine. Philadelphia: Lippincott Williams & Wilkins; 2006. p. 98–136.

repetitive, stereotyped limb movements occurring in sleep, typically involving the lower extremities. Diagnosis is based on PSG, which demonstrates the stereotyped repetitive movements on limb EMG during non-REM sleep.[5,91]

Management

What are the current treatment options for restless legs syndrome?

Dopaminergic medications are first-line treatment of RLS, and the dopamine agonists ropinirole and pramipexole are FDA approved for this indication (**Table 4**).[69,91–99] Levodopa may also be used but may cause augmentation, a phenomenon in which RLS symptom severity worsens and occurs earlier in the day in some patients.[91,100] Second-line medications include gabapentin, benzodiazepines, clonidine, or opiates, such as oxycodone.[69] Patients who have iron deficiency anemia–associated RLS should also be treated with iron supplements as adjunctive therapy.[86]

SUMMARY

Sleep disorders are prevalent in the general population and can significantly affect physical and mental health and emotional well-being. There is a broad range of sleep disorders with varied clinical presentations. Physicians of all specialties should screen for the presence of disturbed sleep and consider referral to a sleep specialist when indicated.

REFERENCES

1. Thorpy MJ. Approach to the patient with a sleep complaint. Semin Neurol 2004; 24(3):225–35.
2. Breslau N, Roth T, Rosenthal L, et al. Sleep disturbance and psychiatric disorders: a longitudinal epidemiological study of young adults. Biol Psychiatry 1996;39(6):411–8.
3. Lockley SW, Barger LK, Ayas NT, et al. Effects of health care provider work hours and sleep deprivation on safety and performance. Jt Comm J Qual Patient Saf 2007;33(11 Suppl):7–18.
4. Copinschi G. Metabolic and endocrine effects of sleep deprivation. Essent Psychopharmacol 2005;6(6):341–7.
5. American Academy of Sleep Medicine, A. The international classification of sleep disorders. In: Sateia M, editor. Diagnostic and coding manual. 2nd edition. Westchester (IL): American Academy of Sleep Medicine; 2005. p. 1–297.
6. Hailey D, Tran K, Dales R, et al. Recommendations and supporting evidence in guidelines for referral of patients to sleep laboratories. Sleep Med Rev 2006; 10(4):287–99.
7. Bae C, Avidan A. Evaluation and testing of the sleepy patient. In: Smith HR, Comella CL, Birgit H, editors. Sleep medicine. Cambridge (UK): Cambridge University Press; 2008. p. 25–46.
8. Johns MW. A new method for measuring daytime sleepiness: the Epworth sleepiness scale. Sleep 1991;14(6):540–5.
9. Boeve BF, Silber MH, Ferman TJ. REM sleep behavior disorder in Parkinson's disease and dementia with Lewy bodies. J Geriatr Psychiatry Neurol 2004; 17(3):146–57.
10. Schenck CH, Bundlie SR, Mahowald MW. Delayed emergence of a parkinsonian disorder in 38% of 29 older men initially diagnosed with idiopathic rapid eye movement sleep behaviour disorder. Neurology 1996;46(2):388–93.
11. Littner MR, Kushida C, Wise M, et al. Practice parameters for clinical use of the multiple sleep latency test and the maintenance of wakefulness test. Sleep 2005; 28(1):113–21.

12. Kushida CA, Morgenthaler TI, Littner MR, et al. Practice parameters for the indications for polysomnography and related procedures: an update for 2005. Sleep 2005;28(4):499–521.
13. Silber M. Insomnia. Continuum Lifelong Learning Neurol 2007;13(3):85–100.
14. Benca RM. Insomnia. In: Avidan AY, Zee PC, editors. Handbook of sleep medicine. Philadelphia: Lippincott Williams & Wilkins; 2006. p. 36–69.
15. National Institutes of Health State of the Science Conference statement on manifestations and management of chronic insomnia in adults, June 13–15, 2005. Sleep 2005;28(9):1049–57.
16. Ohayon MM. Epidemiology of insomnia: what we know and what we still need to learn. Sleep Med Rev 2002;6(2):97–111.
17. Ohayon MM, Roth T. What are the contributing factors for insomnia in the general population? J Psychosom Res 2001;51(6):745–55.
18. Ohayon MM, Zulley J, Guilleminault C, et al. How age and daytime activities are related to insomnia in the general population: consequences for older people. J Am Geriatr Soc 2001;49(4):360–6.
19. Smith MT, Klick B, Kozachik S, et al. Sleep onset insomnia symptoms during hospitalization for major burn injury predict chronic pain. Pain 2008;138(3):497–506.
20. Stiefel F, Stagno D. Management of insomnia in patients with chronic pain conditions. CNS Drugs 2004;18(5):285–96.
21. Gottlieb DJ, Punjabi NM, Newman AB, et al. Association of sleep time with diabetes mellitus and impaired glucose tolerance. Arch Intern Med 2005;165(8):863–7.
22. Phillips B, Mannino DM. Do insomnia complaints cause hypertension or cardiovascular disease? J Clin Sleep Med 2007;3(5):489–94.
23. Sallinen M, Holm J, Hirvonen K, et al. Recovery of cognitive performance from sleep debt: do a short rest pause and a single recovery night help? Chronobiol Int 2008;25(2):279–96.
24. Pj H. Primary insomnia. 2003.
25. Fetveit A, Straand J, Bjorvatn B. Sleep disturbances in an arctic population: The Tromso Study. BMC Health Serv Res 2008;8:117–25.
26. Nofzinger EA, Buysse DJ, Germain A, et al. Functional neuroimaging evidence for hyperarousal in insomnia. Am J Psychiatry 2004;161(11):2126–8.
27. Morin CM, Rodrigue S, Ivers H. Role of stress, arousal, and coping skills in primary insomnia. Psychosom Med 2003;65(2):259–67.
28. Durmer J, Chervin R. Pediatric sleep medicine. Continuum Lifelong Learning Neurol 2007;13(3):153–200.
29. Rybarczyk B, Stepanski E, Fogg L, et al. A placebo-controlled test of cognitive-behavioral therapy for comorbid insomnia in older adults. J Consult Clin Psychol 2005;73(6):1164–74.
30. Sivertsen B, Omvik S, Pallesen S, et al. Cognitive behavioral therapy vs zopiclone for treatment of chronic primary insomnia in older adults: a randomized controlled trial. JAMA 2006;295(24):2851–8.
31. Irwin MR, Cole JC, Nicassio PM. Comparative meta-analysis of behavioral interventions for insomnia and their efficacy in middle-aged adults and in older adults 55+ years of age. Health Psychol 2006;25(1):3–14.
32. Edinger JD, Means MK. Cognitive-behavioral therapy for primary insomnia. Clin Psychol Rev 2005;25(5):539–58.
33. Wu R, Bao J, Zhang C, et al. Comparison of sleep condition and sleep-related psychological activity after cognitive-behavior and pharmacological therapy for chronic insomnia. Psychother Psychosom 2006;75(4):220–8.

34. Edinger JD, Wohlgemuth WK, Radtke RA, et al. Dose-response effects of cognitive-behavioral insomnia therapy: a randomized clinical trial. Sleep 2007; 30(2):203–12.
35. Lieberman JA. Update on the safety considerations in the management of insomnia with hypnotics: incorporating modified-release formulations into primary care. Prim Care Companion J Clin Psychiatry 2007;9(1):25–31.
36. Zammit G, Erman M, Wang-Weigand S, et al. Evaluation of the efficacy and safety of ramelteon in subjects with chronic insomnia. J Clin Sleep Med 2007; 3(5):495–504.
37. Buscemi N, Vandermeer B, Hooton N, et al. The efficacy and safety of exogenous melatonin for primary sleep disorders. A meta-analysis. J Gen Intern Med 2005;20(12):1151–8.
38. Buscemi N, Vandermeer B, Hooton N, et al. Efficacy and safety of exogenous melatonin for secondary sleep disorders and sleep disorders accompanying sleep restriction: meta-analysis. BMJ 2006;332(7538):385–93.
39. Banno K, Kryger MH. Sleep apnea: clinical investigations in humans. Sleep Med 2007;8(4):400–26.
40. White DP. Sleep apnea. Proc Am Thorac Soc 2006;3(1):124–8.
41. Tabba MK, Johnson JC. Obstructive sleep apnea: a practical review. Mo Med 2006;103(5):509–13.
42. Chan A, Kushida C. Sleep-disordered breathing. Continuum Lifelong Learning Neurol 2007;13(3):139–52.
43. Sewell-Scheuermann S, Phillips B. Sleep-disordered breathing. In: Avidan AY, Zee PC, editors. Handbook of sleep medicine. Philadelphia: Lippincott Williams & Wilkins; 2006. p. 13–35.
44. Young T, Palta M, Dempsey J, et al. The occurrence of sleep-disordered breathing among middle-aged adults. N Engl J Med 1993;328(17):1230–5.
45. Tishler PV, Larkin EK, Schluchter MD, et al. Incidence of sleep-disordered breathing in an urban adult population: the relative importance of risk factors in the development of sleep-disordered breathing. JAMA 2003;289(17):2230–7.
46. Hudgel DW. Mechanisms of obstructive sleep apnea. Chest 1992;101(2):541–9.
47. Mehra R, Stone KL, Blackwell T, et al. Prevalence and correlates of sleep-disordered breathing in older men: osteoporotic fractures in men sleep study. J Am Geriatr Soc 2007;55(9):1356–64.
48. Alchanatis M, Zias N, Deligiorgis N, et al. Comparison of cognitive performance among different age groups in patients with obstructive sleep apnea. Sleep Breath 2007;12(1):17–24.
49. Weaver TE, Chasens ER. Continuous positive airway pressure treatment for sleep apnea in older adults. Sleep Med Rev 2007;11(2):99–111.
50. Guilleminault C, Abad VC. Obstructive sleep apnea syndromes. Med Clin North Am 2004;88:611–30.
51. Lavie L. Sleep-disordered breathing and cerebrovascular disease: a mechanistic approach. Neurol Clin 2005;23(4):1059–75.
52. Weaver TE, Grunstein RR. Adherence to continuous positive airway pressure therapy: the challenge to effective treatment. Proc Am Thorac Soc 2008;5(2):173–8.
53. Sundaram S, Bridgman SA, Lim J, et al. Surgery for obstructive sleep apnoea. Cochrane Database Syst Rev 2005;(4):CD001004.
54. Sher A, Goldberg A. Upper airway surgery for obstructive sleep apnea. Sleep apnea pathogenesis diagnosis and treatment. In: Pack A, editor. Sleep apnea. New York: Marcel Dekker; 2002. p. 575–605.

55. Pillar G, Schnall R, Peled R, et al. Surgical treatment of sleep apnea syndrome. Isr J Med Sci 1996;32(9):710–5.
56. Thorpy MJ. Narcolepsy. Continuum Lifelong Learning Neurol 2007;13(3):101–14.
57. Dauvilliers Y, Arnulf I, Mignot E. Narcolepsy with cataplexy. Lancet 2007; 369(9560):499–511.
58. Hoban T, Chervin R. Hypersomnia and narcolepsy. In: Avidan A, Zee PC, editors. Handbook of sleep medicine. Philadelphia: Lippincott Williams & Wilkins; 2006. p. 70–97.
59. The international classification of sleep disorders pocket version: diagnostic & coding manual. 2nd editon. West (IL): American Academy of Sleep Medicine; 2006.
60. Black JL 3rd. Narcolepsy: a review of evidence for autoimmune diathesis. Int Rev Psychiatry 2005;17(6):461–9.
61. Broughton RJ, Fleming JA, George CA, et al. Randomized, double-blind, placebo-controlled crossover trial of modafinil in the treatment of excessive daytime sleepiness in narcolepsy. Neurology 1997;49(2):444–51.
62. Randomized trial of modafinil as a treatment for the excessive daytime somnolence of narcolepsy: US Modafinil in Narcolepsy Multicenter Study Group. Neurology 2000;54(5):1166–75.
63. Thorpy M. Therapeutic advances in narcolepsy. Sleep Med 2007;8(4):427–40.
64. Wise MS, Arand DL, Auger RR, et al. Treatment of narcolepsy and other hypersomnias of central origin. Sleep 2007;30(12):1712–27.
65. Okawa M, Uchiyama M. Circadian rhythm sleep disorders: characteristics and entrainment pathology in delayed sleep phase and non-24-h sleep-wake syndrome. Sleep Med Rev 2007;11(6):485–96.
66. Lu B, Manthena P, Zee PC. Circadian rhythm sleep disorders. In: Avidan A, Zee PC, editors. Handbook of sleep medicine. Philadelphia: Lippincott Williams & Wilkins; 2006. p. 137–64.
67. Reid KJ, Zee PC. Circadian rhythm disorders. Semin Neurol 2004;24(3):315–25.
68. Morgenthaler TI, Lee-Chiong T, Alessi C, et al. Practice parameters for the clinical evaluation and treatment of circadian rhythm sleep disorders. An American Academy of Sleep Medicine report. Sleep 2007;30(11):1445–59.
69. Avidan A. Motor disorders of sleep and parasomnias. In: Avidan A, Zee PC, editors. Handbook of sleep medicine. Philadelphia: Lippincott Williams & Wilkins; 2006. p. 98–136.
70. Vaughn BV, D'Cruz ON. Parasomnias and other nocturnal events. American Academy of Neurology Continuum: lifelong learning in neurology. Sleep Disorders 2007;13(3):225–47.
71. Zaiwalla Z. Parasomnias. Clin Med 2005;5(2):109–12.
72. Lee-Chiong TL Jr. Parasomnias and other sleep-related movement disorders. Prim Care 2005;32(2):415–34.
73. Ferini-Strambi L, Fantini ML, Zucconi M, et al. REM sleep behaviour disorder. Neurol Sci 2005;26(Suppl 3):s186–92.
74. Mahowald MW, Bornemann MC, Schenck CH. Parasomnias. Semin Neurol 2004; 24(3):283–92.
75. Farid M, Kushida CA. Non-rapid eye movement parasomnias. Curr Treat Options Neurol 2004;6(4):331–7.
76. Leo G. Parasomnias. WMJ 2003;102(1):32–5.
77. Sheldon SH. Parasomnias in childhood. Pediatr Clin North Am 2004;51(1):69–88, vi.
78. Ferini-Strambi L, Zucconi M. REM sleep behavior disorder. Clin Neurophysiol 2000;111(Suppl 2):S136–40.

79. Matsurnoto M, Mutoh F, Naoe H, et al. The effects of imipramine on REM sleep behavior disorder in 3 cases. Sleep Res 1991;20A:351.
80. Nash JR, Wilson SJ, Potokar JP, et al. Mirtazapine induces REM sleep behavior disorder (RBD) in parkinsonism. Neurology 2003;61(8):1161.
81. Stolz SE, Aldrich MS. REM sleep behavior disorder associated with caffeine abuse. Sleep Res 1991;20:341.
82. Boeve BF, Silber MH, Ferman TJ. Melatonin for treatment of REM sleep behavior disorder in neurologic disorders: results in 14 patients. Sleep Med 2003;4(4):281–4.
83. Boeve B. Melatonin for treatment of REM sleep behavior disorder: response in 8 patients. Sleep 2001;24(Suppl):A35.
84. Ringman JM, Simmons JH. Treatment of REM sleep behavior disorder with donepezil: a report of three cases. Neurology 2000;55(6):870–1.
85. Bamford CR. Carbamazepine in REM sleep behavior disorder. Sleep 1993; 16(1):33–4.
86. Walters AS. Restless legs syndrome and periodic limb movements in sleep. American Academy of Neurology Continuum: lifelong learning in neurology. Sleep Disorders 2007;13(3):115–38.
87. Trenkwalder C, Paulus W, Walters AS. The restless legs syndrome. Lancet Neurol 2005;4(8):465–75.
88. Benes H, Walters AS, Allen RP, et al. Definition of restless legs syndrome, how to diagnose it, and how to differentiate it from RLS mimics. Mov Disord 2007; 22(Suppl 18):S401–8.
89. Allen RP, Picchietti D, Hening WA, et al. Restless legs syndrome: diagnostic criteria, special considerations, and epidemiology. A report from the restless legs syndrome diagnosis and epidemiology workshop at the National Institutes of Health. Sleep Med 2003;4(2):101–19.
90. Rama AN, Kushida CA. Restless legs syndrome and periodic limb movement disorder. Med Clin North Am 2004;88(3):653–67, viii.
91. Lesage S, Hening WA. The restless legs syndrome and periodic limb movement disorder: a review of management. Semin Neurol 2004;24(3):249–59.
92. Winkelman JW, Sethi KD, Kushida CA, et al. Efficacy and safety of pramipexole in restless legs syndrome. Neurology 2006;67(6):1034–9.
93. Littner MR, Kushida C, Anderson WM, et al. Practice parameters for the dopaminergic treatment of restless legs syndrome and periodic limb movement disorder. Sleep 2004;27(3):557–9.
94. Lesage S, Earley CJ. Restless legs syndrome. Curr Treat Options Neurol 2004; 6(3):209–19.
95. Hening WA, Allen RP, Earley CJ, et al. An update on the dopaminergic treatment of restless legs syndrome and periodic limb movement disorder. Sleep 2004; 27(3):560–83.
96. Cheer SM, Bang LM, Keating GM. Ropinirole: for the treatment of restless legs syndrome. CNS Drugs 2004;18(11):747–54 [discussion 755–6].
97. Allen R, Becker PM, Bogan R, et al. Ropinirole decreases periodic leg movements and improves sleep parameters in patients with restless legs syndrome. Sleep 2004;27(5):907–14.
98. Adler CH, Hauser RA, Sethi K, et al. Ropinirole for restless legs syndrome: a placebo-controlled crossover trial. Neurology 2004;62(8):1405–7.
99. Wetter TC, Winkelmann J, Eisensehr I. Current treatment options for restless legs syndrome. Expert Opin Pharmacother 2003;4(10):1727–38.
100. Trenkwalder C, Hogl B, Benes H, et al. Augmentation in restless legs syndrome is associated with low ferritin. Sleep Med 2007;9(5):572–4.

Neurological Aspects of Syncope and Orthostatic Intolerance

Louis H. Weimer, MD*, Pezhman Zadeh, MD

KEYWORDS

- POTS • Orthostatic hypotension • Vasovagal
- Vasodepressor • Carotid sinus syndrome
- Autonomic neuropathy • Multiple system atrophy

A sudden, unexpected loss of consciousness is one of the more dramatic and anxiety-provoking symptoms encountered by patients. Syncope, however, is a common manifestation of numerous disorders of varied mechanisms. The final common pathway in most, however, is insufficient cerebral perfusion to maintain consciousness. Symptoms short of frank syncope (presyncope) are also common and may appear relatively non-specific in isolation or out of context. A current view is to consider one's capacity for postural and similar challenges as *orthostatic tolerance* that can be impaired by a wide variety of disorders and may become symptomatic under certain conditions. For diagnosis syncope must be differentiated from other processes with paroxysmal onset and altered consciousness such as seizures, drop attacks, metabolic disturbances, or psychiatric events. After many events, no residual abnormalities are evident on examination or on initial studies to prove a specific diagnosis. More than most areas of medicine, this lack of objective residua makes a detailed and accurate history the most important aspect of diagnosis. The distinction is vital for clinical decision-making and effective treatment. Once a designation is made, alternative diagnoses may be inadequately considered at later assessments, even if correct.

This review focuses on syncope from the perspective of the neurologist and the disorders generally considered in the setting of acute, transient loss of consciousness. The numerous and important causes of syncope related to primary cardiac and pulmonary dysfunction (cardiac syncope) mostly due to insufficient cardiac output despite adequate venous supply including valvular disease, sustained arrhythmias, myocardial disease and heart failure, and structural heart and lung disease are not discussed. Many of these cardiac etiologies are clearly evident with pertinent signs on examination, other historical details, prior history, or abnormalities with initial

---

The Neurological Institute of New York, 710 West 168th Street, Unit 55, New York, NY 10032, USA
* Corresponding author.
E-mail address: lhw1@columbia.edu (L.H. Weimer).

Med Clin N Am 93 (2009) 427–449
doi:10.1016/j.mcna.2008.10.002
0025-7125/08/$ – see front matter © 2009 Elsevier Inc. All rights reserved.

investigations such as electrocardiography (ECG) that lead to additional testing.[1] Also important to recognize are neurogenic orthostatic hypotension and orthostatic tachycardia, which may prompt evaluation of autonomic failure or other orthostatic intolerance syndromes.

In some cases an accurate history and examination is sufficiently diagnostic, such as a lone episode of reflex syncope with a clear precipitant in an otherwise healthy person; however, many confounding factors can arise. Tonic or myoclonic movements associated with syncope are common.[1,2] Patients may have minimal or no warning before an episode or have brief amnesia after an unwitnessed event, negating vital aspects of the history. Witnesses may be unavailable or provide inadequate or inaccurate observations. Also, mild cardiac disease, relatively benign arrhythmias, or asymptomatic orthostatic hypotension may be found and be of uncertain severity to produce syncope.

WHEN SHOULD REFLEX CAUSES OF SYNCOPE BE CONSIDERED AND WHAT ARE THE MAJOR FORMS?

Reflex syncope should be considered if a characteristic precipitating factor is temporally associated with events (**Box 1**). Major categories include neurally mediated (vasovagal), carotid sinus hypersensitivity, and situational syncopes. All share certain similarities and likely some mechanisms. Most forms are benign; however, recurrent events can have a significant impact on patient quality of life if frequent or lead to injury.[3]

WHAT IS THE MOST COMMON FORM OF REFLEX SYNCOPE?

Neurally mediated or vasovagal types are the most common and most benign forms of syncope and demonstrate sudden hypotension and frequent bradycardia.[1,4,5] Other often indiscriminately applied terms include vasodepressor, neurovascular, neurocardiogenic, and vasomotor syncope. More severe and recurrent spells, especially those associated with fall-related trauma, are often unfortunately labeled as malignant. In some cases the distinction between vasodepressor and cardioinhibitory subtypes is useful (see later discussion).

Box 1
Orthostatic aggravating factors

Warm environment, hot bath

Post-exercise

Prolonged motionless standing

Large meals (carbohydrate load)

Early morning

Valsalva

Volume depletion

Rising after prolonged bedrest

Rapid postural change

Spaceflight

Alcohol

Medications

IS NEURALLY MEDIATED SYNCOPE RESTRICTED TO THE YOUNG AND HEALTHY?

Most patients are young and otherwise healthy, but the process also occurs at later ages, including the elderly, and in patients with cardiac, neurologic, or autonomic impairment.[6] Elderly patients, however, are more likely to have comorbid conditions, multiple confounding medications, and other complicating factors. Therefore the outcome is less benign. Familial forms are also known, in some cases attributed to specific genetic defects.[7]

WHAT TRIGGERS THE PHENOMENON?

The cause is an aberrant reflex that can be triggered by a variety of conditions, especially in the setting of emotionally charged situations such as fear and pain, possibly resembling primitive "playing dead" fainting defenses. Following a period of increased sympathetic tone, a sudden sympathetic withdrawal is triggered, leading to paradoxical vasodilation and hypotension. This effect is supported by studies that captured a sharp decrease in sympathetic nerve traffic to the legs during this period.[8] An associated vagal surge often produces relative or marked bradycardia. If cerebral perfusion drops sufficiently, loss of consciousness results. Lewis[9] observed long ago that, although the accompanying bradycardia was reversed by atropine, hypotension, and the altered level of consciousness persisted and early pacing attempts to prevent bradycardia in an unselected vasovagal group did not prevent syncope.[10]

Attacks occur with upright posture and often with one or more aggravating conditions present (see **Box 1**). Prodromal symptoms often include a feeling of warmth or cold, sweating, lightheadedness, nausea, yawning, and visual dimming. However, warnings may be brief or absent altogether. If the patient does not voluntarily recline, the syncopal fall will accomplish a horizontal position, allowing a rapid restoration of cerebral perfusion. Recovery is usually rapid without confusion, headache, or focal neurologic symptoms, though fatigue is frequent. Complications such as convulsive syncope can result if recumbency is prevented, usually by well-intentioned bystanders.

ISN'T THE VASOVAGAL SYNCOPE MECHANISM WELL ESTABLISHED?

It has long been assumed that the mechanism for suddenly converting from vasoconstriction to vasodilation and bradycardia is excessive stimulation of mechanoreceptors due to forceful contractions of an underfilled left ventricle, leading to paradoxical signals to the central nervous system pathways, hence the term *neurocardiogenic* supported by work in a small number of cats.[11] However, significant evidence against this Bezold-Jarisch phenomenon as an important etiology persists, and other mechanisms such as aberrant autonomic regulation, endogenous vasodilators, disordered baroreflex function, and paradoxical cerebral autoregulation may play a role and are likely to be targets of future treatment approaches. Norcliffe-Kaufmann and colleagues[12] recently demonstrated that individuals prone to neurally mediated syncope had a greater reduction in cerebral blood flow and a greater dilatation of the forearm vasculature in response to hypocapnia compared with healthy control subjects. This enhanced vascular sensitivity to CO_2, both in the cerebral and peripheral vasculature, may at least partly explain why some individuals are more susceptible to this phenomenon. Overall, however, the full explanation remains unproven.[8] The underlying purpose of this phenomenon has generated much speculation and discussion. Vasovagal syncope is considered to be a normal reflex triggered at unintended situations, especially in younger individuals. The tendency may have conferred some selection advantage in earlier times, such as "appearing dead" in highly dangerous situations and lowering blood pressure and heart rate in the setting of hemorrhagic shock to allow increased time for blood clotting.[13]

WHAT IS CAROTID SINUS HYPERSENSITIVITY?

Minor local stimulation of the carotid region (eg, from a tight collar, neck pressure from head turning or shaving) can trigger bradycardia, hypotension, or both. This tendency, termed *carotid sinus hypersensitivity* (CSH) or *carotid sinus syndrome*, should be considered in older patients with syncope or unexplained falls, even without a classical history. Some are also misdiagnosed to have treatment-resistant epilepsy.[14]

High-pressure mechanoreceptors in the carotid sinus are traditionally thought to be overly susceptible to stimulation, especially in stiffened, atherosclerotic blood vessels providing erroneous afferent signals to the brainstem. The true site of abnormality, however, remains unclear, whether local or in brainstem integration centers.

IS CAROTID SINUS HYPERSENSITIVITY UNDER- OR OVERDIAGNOSED?

Many authors advocate expanded diagnostic carotid sinus massage because of concerns regarding underdiagnosis.[15] A 3-second pause or ≥50 mmHg systolic drop on stimulation is considered to be positive. Responses are divided into three categories:

(1) predominantly cardioinhibitory with marked, transient bradycardia or asystole;
(2) vasodepressor with hypotension without bradycardia; and
(3) mixed (most common) with features of both.[16]

The distinction is therapeutically relevant because predominantly cardioinhibitory syncope patients may benefit from pacing, unlike most patients with a vasodepressor pattern.[17] The incidence appears to increase progressively with age, and positive responses to manual massage appear to be commonplace in elderly patients, especially those with nonaccidental falls. The incidence was 45% in one series compared with 13% of healthy controls, although only fallers developed syncope during testing.[15] Care must be taken not to designate a disease simply based on a clinical sign; moreover, the importance of this sign is not yet firmly established.[18] No firm clinical–pathologic correlations are known, although the incidence appears to be increased in certain degenerative neurologic conditions that affect brainstem nuclei, such as diffuse Lewy body dementia and idiopathic Parkinson's disease, but these conditions are also strongly associated with neurogenic orthostatic hypotension from autonomic failure (see later discussion). Other dementias have much lower incidence, including Alzheimer's disease and vascular dementia.[19,20]

Pacing remains a controversial topic, but in one placebo-controlled trial, pacing reduced the total number of falls by 70%, syncopal events by 53%, and injuries by 70%.[21] Carotid massage should be performed with caution and avoided in patients with carotid bruits, prior stroke, or cerebrovascular disease.[22]

WHAT SPECIAL SITUATIONAL CONDITIONS CAN TRIGGER SYNCOPE?

Situational syncope triggers are varied but many are associated with a concomitant Valsalva maneuver, during which transthoracic pressure increases, venous return is curtailed, and respiratory patterns change. Examples include, cough, micturition, defecation, instrumentation (eg, colonoscopy), swallow, postexercise, sneeze, diving, and pain (glossopharyngeal neuralgia) -related syncope.

WHAT IS TUSSIVE SYNCOPE?

Cough (tussive) syncope and *laughter-associated syncope* are most common in obese men over 40, smokers with chronic cough and emphysema, and children with asthma.[23,24] Syncope often follows coughing spells or prolonged laughter with associated intrathoracic pressure surges. Diaphragm contraction further impedes venous return by vena caval compression, raised intracranial pressure, and blunted cerebral perfusion, usually without bradycardia or vagal signs.[24] In asthmatic children, cough syncope often occurs shortly after falling asleep, abruptly waking the child, and may resemble a seizure.[23] Other examples have been misdiagnosed as epilepsy.[25] Recovery is fast without postevent confusion, and the patient may be amnestic of the episode other than the inciting trigger. Breath-holding spells may cause syncope by similar means, particularly after hyperventilation.

IS MICTURITION SYNCOPE LIMITED TO ELDERLY MEN?

Syncope associated with urination was originally described in young healthy men,[26,27] but more commonly occurs in older patients with multiple medical problems.[28] Micturition syncope usually occurs in the early morning during or immediately following urination. The mechanism remains unproven, but prime factors include nocturnal blood pressure decline, Valsalva during urination, warm environment, standing position, and vagal afferent stimulation by rapid emptying of a distended bladder.[28] Especially in the elderly, underlying orthostatic hypotension and medications may be predisposing factors. Sitting during urination may benefit recurrent events.

ARE CERTAIN TYPES OF PAIN MORE PRONE TO TRIGGERING SYNCOPE?

Severe, acute pain can trigger syncope, notably glossopharyngeal neuralgia, which is characterized by paroxysms of stabbing pain of the posterior tongue and throat. Syncope with severe bradycardia or asystole usually follows a painful paroxysm.[29,30] The syncope can be treated separately in some cases from the painful paroxysms. Aberrant spread of glossopharyngeal nerve afferent impulses to the brainstem is presumed to play a role.[30]

IS SYNCOPE ASSOCIATED WITH SEIZURE-LIKE ACTIVITY?

Stiffening, myoclonic, or limited clonic movements associated with syncope, termed *convulsive syncope*, can mimic seizures and are a frequent source of epilepsy center referrals as well as a common reason for seizure misdiagnosis.[31] Consequences of misdiagnosis have medical and social implications for the patient. Usual syncope clues such as brief duration, aggravating conditions or triggers, rapid recovery, and lack of postictal phenomena are usually present, although patients occasionally have incontinence. Attacks are generally brief and show multifocal or 1–2 clonic jerks rather than typical rhythmic clonic movements seen with many generalized seizures; they also lack significant postictal confusion. Movements are generally during the episode and not at outset.

WHAT CAUSES CONVULSIVE SYNCOPE?

Convulsive syncope is a manifestation of prolonged cerebral hypoperfusion. EEG changes during syncope have been long recognized, and landmark studies have demonstrated that short cardiac pauses (3–6 seconds) have no observable consequences. Longer pauses (7–13 seconds) initially show mild generalized cerebral slowing on

EEG, followed by high voltage frontal delta activity with altered consciousness.[32] If hypoperfusion persists (>14 seconds), the EEG begins to flatten and convulsive movements or stiffening resembling posturing develops. Regardless of the syncope cause, EEG findings are similar.[33] Lempert and colleagues[2] induced complete syncope in 42 normal subjects, 90% of whom developed multifocal arrhythmic movements or generalized myoclonus.

DOES CONVULSIVE SYNCOPE IMPLY A MORE SERIOUS UNDERLYING CONDITION?

Uncomplicated reflex syncope may account for many cases, especially in children, and have similar triggers as other reflex causes.[34,35] When a reflex form is the cause, the risk of death remains remote, but the chance of injury is increased. When triggered by a reflex cause, the phenomenon is also descriptively known as reflex anoxic seizures or reflex asystolic syncope. However, convulsive syncope may also be cardiac in origin (convulsive arrhythmic syncope) and occur at any age.[36]

Tilt testing or prolonged epilepsy monitoring is sometimes useful in distinguishing difficult cases.[34] In one study, nine children previously diagnosed with seizures, but with clinical records suggestive of convulsive syncope, showed positive tilt table testing, with reproduction of symptoms previously considered part of the epileptic attacks.[37] Simultaneous tilt, EEG, and transcranial Doppler testing can aid in distinguishing difficult cases.[38]

HOW COMMON ARE THESE PHENOMENA?

The incidence is not clearly known, but all of the reflex phenomena discussed are common. One review of a cohort of Dutch medical students found that nearly 40% reported at least one bout of vasovagal syncope in their lifetime.[39] Prolonged standing, warm environment, illness, and pain were the most common triggers in women; alcohol was the most common trigger in men followed by similar ones as women, except for pain-induced syncope. Only 3% of episodes were labeled as unknown. The incidence of carotid sinus hypersensitivity and reflex syncope in the elderly is controversial, especially because some falls attributed to other causes may be triggered syncope examples.

WHAT IS THE BASIC APPROACH TO DIAGNOSTIC TESTING?
Basic Laboratory Testing

Basic laboratory testing is indicated to uncover volume retraction or metabolic causes such as hypoglycemia if suspected. In series that also included seizure patients, abnormal findings such as hyponatremia, hypoglycemia, and renal failure were found in only 2% to 3% of patients.[40] ECG has been advocated in virtually all cases.[40,41] Although ECG is abnormal in approximately half of patients evaluated with syncope, abnormalities are diagnostic in less than 5% of cases but can prompt diagnostic cardiac evaluation.[1,41,42] The application of these tests, including echocardiography, cardiac electrophysiology, and prolonged ECG monitoring (Holter monitoring and external and implanted loop recorders), are reviewed in detail elsewhere.[41]

Carotid Sinus Massage

Carotid sinus massage with ECG monitoring can be applied in both the supine and upright positions, usually on a tilt table. The incidence of positive tests increases with age. Continuous blood pressure monitoring is desirable to capture a rapid vasodepressor response. Upright massage has a higher positive rate and is a stronger stimulus for vasodepression. As noted earlier, pacing is generally less effective in mixed forms with a significant vasodepressor component than in predominantly cardioinhibitory forms.[43] The European Society of Cardiology guidelines recommend testing for carotid sinus hypersensitivity in all patients over 40 with syncope of unknown cause; however, this recommendation has been challenged because of low rates of positive tests.[44] The maneuver is performed much less commonly in the United States.

Tilt Table Testing

Tilt table testing is a standard and widely available method of assessing recurrent unexplained syncope or lone episodes in high-risk individuals or settings.[45] A gravitational shift of blood (500–800 cc) into venous capacitance systems of the legs and pelvis occurs with active standing, reducing venous return.[8,46] Upright tilting provides a similar but not identical orthostatic stress, primarily from lesser muscle activation. Prolonged motionless standing causes further stress in part by fluid movement into interstitial spaces and blunted venous return because of a lack of muscular pumping.

During passive tilt testing, roughly half of patients develop delayed syncope compared with 10% or less of controls.[42] However, much variability in patient populations and test protocols employed have made precise values for sensitivity and specificity problematic, especially without a gold standard for comparison.[47] Reproducibility is also variable and laboratory dependent.[42] Pharmacologic provocation including isoproterenol or nitroglycerin can further increase the chance of syncope in both patient and control groups and is consequently not used in some centers. Some protocol differences include tilt angles (60–90°), test duration (20–60 minutes), patient preparation, and provocative drug use. Consensus panels have tried to better standardize protocols.[43,48] Recommendations include a 2-hour fast before testing, a supine position of up to 45 minutes before tilting, beat-to-beat arterial blood pressure monitoring, and a 60–70° tilt angle. Further classification of positive tilt responses based on the timing and degree of HR cardioinhibitory responses, presence of vasodepression, or mixed findings was proposed by Sutton.[13,49]

Tilt testing is an extremely safe procedure with a very low complication rate. Life-threatening ventricular arrhythmia after isoproterenol in the presence of heart disease has been reported rarely.[50]

Electroencephalography

Electroencephalography (EEG) is useful in patients with a relative likelihood of epilepsy, such as a history of seizures, abnormal neurologic examination, prolonged postevent confusion, or abnormal movements preceding other events. In typical syncope cases the yield is extremely low.[51] EEG can distinguish syncope from seizure-related cerebral hypoperfusion in the event of a recorded spell during testing or provoked by tilt testing.[38]

Neuroimaging

Head CT is relevant mostly in patients with neurologic signs or possible seizures. The measured yield of CT was low (4%) in most series with positive scans predominantly restricted to those with focal neurologic signs or a witnessed seizure.[1] MRI, transcranial, or carotid Doppler studies have not demonstrated general usefulness in the usual syncope evaluation.[1] However, a careful history and neurologic examination is necessary to draw these conclusions before decision making on neurologic testing.

WHAT IS THE APPROACH TO TREATMENT AND WHICH MEDICATIONS HAVE BEEN SHOWN TO BE EFFICACIOUS IN CONTROLLED TRIALS?

Treatment should be proportional to the episode frequency and severity. General educational measures such as avoidance of triggering conditions and reassurance about the generally benign nature of the disorder may be adequate. Salt and water supplements are the cornerstone of treatment and both independently appear to improve orthostatic tolerance.[52,53] For more severe or recurrent cases a plethora of prophylactic agents have been tested in uncontrolled small series, but relatively few placebo-controlled trials have been conducted.[54]

β-Adrenergic blocking agents have been widely used and efficacy supported in some large uncontrolled trials[55,56] and one older randomized placebo-controlled trial of 42 patients.[57] More recent trials, however, failed to reproduce a significant benefit in symptomatic patients using atenolol or metoprolol.[58,59] The mineralocorticoid fludrocortisone is another often-used agent despite a lack of placebo-controlled trial evidence of efficacy. A large controlled multicenter trial is ongoing (POST II).[60] The only other agents to date to demonstrate efficacy in at least one prospective, randomized placebo-controlled clinical trial are the α-agonist midodrine and the selective serotonin reuptake inhibitor (SSRI) paroxetine.[56,61,62] Randomized trials on disopyramide and another α-agonist etilefrine showed no significant differences and neither are considered first-line agents.[63,64] Other agents used empirically with favorable responses in uncontrolled studies include theophylline, other β-blockers (metoprolol), anticholinergics (scopolamine), other SSRIs (fluoxetine, sertraline), verapamil, other α-agonists, clonidine, central stimulants (methylphenidate), and numerous others.[4,54] Combinations of agents with differing mechanisms are also frequently employed. Exercise programs, sleeping with a slight head-up tilt (>10°), and tilt training may also be of benefit.[65] More recent attention has focused on physical countermaneuvers, such as leg crossing and squatting, to reduce hypotension.[66,67] Squatting is a potent physical maneuver to prevent syncope; however, standing up afterward is a large hemodynamic stressor that often reproduces presyncopal symptoms. Tensing of lower body muscles while standing is shown to reduce the systolic blood pressure (BP) decline on standing by over 20 mmHg.[68]

IS A PACEMAKER AN OPTION IN REFRACTORY PATIENTS?

Cardiac pacing appears to be beneficial in selected patients with predominantly cardioinhibitory forms of syncope but remains highly controversial as a widespread application, especially in cases with an otherwise excellent prognosis.[17] Pacing goals are to override transient bradycardia and provide enough HR support to minimize hypotensive effects, which is generally insufficient in patients with a significant vasodepressor response. Randomized controlled studies have demonstrated the benefit of pacing over medical therapy in certain settings. The North American Vasovagal Pacemaker Study (VPS) randomized 54 patients with a bradycardic tilt response and at least six syncopal episodes to receive a pacemaker with rate drop response or best medical therapy. A lower rate of recurrence was seen among the paced (22%) compared with medically treated patients (70%) at 1 year.[69] The Vasovagal Syncope International Study (VASIS) randomized 42 patients with three or more syncopes over 2 years and a positive cardioinhibitory tilt response to either a dual chamber pacemaker or not. A lower recurrence rate was seen in the pacemaker group over 3.7 years.[17] A larger study of 93 patients randomized to dual chamber pacing with rate-drop response or atenolol was stopped because of a significantly favorable effect in the pacemaker group.[70] However, the largest and only blinded trial to date, which randomized

100 patients (VPS II) reported a much less favorable response to pacing than its pre-decessor and did not recommend pacing as a first-line treatment.[71] An Italian study in 2004 placed pacemakers in 29 subjects with unspecified recurrent vasovagal syncope and studied the benefit of active versus inactive pacemakers; no significant effect was found.[72] The importance of a potential expectation (placebo) effect in earlier uncontrolled trials is highlighted.[73] Pacemakers may be considered for patients with recurrent, medically refractory, neurally mediated syncope with a documented cardioinhibitory tilt-testing response.[17]

WHAT ARE SOME IMPORTANT CONSIDERATIONS FOR SEPARATING SEIZURES FROM SYNCOPE?

Seizures are also common, paroxysmal events that impair consciousness. Analogous to a syncopal episode, a seizure is a lone symptomatic event that does not necessarily imply a tendency for recurrent epilepsy. A reliable history and examination are often sufficient to distinguish the two in the majority of cases. However, instances with inadequate details including past history and prior events and lack of neurologic or cardiac signs can lead to uncertainty. Generalized seizures cause some amnesia that obscures patient recollections, thus eyewitnesses are vital if available. Basic indicators suggestive of a seizure include a characteristic aura, nonpostural tonic, and clonic or myoclonic movements, especially if onset precedes loss of consciousness, confusion and delayed recovery, headache, trauma to the side and not tip of the tongue, and incontinence.

CAN SEIZURES DIRECTLY PRODUCE TRUE SYNCOPE?

As in most areas of medicine, exceptions occur. Although spontaneous movements associated with syncope are not unusual, seizures that directly induce true syncope are rarely seen and are a potential cause of unexplained death.[74–76] Sinus tachycardia is a typical seizure marker but is generally insufficient to cause cardiovascular instability.[77] Rarely, bradycardia or asystole severe enough to cause syncope during a complex partial seizure is seen (ictal bradycardia syndrome).[75] If identified, patients may benefit from anticonvulsants, cardiac pacing, or both in individual cases.[75,76,78] Routine use of an ECG channel during EEG recordings is advocated but is not universal. In some cases an arrhythmia will be detected during prolonged epilepsy monitoring, but more commonly unrecognized partial seizures will be recorded.[79] More malignant, autonomically mediated rhythms are suspected but not proven as a primary cause of the increased risk of sudden unexpected death in epilepsy patients.[75]

HOW COMMONLY ARE PATIENTS WITH EPILEPSY INITIALLY MISDIAGNOSED?

Cases of refractory epilepsy without identifiable cause and frequent apparent seizures despite therapeutic anticonvulsant levels should at least be considered for the possibility of cardiogenic or reflex syncope or psychiatric cause. In several English series of patients referred to specialist clinics or neurologists with the diagnosis of epilepsy by primary care physicians, 20%–42% were misdiagnosed depending on the populations selected, most commonly with syncope and nonepileptic seizures.[31,80–82] Incomplete histories and misinterpretation of normal variant EEG patterns were most commonly implicated followed by lack of a witnessed account, misinterpretation of motor phenomena, and lack of consideration of prior medical history.[82]

WHEN SHOULD NEUROGENIC ORTHOSTATIC HYPOTENSION BE CONSIDERED AND HOW COMMON IS IT?

Postural or orthostatic hypotension (OH) is a prevalent clinical sign seen in numerous and diverse neurologic and nonneurologic conditions. Syncope from marked orthostatic hypotension (OH) is not uncommon in advanced cases of autonomic failure and is a potentially serious complication.[83,84] Shibao and colleagues[85,86] estimated over 80,000 orthostatic hypotension-related hospitalizations in the United States in 2004; OH was the primary diagnosis in 35%. One consensus agreement defines OH as a fall in systolic blood pressure of 20 mmHg or 10 mmHg diastolic within 3 minutes of standing or similar orthostatic challenge, such as upright tilt, although some require a 30-mmHg decline. OH, however, may be asymptomatic, especially in the elderly, and varies according to underlying conditions or confounding factors.

Impairment of autonomic control at a number of anatomic levels can be sufficient to disrupt the postural reflexes necessary to maintain cerebral perfusion. Syncope is especially prevalent in elderly patients with multiple underlying reasons for having OH.[87] These patients especially may have little to no recognizable symptoms or simply vague difficulty with concentration or cognition, pure vertigo, or "coat-hanger" pattern shoulder pain (muscle hypoperfusion) just before frank syncope.[87,88] Usually, however, a clear postural pattern is evident on questioning and a postural drop on supine to standing BP after 2 minutes is measurable. The process may develop with enough rapidity to be confused with drop attacks or simple falls. Elderly patients may erroneously report syncope as a simple fall as well.[15] Less commonly, the BP declines slowly and progressively for 5 minutes or longer and is missed on routine 1- to 2-minute standing bedside measurements but detected on tilt or autonomic studies.[89] Measurable OH is common in the elderly (10%–30%), but may be asymptomatic or manifest only under aggravating conditions (see **Box 1**). Multiple contributing factors have been implicated.

Nonautonomic conditions can produce OH, most importantly adrenal failure and pheochromocytoma. Paroxysmal surges in BP are a primary pheo characteristic, but OH is also present and can lead to syncope.[90] Screening for both conditions is warranted in newly diagnosed OH cases of uncertain cause. Other common factors including hypovolemia and medication effects are important considerations. Some of the more important and prevalent causes of OH are discussed.

WHICH CAUSES OF PERIPHERAL NEUROPATHY HAVE AUTONOMIC INVOLVEMENT?

Of the many scores of known peripheral neuropathy causes, the majority have some degree of autonomic involvement, often limited to distal sweating and vasomotor control. Dysfunction is generally not severe enough to impair peripheral vasoconstriction or postural reflexes to the degree necessary to lead to symptomatic OH and even less often to frank syncope, even if mild OH is measurable. A minority of causes, however, can lead to more severe or targeted autonomic dysfunction and produce frank autonomic failure and symptomatic OH. Particularly noteworthy causes include diabetes, amyloidosis, paraneoplastic neuropathies, some hereditary and toxic neuropathies, and rare genetic conditions such as dopamine β-hydoxylase deficiency.[84,90,91] Some of the more prominent examples are listed in **Box 2**.

WHAT IS THE MOST COMMON CAUSE OF AUTONOMIC NEUROPATHY?

Diabetic autonomic neuropathy (DAN) is the most common and clinically important cause of autonomic neuropathy in the U.S. and the most extensively examined.

Box 2
Selected syncope causes

Cardiac arrhythmia, structural (organic) myocardial or valvular disease, obstruction

Reflex syncope

Vasovagal (neurally mediated)

Situational

Carotid sinus hypersensitivity

Autonomic failure (orthostatic hypotension)

Pure autonomic failure

Multiple system atrophy (MSA) (Shy-Drager syndrome)

Parkinson's disease with autonomic failure

Dopamine β-hydroxylase deficiency

Baroreflex failure or injury (bilateral)

Chronic autonomic neuropathy

    (diabetes, amyloidosis, hereditary, toxin- or medication-induced, HIV, uremia)

Acute/subacute autonomic neuropathy

   Immune-mediated and idiopathic

   Paraneoplastic

   Guillain-Barré syndrome

Spinal cord injury

Other: adrenal failure, pheochromocytoma, hypovolemia

Reduced orthostatic tolerance

Postural orthostatic tachycardia syndrome (orthostatic intolerance), mitral valve prolapse syndrome, prolonged bedrest or weightlessness, Chiari I

Mimics

Atypical seizures

Seizures with bradycardia

Psychiatric events

Drop attacks

Acute intracranial pressure surges

Medication effects

Anticholinergics: tricyclic antidepressants, atropine, oxybutynin

β-Adrenergic blockers: propranalol and others

a_2 Agonists: clonidine, prazosin, alpha methyl-dopa, terazosin, doxazosin

a_1 Antagonists: phentolamine, phenoxybenzamine, guanabenz

Ganglionic blockers: guanethidine, hexamethonium, mecamylamine

Other agents: hydralazine, nitrates, diuretics, calcium channel blockers, ACE inhibitors, antihistamines, combination preparations, antipsychotics, antiparkinsonian, narcotics, sildenafil, tadalafil, tamsulosin, amifostine.

Syncope is usually limited to the most severely affected cases and numerous other symptoms of dysautonomia are generally present when the disorder progresses to symptomatic OH, but the condition may be easily overlooked and may be present in the absence of severe diabetes.

What Precautions Should Patients Take and How Should they be Informed?

A number of exacerbating factors are important for the both the patient and physician to consider to take appropriate precautions or avoid certain situations (see **Box 1**). Prominent examples include factors that promote vasodilation such as a warm environment, hot bath, fever, and alcohol ingestion. Additionally, large meals (especially if high in carbohydrates—pasta, pancakes, etc.), prolonged standing (especially after recumbency), prolonged bedrest, early morning, relative volume depletion, and medication effects may play a role. Arising in stages can minimize an exercise-induced reflex, in part responsible for the immediate BP drop on active standing. Patients with chronic, symptomatic OH may learn to recognize these conditions and take precautions, but often need some advance physician instruction.[92,93]

How Ominous is a DAN Diagnosis?

Much attention has focused on the significance of diabetic autonomic dysfunction on long-term prognosis and survival.[94,95] Ewing and colleagues[94] found 56% of 73 patients with DAN died within 5 years, but many deaths were due to non-autonomic complications, such as renal failure. Other studies have shown an increased but less ominous mortality rate in diabetics with DAN but not other complications at the outset (23% at 8 years) compared with diabetics without DAN and similar disease duration (3% at 8 years).[95,96]

Other important entities to consider because of the severity of autonomic failure are hereditary and acquired amyloidosis. Although much less frequent, early recognition is important so symptomatic treatment and potential interventions such as hepatic or bone marrow transplantation can be considered.[97] Other forms of autonomic neuropathy with known symptomatic OH are listed in **Box 2**.

Is There a Subacute Onset Form of Autonomic Neuropathy that can Produce Syncope?

An unusual but notable entity with acute or subacute onset is acute autonomic neuropathy, which may target cholinergic, adrenergic nerves, or both (acute pandysautonomia). A viral syndrome precedes roughly half, slightly less than the analogous disorder–Guillain-Barré syndrome.[92,98,99] Patients develop generalized or partial autonomic failure, frequently including marked, symptomatic OH, except in the restricted cholinergic form (25%). Attack on enteric neurons is common and can lead to confusion with gastroenteritis or in severe cases, an acute abdomen prompting surgical exploration (pseudo-obstruction). An attenuated form has been proposed to underlie many cases of orthostatic intolerance discussed later.[100] A paraneoplastic form is indistinguishable on clinical or laboratory grounds. The cause is presumably immune-mediated and anti-autonomic ganglia acetylcholine receptor antibodies are found in roughly 40% of cases as well as 10% of orthostatic intolerance patients.[101,102] Anecdotal reports of improvement with intravenous immune globulin are known.[103,104] Brady- and tachyarrhythmias and orthostatic hypotension are also common in typical Guillain-Barré syndrome patients, especially in more severe cases.[105]

Can Syncope be a Sign of a Paraneoplastic Syndrome?

Although uncommon, recognition of paraneoplastic syndromes is crucial to prompt an early search for the underlying malignancy. Several syndromes have prominent autonomic involvement, some with OH severe enough to cause syncope. This phenomenon should be considered in adult cases with new onset OH or autonomic failure, especially with acute or subacute onset. Cases are most commonly but not exclusively associated with small cell lung cancer and the neuropathy onset typically precedes tumor detection; a variety of associated antibodies are known, including anti-Hu (ANNA-1) antibodies.[99,106]

WHAT ARE IMPORTANT CONSIDERATIONS WITH PARKINSONISM AND AUTONOMIC FAILURE?

Marked autonomic failure (AF) is frequent in patients with multiple system atrophy (MSA) previously known as the Shy-Drager syndrome.[107] MSA is a group of disorders with overlapping neuropathology and may have autonomic, parkinsonian, or cerebellar onset. Other manifestations include sleep apnea, incontinence, impotence, dystonia, inspiratory stridor, lack of rest tremor, and no significant or sustained L-dopa response. The disorder is common and increasingly recognized because of better awareness of the condition.[108] Syncope from OH in these patients is not uncommon and can be an initial complaint.

Many idiopathic Parkinson's disease (IPD) patients, however, have autonomically mediated complaints, most commonly constipation, but OH if present is usually asymptomatic. Exacerbation or inducement of OH from medications such as L-dopa is recognized. A small subset of patients with otherwise typical PD has severe autonomic failure including symptomatic OH and is separately designated as PD with autonomic failure. However, increased numbers of Parkinson patients are recognized to have separate autonomic failure, most notably cardiac sympathetic denervation, demonstrated by abnormal cardiac [18]fluorodopamine PET studies.

WHAT IS PURE AUTONOMIC FAILURE?

Pure autonomic failure (PAF) or Bradbury-Eggleston syndrome is a separate disorder previously known as idiopathic orthostatic hypotension.[109] The disorder is a profound, slowly progressive disorder with disabling OH, usually with onset after age 50. By definition, no other neurologic impairment is seen, and the ultimate diagnosis is often delayed for 3–5 years to ensure that MSA does not emerge. Autopsies show a similar pattern of Lewy body inclusions in autonomic and enteric ganglia as Parkinson's disease with AF and diffuse Lewy body dementia. The relationship between IPD and PAF is not clear, but shared neurodegenerative mechanisms are likely.[92,110]

Dopamine β-hydroxylase deficiency is a rare but treatable entity with severe OH and syncope and nearly undetectable norepinephrine and epinephrine and elevated dopamine levels that fail to change with upright posture.[111] If recognized, treatment with the norepinephrine precursor L-threo-dihydroxyphenylserine (droxidopa) can be beneficial.[109] Benefit from this orphan drug has also been shown in patients with other forms of autonomic failure and is currently undergoing phase III clinical trials.[112]

Numerous other common and uncommon disorders affecting the brain and spinal cord affect autonomic function but less commonly cause symptomatic OH unless provoked by aggravating conditions.

HOW CAN AUTONOMIC FAILURE BE BETTER DOCUMENTED IN SUSPECTED CASES?

Measurable OH on standing is a clinical sign but not proof of autonomic dysfunction assuming confounding factors such as hypovolemia, hemorrhage, and medication effects are absent. Current consensus specifies at least a 20-mmHg systolic or 10-mmHg diastolic drop within 3 minutes.[113] Orthostatic hypotension is also prevalent but asymptomatic under most conditions in the elderly. Confirmation by formal autonomic testing is desirable, if available, to document the systems involved and severity under the more controlled conditions dictated by these laboratories.[114] Laboratories and trained physicians are increasingly available. Standard and well-established tests most commonly used and most extensively examined are responses to controlled perturbations of cardiovagal (parasympathetic), adrenergic, and sudomotor (sweating) reflexes, but numerous other measures are known and employed as well.[113] Tilt table studies are only one aspect of testing and provide a more uniform and controlled orthostatic stress than standing.

HOW IMPORTANT ARE MEDICATION EFFECTS IN CAUSING OR EXACERBATING SYNCOPE?

Numerous mediations are known to exacerbate or induce OH, especially in the elderly, who may have altered pharmacodynamics and other reasons for enhanced toxicity and are often on numerous medications. Prominent examples include drugs with antihypertensive action, notably vasodilators. In addition, antiparkinsonian drugs, antidepressants, erectile dysfunction agents, and antipsychotics are known to produce or enhance OH (see **Box 2**). It is not unusual to evaluate patients with recurrent OH or syncope and find them taking several BP-lowering medications.

HOW IS SYMPTOMATIC ORTHOSTATIC HYPOTENSION TREATED?

Numerous pharmacologic and nonpharmacologic interventions are used to improve OH and orthostatic tolerance.[115] In mild forms, adequate precautions and avoidance of precipitating factors may be adequate, but lesser indicators of hypoperfusion without imminent syncope need to be considered such as postural "coat-hanger" pattern shoulder fatigue and headache (local muscle ischemia), pure vertigo, postprandial fatigue, and cognitive slowing. An increase in sodium and fluid intake may be adequate to reduce mild symptomatic OH. Simple water intake and salt supplements are independently shown to be beneficial.[53,116] Other simple initial measures include raising the head of the bed with blocks (4–6 inches) to partially stimulate baroreceptors and decrease nocturnal diuresis. Measures such as leg crossing, squatting, stooping, avoidance of prolonged motionless standing, and arising in stages are helpful if able to perform, as discussed earlier. Isotonic exercise and avoidance of straining, coughing, and isometric exercise may be beneficial. More recently noted are certain respiratory countermaneuvers that can lessen OH.[117] Compressive garments are less commonly used and should include abdominal compression for effect, often making them too cumbersome to expect compliance. Meal adjustments with small, more frequent meals low in carbohydrates are helpful in patients with postprandial hypotension. Re-evaluation of the need for prescribed BP-lowering and autonomically active agents should be considered as discussed earlier. If not sufficient, first-line medications include fludrocortisone or the α-adrenergic agonist midodrine or both.[115,118] Midodrine is relatively short-acting and must be dosed to cover the most vulnerable periods, especially early morning, and should not be taken after 6 PM. Concerns of excessive fluid retention and heart failure must be addressed, especially in the elderly. Relative anemia can exacerbate OH. Rarely, supine hypertension is severe enough to cause concern, and a small dose of an antihypertensive overnight is used unless morning BP is excessively affected or overnight bathroom trips cause syncope. Moderate supine hypertension is generally accepted in these patients to reduce syncope risk, but concerns have been raised about long-term consequences.[119] Second-line agents are numerous and are sometimes effective if earlier agents have failed. Pyridostigmine, an acetylcholinesterase inhibitor, has shown significant improvement in standing BP in patients with orthostatic hypotension without notable worsening of supine hypertension.[120] Other examples include nonsteroidal anti-inflammatories, other sympathomimetics, some SSRIs, caffeine, octreotide, and vasopressin analogs.[115] Third-line agents, including dihydroergotamine, the β-blockers pindolol and xamoterolol, clonidine, and yohimbine, can be tried in refractory cases.

WHAT OTHER PHENOMENA CAN MIMIC SYNCOPE?

Brief mention should be made of other phenomena that can mimic syncope. Drop attacks are an acute loss of postural tone with or without loss of consciousness. Episodes with clearly unaltered consciousness should be easily distinguished. Vascular events such as vertebrobasilar or less commonly bilateral anterior circulation ischemia may lead to drop attacks that can impair consciousness. Neurologic markers, for example diplopia, ataxia, and weakness are often present at least transiently to help distinguish. Processes that cause an abrupt surge in intracranial pressure such as a ruptured aneurysm or ventricular system blockage can lead to abrupt loss of consciousness, but not generally rapid recovery.

Psychiatric events can mimic both seizures (pseudoseizures or nonepileptogenic seizures) and syncope. Frequent atypical or unwitnessed events without corroborating clinical or laboratory evidence may be an indication. A significant prior psychiatric history may raise suspicion, but is not diagnostic in isolation.

CAN SEVERE PRESYNCOPAL SYMPTOMS DEVELOP WITHOUT A SIGNIFICANT DROP IN BLOOD PRESSURE?

All forms of syncope including reflex syncope, orthostatic hypotension, and cardiac causes can technically be considered forms of orthostatic intolerance. However, usually implied by the term is a group of disorders with chronic, consistent orthostatic symptoms without significant OH in contrast to the episodic neurally mediated and reflex disorders.[121–123]

WHAT IS POSTURAL ORTHOSTATIC TACHYCARDIA SYNDROME?

A group of disorders with heterogeneous mechanisms and even more designations including postural orthostatic tachycardia syndrome (POTS) and idiopathic orthostatic intolerance (OI) has gathered attention in recent years.[121–123] The incidence is unknown but similar patients are commonly referred to autonomic disorder clinics as well as syncope centers. The hallmark is a combination of posturally induced symptoms and robust tachycardia without significant BP decline. Criteria for the degree of tachycardia necessary for diagnosis are currently an increase of 30 beats per minute within 5 minutes of standing or tilt and/or an absolute level over 120, assuming secondary causes such as hypovolemia, recent illness, or prolonged recumbency are excluded. Symptoms, many of which are due to cerebral hypoperfusion, include lightheadedness or dizziness, blunted cognition, palpitations, blurred vision, fatigue, exercise intolerance, and numerous others. Symptoms are usually fully or partially relieved by sitting or lying down. Similar patients have been long recognized under multiple other names (irritable heart syndrome, Soldier's heart, mitral valve prolapse syndrome) but many remain undiagnosed or dismissed as functional, in part due to the relative lack of specificity of the complaints and possibly the higher prevalence in young, otherwise healthy women.

WHAT ARE THE SUSPECTED MECHANISMS TO THIS PARADOXICAL GROUP OF DISORDERS?

Mechanisms explored are multiple, none of which are evident in all patients but each may be a contributant to orthostatic intolerance in individual cases. Examples include diminished plasma volume or red cell mass despite adequate attempts at repletion, exaggerated venous pooling, circulating vasodilators, partial lower limb autonomic denervation, brainstem dysfunction leading to aberrant cerebral autoregulation, altered baroreflex sensitivity, and β-adrenoreceptor hypersensitivity. Symptoms often begin subacutely, and in retrospect an attenuated bout of acute autonomic neuropathy may have occurred in roughly 30%.[100] Peripheral impairment of vasoconstriction with excessive venous pooling is common in these patients and some show postural swelling and purplish color changes in dependent areas as a marker. In support, laboratory evidence of distal autonomic neuropathy, other autonomic symptoms, and a prior viral prodrome has been found in a large subset of patients.

Many patients also have evidence of increased sympathetic activation including an exaggerated plasma norepinephrine increase on standing and an augmented HR increase to isoproterenol. Prior names have focused on this aspect and included descriptive terms such as *sympathotonic*, *hyperadrenergic*, and *hyperdynamic β-adrenergic*. Neurally mediated syncope can also occur in these patients and the incidence may be as high as 40%.[122] Interestingly, genetic defects in a norepinephrine transporter gene manifests a phenotype with many overlapping clinical features with OI and blocking this transporter with reboxetine reproduced many OI symptoms and signs in normal subjects.[124,125]

Not surprisingly, many patients are inappropriately diagnosed, sometimes as chronic fatigue syndrome (CFS) or panic disorder, but the clear postural triggers, not social or situational triggers or chronic symptoms irrespective of orthostatic stress and other features, should separate these disorders. Fatigue, presumably from recurrent bouts of hypoperfusion, is also a common complaint in patients with recurrent vasovagal syncope.[126] Moreover, all three conditions occur in similar patient populations. The finding of an increased incidence of positive tilt tests of CFS patients previously complicated the distinction, but the importance of orthostatic intolerance as a common cause of CFS-related fatigue remains controversial.[127,128] One randomized trial of fludrocortisone showed no significant benefit in one CFS population.[129] A minority of patients (including those with CFS diagnoses) referred for tilt testing will demonstrate orthostatic tachycardia and signs of orthostatic intolerance instead.

There is an overrepresentation of this syndrome in patients with mitral valve prolapse and the so-called mitral valve prolapse syndrome shares many clinical features.[130] Anecdotal reports of patients with grade I Chiari malformations have been noted and popularized in the media, but no controlled scientific data are available yet to confirm an association.[131]

HOW ARE THESE PATIENTS TREATED?

Rational treatment of OI is ideally dependent on dissecting out which mechanism discussed is the most likely cause based on clinical grounds and results of autonomic and cardiologic testing. In some cases, specialized evaluation at a center with additional capabilities may be necessary. In general, the options overlap with both neurally mediated syncope and orthostatic hypotension interventions and medications. Beta-blockade is often empirically tried before diagnosis to block the tachycardia, but may be detrimental in patients where the HR increase is an important adaptive response and not a primary abnormality. Intravenous fluids are usually much more efficacious than sedation in acute situations.

SUMMARY

Syncope and orthostatic intolerance remain common and significant clinical problems with many undocumented, misdiagnosed, or cryptogenic cases. Careful clinical assessment and application of advancing laboratory support can further improve diagnosis and treatment. Despite the depth of existing research into these common problems, many underlying mechanisms remain unproven.

REFERENCES

1. Kapoor WN. Syncope. N Engl J Med 2000;343:1856–62.
2. Lempert T, Bauer M, Schmidt D. Syncope: a videometric analysis of 56 episodes of transient cerebral hypoxia. Ann Neurol 1994;36:233–7.
3. Raj SR, Sheldon RS. Permanent cardiac pacing to prevent vasovagal syncope. Curr Opin Cardiol 2002;17:90–5.
4. Kaufmann H. Neurally mediated syncope: pathogenesis, diagnosis, and treatment. Neurology 1995;45(Suppl 5):S12–8.
5. Abboud FM. Neurocardiogenic syncope. N Engl J Med 1993;328:1117–20.
6. Bloomfield D, Maurer M, Bigger JT Jr. Effects of age on outcome of tilt-table testing. Am J Cardiol 1999;83:1055–8.
7. Mathias CJ, Deguchi K, Bleasedale-Barr K, et al. Familial vasovagal syncope and pseudosyncope: observations in a case with both natural and adopted siblings. Clin Auton Res 2000;10:43–5.
8. Mosqueda-Garcia R, Furlan R, Tank J, et al. The elusive pathophysiology of neurally mediated syncope. Circulation 2000;102:2898–906.
9. Lewis T. Vasovagal syncope and the carotid sinus mechanism. Br Med J 1932;1:873–6.
10. El-Bedawi KM, Wahbha MA, Hainsworth R. Cardiac pacing does not improve orthostatic tolerance in patients with vasovagal syncope. Clin Auton Res 1994;4:233–7.
11. Oberg B, Thoren P. Increased activity in the left ventricular receptors during hemorrhage or occlusion of caval veins in the cat; a possible cause of the vasovagal reaction. Acta Physiol Scand 1972;85:164–73.
12. Norcliffe-Kaufmann LJ, Kaufmann H, Hainsworth R. Enhanced vascular responses to hypocapnia in neurally mediated syncope. Ann Neurol 2008;63(3):288–94.
13. Alboni P, Alboni M, Bertorelle G. The origin of vasovagal syncope: to protect the heart or to escape predation? Clin Auton Res 2008;18(4):170–8.
14. Parry SW, Kenny RA. Carotid sinus syndrome masquerading as treatment resistant epilepsy. Postgrad Med J 2000;76:656–8.
15. Davies AJ, Steen N, Kenny RA. Carotid sinus hypersensitivity is common in older patients presenting to an accident and emergency department with unexplained falls. Age Ageing 2001;30:289–93.
16. Sutton R, Petersen M, Brignole M, et al. Proposed classification for tilt induced vasovagal syncope. Eur J Card Pacing Electrophysiol 1992;3:180–3.
17. Sutton R, Brignole M, Menozzi C, et al. Dual chamber pacing in the treatment of neurally mediated tilt positive cardioinhibitory syncope. Pacemaker versus no

therapy- a multicenter randomized study. The vasovagal syncope international study (VASIS) investigators. Circulation 2000;102:294–9.

18. O'Mahony D. Carotid sinus hypersensitivity in old age: clinical syndrome or physical sign? Age Ageing 2001;30:273–4.

19. Allan LM, Ballard CG, Allen J, et al. Autonomic dysfunction in dementia. J Neurol Neurosurg Psychiatr 2007;78(7):671–7.

20. Kenny RA, Shaw FE, O'Brien JT, et al. Carotid sinus syndrome is common in dementia with Lewy bodies and correlates with deep white matter lesions. J Neurol Neurosurg Psychiatr 2004;75(7):966–71.

21. Kenny RA. Carotid sinus syndrome: a modifiable risk factor for nonaccidental falls in older adults (SAFE PACE). J Am Coll Cardiol 2001;38:1491–6.

22. Hilal H, Massumi R. Fatal ventricular fibrillation during carotid sinus stimulation. N Engl J Med 1966;275:157–8.

23. Haslam RH, Freigang B. Cough syncope mimicking epilepsy in asthmatic children. Can J Neurol Sci 1985;12:45–7.

24. Mattle HP, Nirkko AC, Baumgartner RW, et al. Transient cerebral circulatory arrest coincides with fainting in cough syncope. Neurology 1995;45: 498–501.

25. Gelisse P, Genton P. Cough syncope misinterpreted as epileptic seizure. Epileptic Disord 2008;10(3):223–4.

26. Lyle CB, Monroe JT, Flinn DE, et al. Micturition syncope: a report of 24 cases. N Engl J Med 1961;265:982–6.

27. Proudfit WL, Forteza ME. Micturition syncope. N Engl J Med 1959;260:328–31.

28. Kapoor WN, Peterson JR, Karpf M. Micturition syncope: a reappraisal. JAMA 1985;253:796–8.

29. Riley HA, German WJ, Wortis H, et al. Glossopharyngeal neuralgia initiating or associated with cardiac arrest. Trans Am Neurol Assoc 1942;68:28–9.

30. Wallin BG, Westerberg C, Sundlof G. Syncope induced by glossopharyngeal neuralgia. Sympathetic outflow to muscle. Neurology 1984;34:522–4.

31. Zaidi A, Clough P, Cooper P, et al. Misdiagnosis of epilepsy: many seizure-like attacks have a cardiovascular cause. J Am Coll Cardiol 2000;36:181–4.

32. Gastaut H, Fischer-Williams M. Electroencephalographic study of syncope: its differentiation from epilepsy. Lancet 1957;2:1018–25.

33. Brenner RP. Electroencephalography in syncope. J Clin Neurophysiol 1997;14: 197–209.

34. Grubb BP, Gerard G, Roush K, et al. Differentiation of convulsive syncope and epilepsy with head-up tilt testing. Ann Intern Med 1991;115:871–6.

35. Lin JT, Zeigler DK, Lai CW Bayer W. Convulsive syncope in blood donors. Ann Neurol 1982;11:523–8.

36. Patel SJ, Jackson G, Marshall A. Convulsive syncope in young adults: think of a cardiac cause. Int J Clin Pract 2001;55:639–40.

37. Eiris-Punal J, Rodriguez-Nunez A, Fernandez-Martinez N, et al. Usefulness of head-upright tilt test for distinguishing between syncope and epilepsy in children. Epilepsia 2001;42:709–13.

38. Vicenzini E, Pro S, Strano S, et al. Combined transcranial Doppler and EEG recording in vasovagal syncope. Eur Neurol 2008;60(5):258–63.

39. Ganzeboom KS, Colman N, Reitsma JB, et al. Prevalence and triggers of syncope in medical students. Am J Cardiol 2003;91:1006–8.

40. Linzer M, Yang EH, Estes NA 3rd, et al. Part 1. Value of history, physical examination and electrocardiography. Clinical efficacy assessment project of the American College of Physicians. Ann Intern Med 1997;126:989–96.

41. Schnipper JL, Kapoor WN. Diagnostic evaluation and management of patients with syncope. Med Clin North Am 2001;85:423–56.
42. Brignole M, Alboni P, Benditt D, et al. Task force on syncope, European Society of Cardiology. Part 2. Diagnostic tests and treatment: summary of recommendations. Europace 2001;3:261–8.
43. Brignole M, Menozzi C, Lolli G, et al. Long-term outcome of paced and non-paced patients with severe carotid sinus syndrome. Am J Cardiol 1992;69: 1039–43.
44. Humm AM, Mathias CJ. Unexplained syncope–is screening for carotid sinus hypersensitivity indicated in all patients aged >40 years? J Neurol Neurosurg Psychiatr 2006;77(11):1267–70.
45. Kenny RA, Ingram A, Bayliss J, et al. Head-up tilt: a useful test for investigating unexplained syncope. Lancet 1986;1:1352–5.
46. Schondorf R, Benoit J, Stein R. Cerebral autoregulation in orthostatic intolerance. Ann N Y Acad Sci 2001;940:514–26.
47. Gatzoulis KA, Toutouzas PK. Neurocardiogenic syncope, aetiology and management. Drugs 2001;61:1415–23.
48. Benditt DG, Ferguson DW, Grubb BP, et al. Tilt table testing for assessing syncope. American College of Cardiology expert consensus document. J Am Coll Cardiol 1996;28:263–75.
49. Sutton R. How and when to pace in vasovagal syncope. J Cardiovasc Electrophysiol 2002;13(Suppl 1):S4–16.
50. Leman RB, Clarke E, Gillette P. Significant complications can occur with ischemic heart disease and tilt table testing. Pacing Clin Electrophysiol 1999;22:675–7.
51. Davis TL, Freemon FR. Electroencephalography should not be routine in the evaluation of syncope in adults. Arch Intern Med 1990;150:2027–9.
52. El-Sayed H, Hainsworth R. Salt supplement increases plasma volume and orthostatic tolerance in patients with unexplained syncope. Heart 1996;75:134–40.
53. Shannon JR, Diedrich A, Biaggioni I, et al. Water drinking as a treatment for orthostatic syndromes. Am J Med 2002;112:355–60.
54. Calkins H. Pharmacological approaches to therapy for vasovagal syncope. Am J Cardiol 1999;84:20Q–5Q.
55. Cox MM, Perlman BA, Mayor MR, et al. Acute and long-term beta-adrenergic blockade for patients with neurocardiogenic syncope. J Am Coll Cardiol 1995; 26:1293–8.
56. Natale A, Sra J, Dhala A, et al. Efficacy of different treatment strategies for neurocardiogenic syncope. Pacing Clin Electrophysiol 1995;18:655–62.
57. Mahanonda N, Bhuripanyo K, Kangkagate C, et al. Randomized double-blind, placebo-controlled trial of oral atenolol in patients with unexplained syncope and positive upright tilt table test results. Am Heart J 1995;130:1250–3.
58. Madrid AH, Ortega J, Rebollo JG, et al. Lack of efficacy of atenolol for the prevention of neurally mediated syncope in a highly symptomatic population: a prospective, double-blind, randomized and placebo controlled study. J Am Coll Cardiol 2001;37:554–9.
59. Sheldon R, Connolly S, Rose S, et al. Prevention of Syncope Trial (POST): a randomized, placebo-controlled study of metoprolol in the prevention of vasovagal syncope. Circulation 2006;113:1164–70.
60. Raj SR, Rose S, Ritchie D, et al. The second prevention of syncope trial (POST II)–a randomized clinical trial of fludrocortisone for the prevention of neurally mediated syncope: rationale and study design. Am Heart J 2006; 151(6):1186.e11–7.

61. Di Girolamo E, Di Iorio C, Sabatini P, et al. Effects of paroxetine hydrochloride, a selective serotonin reuptake inhibitor, on refractory vasovagal syncope: a randomized, double-blind, placebo-controlled study. J Am Coll Cardiol 1999;33: 1227–30.

62. Ward CR, Gray JC, Gilroy JJ, et al. Midodrine: a role in the management of neurocardiogenic syncope. Heart 1998;79:45–9.

63. Morillo CA, Leitch JW, Yee R, et al. A placebo-controlled trial of intravenous and oral disopyramide for prevention of neurally mediated syncope induced by head-up tilt. J Am Coll Cardiol 1993;22:1843–8.

64. Raviele A, Brignole M, Sutton R, et al. Effect of etilefrine in preventing syncopal recurrence in patients with vasovagal syncope: a double-blind, randomized, placebo-controlled trial. The vasovagal syncope international study. Circulation 1999;99:1452–7.

65. Reybrouck T, Heidbuchel H, Van de Werf F, et al. Tilt training: a treatment for malignant and recurrent neurocardiogenic syncope. Pacing Clin Electrophysiol 2000;23:493–8.

66. Krediet CT, van Dijk N, Linzer M, et al. Management of vasovagal syncope: controlling or aborting faints by leg crossing and muscle tensing. Circulation 2002; 106:1684–9.

67. van Dijk N, Quartieri F, Blanc JJ, et al. Effectiveness of physical counterpressure maneuvers in preventing vasovagal syncope: the physical counterpressure manoeuvres trial (PC-Trial). J Am Coll Cardiol 2006;48:1652–7.

68. Krediet CT, Go-Schön IK, van Lieshout JJ, et al. Optimizing squatting as a physical maneuver to prevent vasovagal syncope. Clin Auton Res 2008;18(4):179–86.

69. Connolly SJ, Sheldon R, Roberts RS, et al. The North American Vasovagal Pacemaker Study (VPS). A randomized trial of permanent cardiac pacing for the prevention of vasovagal syncope. J Am Coll Cardiol 1999;33:16–20.

70. Ammirati F, Colivicchi F, Santini M. Permanent cardiac pacing versus medical treatment for the prevention of recurrent vasovagal syncope: a multicenter, randomized, controlled trial. Circulation 2001;104:52–7.

71. Connolly SJ, Sheldon R, Thorpe KE, et al. Pacemaker therapy for prevention of syncope in patients with recurrent severe vasovagal syncope: second vasovagal pacemaker study (VPS II): a randomized trial. JAMA 2003;289:2224–9.

72. Raviele A, Giada F, Menozzi C, et al. A randomized, double-blind, placebo-controlled study of permanent cardiac pacing for the treatment of recurrent tilt-induced vasovagal syncope. The vasovagal syncope and pacing trial (SYNPACE). Eur Heart J 2004;25:1741–8.

73. Sud S, Massel D, Klein GJ, et al. The expectation effect and cardiac pacing for refractory vasovagal syncope. Am J Med 2007;120(1):54–62.

74. Reeves AL, Nollet KE, Klass DW, et al. The ictal bradycardia syndrome. Epilepsia 1996;37:983–7.

75. Schuele SU, Bermeo AC, Locatelli E, et al. Ictal asystole: a benign condition? Epilepsia 2008;49(1):168–71.

76. Tinuper P, Bisulli F, Cerullo A, et al. Ictal bradycardia in partial epileptic seizures: autonomic investigation in three cases and literature review. Brain 2001;124: 2361–71.

77. Keilson M, Hauser W, Magrill J, et al. ECG abnormalities in patients with epilepsy. Neurology 1987;37:1624–6.

78. Locatelli ER, Varghese JP, Shuaib A, et al. Cardiac asystole and bradycardia as a manifestation of left temporal lobe complex partial seizure. Ann Intern Med 1999;130:581–3.

79. Tatum WO, Winters L, Gieron M, et al. Outpatient seizure identification. Result of 502 patients using computer-assisted ambulatory EEG. J Clin Neurophysiol 2001;18:14–9.
80. Chadwick D, Smith D. The misdiagnosis of epilepsy. Br Med J 2002;24:495–6.
81. Scheepers B, Clough P, Pickles C. The misdiagnosis of epilepsy: findings of a population study. Seizure 1998;5:403–6.
82. Smith D, Defalla BA, Chadwick DW. The misdiagnosis of epilepsy and the management of refractory epilepsy in a specialist clinic. QJM 1999;92:15–23.
83. Grubb BP, Kosinski DJ. Syncope resulting from autonomic insufficiency syndromes associated with orthostatic intolerance. Med Clin North Am 2001;85: 457–72.
84. Mathias CJ. Orthostatic hypotension: causes, mechanisms, and influencing factors. Neurology 1995;45(Suppl 5):S6–11.
85. Shibao C, Grijalva CG, Raj SR, et al. Orthostatic hypotension-related hospitalizations in the United States. Am J Med 2007;120:975–80.
86. Consensus statement on the definition of orthostatic hypotension, pure autonomic failure, and multiple system atrophy. The consensus committee of the American Autonomic Society and the American Academy of Neurology. Neurology 1996;46:1470.
87. Low PA. The effect of aging on the autonomic nervous system. In: Low PA, editor. Clinical autonomic disorders. 2nd edition. Philadelphia: Lippincott-Raven; 1997. p. 161–75.
88. Robertson D, Kincaid DW, Haile V, et al. The head and neck discomfort of autonomic failure: an unrecognized aetiology of headache. Clin Auton Res 1994;4: 99–103.
89. Gibbons CH, Freeman R. Delayed orthostatic hypotension: a frequent cause of orthostatic intolerance. Neurology 2006;67:28–32.
90. Streeten DH, Anderson GH. Mechanisms of orthostatic hypotension and tachycardia in patients with pheochromocytoma. Am J Hypertens 1996;9:760–9.
91. Freeman R. Autonomic peripheral neuropathy. Neurol Clin 2007;25(1):277–301.
92. Weimer LH. Neurogenic orthostatic hypotension, autonomic failure, and autonomic neuropathy. In: Rowland LP, Pedley TA, editors. Merritt's neurology. 12th edition. Philadelphia: Lippincott Williams & Wilkins, in press.
93. Weimer LH. Syncope and orthostatic intolerance for the primary care physician. Prim Care 2004;31(1):175–99.
94. Ewing DJ, Campbell IW, Clarke BF. The natural history of diabetic autonomic neuropathy. Q J Med 1980;49:95–108.
95. Rathman W, Ziegler D, Jahnke M, et al. Mortality in diabetic patients with cardiovascular autonomic neuropathy. Diabet Med 1993;10:820–4.
96. Gerritsen J, Dekker JM, TenVoorde BJ, et al. Impaired autonomic function is associated with increased mortality, especially in subjects with diabetes, hypertension, or a history of cardiovascular disease: the hoorn study. Diabetes Care 2001;24:1793–8.
97. Bergethon PR, Sabin TD, Lewis D. Improvement in the polyneuropathy associated with familial amyloid polyneuropathy after liver transplantation. Neurology 1996;47:944–51.
98. Suarez GA, Fealey RD, Camilleri M, et al. Idiopathic autonomic neuropathy: clinical, neurophysiologic, and follow-up studies on 27 patients. Neurology 1994; 44(9):1675–82.
99. Etienne M, Weimer LH. Immune-mediated autonomic neuropathies. Curr Neurol Neurosci Rep 2006;6(1):57–64.

100. Schondorf R, Low PA. Idiopathic postural orthostatic tachycardia syndrome. An attenuated form of acute pandysautonomia? Neurology 1993;43:132–7 [STOP].

101. Vernino S, Adamski J, Kryzer TJ, et al. Neuronal nicotinic ACh receptor antibody in subacute autonomic neuropathy and cancer-related syndromes. Neurology 1998;50:1806–13.

102. Vernino S, Low PA, Fealey RD, et al. Autoantibodies to ganglionic acetylcholine receptors in autoimmune autonomic neuropathies. N Engl J Med 2000;343: 847–55.

103. Heafield MTE, Gammage MD, Nightingale S, et al. Idiopathic dysautonomia treated with intravenous gammaglobulin. Lancet 1996;347:28–9.

104. Smit AAJ, Vermeulen M, Koelman HTM, et al. Unusual recovery from acute panautonomic neuropathy after immunoglobulin therapy. Mayo Clin Proc 1997;72: 333–5.

105. Zochodne DW. Autonomic involvement in Guillain-Barré syndrome: a review. Muscle Nerve 1994;17:1145–55.

106. Camdessanche JP, Antoine JC, Honnorat J, et al. Paraneoplastic peripheral neuropathy associated with anti-Hu antibodies. A clinical and electrophysiological study of 20 patients. Brain 2002;125:166–75.

107. Gilman S, Wenning GK, Low PA, et al. Second consensus statement on the diagnosis of multiple system atrophy. Neurology 2008;71(9):670–6.

108. Magalhães M, Wenning GK, Daniel SE, et al. Autonomic dysfunction in pathologically confirmed multiple system atrophy and idiopathic Parkinson's disease–a retrospective comparison. Acta Neurol Scand 1995;91:98–102.

109. Biaggioni I, Robertson D. Endogenous restoration of noradrenaline by precursor therapy in dopamine-beta-hydroxylase deficiency. Lancet 1987;2:1170–2.

110. Hague K, Lento P, Morgello S, et al. The distribution of Lewy bodies in pure autonomic failure: autopsy findings and review of the literature. Acta Neuropathol 1997;94:192–6.

111. Biaggioni I, Hollister AS, Robertson D. Dopamine in dopamine-beta-hydroxylase deficiency. N Engl J Med 1987;317:1415–6.

112. Mathias CJ, Senard JM, Braune S, et al. L-threo-dihydroxyphenylserine (L-threo-DOPS; droxidopa) in the management of neurogenic orthostatic hypotension: a multi-national, multi-center, dose-ranging study in multiple system atrophy and pure autonomic failure. Clin Auton Res 2001;11:235–42.

113. Assessment: clinical autonomic testing report of the therapeutics and technology assessment subcommittee of the American Association of Neurology. Neurology 1996;46:873–80.

114. Hilz MJ, Dutsch M. Quantitative studies of autonomic function. Muscle Nerve 2006;33(1):6–20.

115. Freeman R. Clinical practice. Neurogenic orthostatic hypotension. N Engl J Med 2008;358(6):615–24.

116. Mathias CJ, Young TM. Water drinking in the management of orthostatic intolerance due to orthostatic hypotension, vasovagal syncope and the postural tachycardia syndrome. Eur J Neurol 2004;11(9):613–9.

117. Thijs RD, Wieling W, van den Aardweg JG, et al. Respiratory countermaneuvers in autonomic failure. Neurology 2007;69(6):582–5.

118. Jankovic J, Gilden JL, Hiner BC, et al. Neurogenic orthostatic hypotension: a double-blind, placebo-controlled study with midodrine. JAMA 1993;95: 38–48.

119. Vagaonescu TD, Saadia D, Tuhrim S, et al. Hypertensive cardiovascular damage in patients with primary autonomic failure. Lancet 2000;355:725–6.

120. Singer W, Sandroni P, Opfer-Gehrking TL, et al. Pyridostigmine treatment trial in neurogenic orthostatic hypotension. Arch Neurol 2006;63:513–8.
121. Low PA, Opfer-Gehrking TL, Textor SC, et al. Postural tachycardia syndrome (POTS). Neurology 1995;45(4):S19–25.
122. Jacob G, Biaggioni I. Idiopathic orthostatic intolerance and postural tachycardia syndromes. Am J Med Sci 1999;317:88–101.
123. Medow MS, Stewart JM. The postural tachycardia syndrome. Cardiol Rev 2007; 15(2):67–75.
124. Shannon JR, Flattem NL, Jordan J, et al. Orthostatic intolerance and tachycardia associated with norepinephrine-transporter deficiency. N Engl J Med 2000; 342(8):541–9.
125. Schroeder C, Tank J, Boschmann M, et al. Selective norepinephrine reuptake inhibition as a human model of orthostatic intolerance. Circulation 2002;105: 347–53.
126. Legge H, Norton M, Newton JL. Fatigue is significant in vasovagal syncope and is associated with autonomic symptoms. Europace 2008;10(9):1095–101.
127. Rowe PC, Bou-Holaigah I, Kan JS, et al. Is neurally mediated hypotension an unrecognized cause of chronic fatigue? Lancet 1995;345:623–4.
128. Jones JF, Nicholson A, Nisenbaum R, et al. Orthostatic instability in a population-based study of chronic fatigue syndrome. Am J Med 2005;118(12):1415.
129. Rowe PC, Calkins H, DeBusk K, et al. Fludrocortisone acetate to treat neurally mediated hypotension in chronic fatigue syndrome: a randomized controlled trial. JAMA 2001;285:52–9.
130. Taylor AA, Davies AO, Mares A, et al. Spectrum of dysautonomia in mitral valve prolapse. Am J Med 1989;86:267–74.
131. Garland EM, Robertson D. Chiari I malformation as a cause of orthostatic intolerance symptoms: a media myth? Am J Med 2001;111:546–52.

Multiple Sclerosis

Ardith M. Courtney, DO[a], Katherine Treadaway, LCSW-ACP[a],
Gina Remington, BSN, RN[a], Elliot Frohman, MD, PhD[a,b,*]

KEYWORDS

- Multiple sclerosis • Disease modifying therapy
- Magnetic resonance imaging • Optic neuritis

EPIDEMIOLOGY AND GENETICS

Multiple sclerosis (MS) affects approximately 350,000 individuals in the United States and more than 1 million individuals worldwide. Although the true onset of disease predates clinical symptoms, MS typically presents between the ages of 18 and 45.[1] The risk of developing the disease seems to be related to genetic and environmental factors. The risk of developing MS is approximately 1 per 1000 (0.1%) in the general population. This risk increases to 20 to 40 per 1000 (2%–4%) when a first-degree relative is affected by MS. In monozygotic twins with one twin affected by the disease, the risk in the second twin increases to 300 per 1000 (30%).[2] Residence in a northern latitude, particularly before the age of 15, is associated with increased risk of developing MS. Perhaps this is related to selective migration of genetically predisposed individuals to these regions. It is known that the presence of the human lymphocyte antigen alleles DR21501B1 is associated with greater susceptibility to MS.[2] Alternately, certain environmental factors may be endemic to northern regions, which trigger disease in genetically susceptible individuals. Recently, low vitamin D levels have been linked to MS,[3,4] an observation that may be partly related to the more tangential projection of sunlight on the earth at more northern latitudes, resulting in a reduced conversion of cutaneous activation of vitamin D.

NATURAL HISTORY

Epidemiologic studies have shown that most patients who have MS exhibit progressive neurologic deterioration without treatment.[1] Ten years after diagnosis, approximately 50% of patients are using a cane to ambulate and 15% require a wheelchair. Approximately half of patients convert to the secondary progressive

Dr. Courtney's fellowship is supported by a grant from the National Multiple Sclerosis Society.
[a] Department of Neurology, University of Texas Southwestern Medical Center at Dallas, 5323 Harry Hines Boulevard, Dallas, TX 75235, USA
[b] Department of Ophthalmology University of Texas Southwestern Medical Center at Dallas, 5323 Harry Hines Boulevard, Dallas, TX 75235, USA
* Corresponding author. Department of Neurology, University of Texas Southwestern Medical Center at Dallas, 5323 Harry Hines Boulevard, Dallas, TX 75235.
E-mail address: elliot.frohman@utsouthwestern.edu (E. Frohman).

Med Clin N Am 93 (2009) 451–476
doi:10.1016/j.mcna.2008.09.014
0025-7125/08/$ – see front matter
medical.theclinics.com

phase of the disease, in which there is acceleration of disability and a paucity of effective therapies.[2] A small percentage of patients have a more benign course, but because there are no reliable predictors to indicate which patients will fall in to this category, these cases can only be recognized in retrospect.[2]

The risk of progression to disability over the first decade may be influenced by several factors.[5] Although MS is more common in women (3:1), men are more likely to have a malignant clinical course.[2] It has been observed that MS relapse rates decrease by 70% in the third trimester of pregnancy, which suggests that hormonal regulation plays a role in immune modulation and expression of the disease.[6–8] Other favorable prognostic factors include infrequent exacerbations, especially in the first year, sensory symptoms predominating over motor or cerebellar dysfunction, and good functional recovery from individual neurologic exacerbations.[2]

It seems that the number of exacerbations or "attacks" that occur in the earliest phase of the disease strongly influences the onset and level of disability.[9] Early recognition and treatment of MS to reduce the risk and mitigate the severity of relapses has the potential to forestall the accrual of disability.[2,10] This concept is supported by observational studies of disease burden on brain MRI at the time of diagnosis.[9] Patients with normal brain MRI results at diagnosis did not accrue significant disability over 14 years, whereas patients with more than ten MRI lesions or a change in lesion load within the first year were significantly more likely to progress to advanced levels of disability (eg, ambulation with a cane or walker) over the same period of time.[9]

DISEASE CLASSIFICATION

MS is divided into various subtypes based on the clinical course. These subtypes are most likely determined by distinctive pathogenic, genetic, and immunologic factors culminating in disease expression.[11] Most (85%) patients initially have a relapsing remitting course. Without treatment, most of these patients transition to the secondary progressive form, which is stereotypically characterized by a steady, insidious neurologic decline with fewer or even no clinically recognized relapses. Primary progressive MS occurs in approximately 10% of patients who have MS and is characterized by a steady decline from onset with predominately myelopathic symptoms. The rarest form is a subtype of progressive relapsing MS in which there is initially a steady progression of dysfunction followed later by the evolution of bona fide exacerbations. These primary progressive forms are notable for fewer inflammatory markers, lower MRI lesional burdens (not always), equal gender predilection (1:1), and older age of onset.

DIAGNOSIS

Classically, the clinical diagnosis of MS has depended on documentation of multiple neurologic events referable to the central nervous system (CNS) and separated by time and (anatomic) space. Advancements in paraclinical investigations, namely MRI, cerebrospinal fluid (CSF) analysis, and visual evoked potential testing, together with the need for confirmation of diagnosis at the earliest point have led to more permissive diagnostic criteria.[12,13] These criteria have resulted in improved sensitivity and specificity of diagnosis and have facilitated earlier recognition and treatment to favorably alter long-term outcome.[10,14,15] Confirmation of a working diagnosis of MS always involves the precondition of excluding (or at least considering) conditions that can mimic MS (of which there are myriad considerations).

MRI findings can aid in making the diagnosis and predicting who will develop clinically definite MS. Patients who present with a clinically isolated inflammatory demyelinating syndrome and have one to three typical periventricular lesions on brain MRI have an 89% chance of developing clinically definite MS over a 14-year period.[12,13] CSF analysis can reveal abnormalities typical—albeit not specific—for MS and can include the presence of oligoclonal immunoglobulin bands unique to the CNS and/or elevation in synthesis of IgG within the CNS, reflected in the CNS IgG index or the IgG synthesis rate. Spinal fluid findings may be important for the purpose of excluding other conditions (eg, infection and other inflammatory conditions) and can be helpful for confirming the diagnosis of MS in cases in which the history, examination, and MRI results are inconclusive.

The new guidelines for CSF analysis recommended isoelectric focusing for detection of oligoclonal immunoglobulin bands, greatly improving the sensitivity.[16] CSF analysis may be entirely normal in 30% of patients who have MS early in the course of the disease.[13,17,18] Visual evoked potentials may be helpful in providing evidence of subclinical disease involving the optic nerves and tracts and confirming spatial dissemination in the nervous system, but abnormal findings are not specific to MS. MS is a heterogeneous disease with a variable presentation and clinical course. It is important to realize that there is still no specific test to confirm the diagnosis of MS and that all available data in any case must be critically evaluated to ensure accurate diagnosis. Conditions that mimic MS must be considered and excluded where appropriate (**Table 1**). This is an abbreviated differential diagnosis and illustrates the need for a thorough history, careful physical examination, and judicious clinical and laboratory investigation.

NEUROPATHOLOGY

MS is fundamentally a chronic, progressive, immune-mediated disease confined to the CNS. The features of its immunopathophysiology are complex, and researchers are only beginning to appreciate the diverse and protean aspects of MS pathology over the course of the disease. The histopathologic hallmark of MS is perivenous inflammation followed by demyelination, axonal injury and transaction, neurodegeneration, and, ultimately, gliotic sclerosis (historically defined as tissue hardening).[19]

The initial trigger of the immune cascade has not been identified. It may involve breakdown of myelin by an infectious agent or immune system dysregulation with failure to recognize and avoid immunologic reactions to self antigens (ie, a failure of tolerance). Lymphocytes are primed through antigen presentation by B cells, macrophages, and microglia. Activated lymphocytes adhere to cerebrovascular endothelium through vascular adhesion molecule interactions.[20] Once stabilized on the vessel surface, these cells release enzymes (metalloproteinases), which break down basement membrane collagen and fibronectin and allow for trafficking of inflammatory cells into the CNS.[20] Once inside the CNS, activated lymphocytes secrete inflammatory cytokines such as tumor necrosis factor and interferon$-\gamma$, leading to further migration into the site, activation of B-cells, complement, free radical, and super oxide release.[19–22] The myelin, axon, and oligodendrocytes are damaged in the process, which culminates in disseminated dying back and wallerian degeneration.

"VIGNETTES"

The following clinical vignettes are meant to illustrate the range of presentations and the types of treatment challenges that confront practitioners who evaluate patients with MS.

1: Clinically Isolated Syndrome

A 24-year-old woman presented to her ophthalmologist with a 2-day history of blurred vision and pain in the left eye. She was ultimately diagnosed with inflammatory optic neuritis.

Table 1
Multiple sclerosis mimics

Condition	Characteristic	Distinction
MS VARIANTS		
Acute disseminated encephalomyelitis	Monophasic demyelination occurring with or just after an infection, vaccine, or other immune-altering event	No infallible method, but it occurs in the setting of an infection or a recent vaccine Unusual neurologic symptoms, such as altered consciousness. MRI lesions may be hemorrhagic and involve gray matter
NMO; Devic's disease	Abrupt onset optic neuritis, transverse myelitis, brainstem tegmentum syndromes (vomiting, ocular motor, vestibular) 10%–50% may have brain lesions	Seropositive for NMO IgG antibody (sensitivity approximately 50%–75%) Presence of antibody is highly specific (approximately 90%) for NMO
INFLAMMATORY		
Bechet's disease	Oral/genital ulcers, arthritis	*CSF pleocytosis without IgG elevation Mucocutaneous ulcer biopsy*
Sarcoidosis	Systemic symptoms usually present, with organ involvement (lung, kidney)	Serum and CSF ACE levels may be elevated. Enhancement of meninges Biopsy of skin, lymph node, or lung diagnostic. Octreotide body scanning
Sjögren's syndrome	Systemic symptoms: dry eyes, dry mouth	+ serology for SS-A (Ro), SS-B (La) autoantibodies
Systemic lupus erythematosus	Multiple systemic involvement: kidney, skin, hematologic system. CSF may be positive for oligoclonal bands and IgG elevation	+ serology ANA, DS-DNA autoantibodies
VASCULAR		
Acute ischemic optic neuropathy	Usually painless vision loss	Older > 50, infarction of the optic nerve, atherosclerotic risk factors Normal CSF, MRI nonspecific aging changes
Susac's disease	Clinical triad: encephalopathy, branch retinal artery occlusion, hearing loss	Fluorescein angiography pathognomonic staining of arterioles proximal to retinal artery occlusion. Biopsy shows autoimmune endothelopathy of microvasculature (brain, retina, cochlea)
Antiphospholipid antibody syndrome	Recurrent brain ischemia Headache, seizures	Skin lesions, arthritis. High titers of antiphospholipid antibody IgG/IgM

Migraine	Focal, transient neurologic deficit usually temporally associated with headache (30–90 min)	CSF and evoked potentials results should be normal. MRI may have some nonspecific white matter changes
INFECTIOUS		
PML	Usually patient is immunocompromised. Death within weeks to months without treatment	Course is progressive rather than relapsing. CSF PCR positive for JC virus. Brain biopsy may be necessary
HTLV-I/II (tropical spastic paraparesis)	Myelopathic symptoms dominate, sometimes associated with dementia. May have white matter lesions on MRI and CSF +oligoclonal bands	+ HTLV-I/II serology
Lyme disease (neuroborreliosis)	Tick exposure, erythema migrans	Western blot positive serology/CSF + PCR
Syphilis	Usually patient is immunocompromised	MRI results usually normal; Negative FTA-ABS results rule out syphilis
Human herpesvirus-6		Positive serology for human herpesvirus-6
Hepatitis C	More commonly affects peripheral nervous system	Serum antibodies are positive There is usually active liver disease
Mycoplasma	Usually in setting of systemic infection (pneumonia)	Serum antibody positive for mycoplasma pneumonia
METABOLIC		
B_{12} deficiency	Rarely cause abnormalities of brain MRI. Myelopathic symptoms dominate	Serum levels of B_{12}/folate are low
Copper deficiency	Myelopathy, peripheral neuropathy, optic neuritis	24-h urine free copper excretion, serum copper level
Zinc deficiency	Diminished taste and smell	Neutrophil zinc determination, 24-h urine zinc excretion
Celiac disease	Ataxia and brainstem involvement dominate	Antigliadin antibody positive Spinal fluid is normal. > 90% human lymphocyte antigen -DQ2 positive
Vitamin E deficiency	Progressive ataxia	Serum vitamin E low, retinal pigmentation
GENETIC		
Wilson's disease	Prominent movement disorder (ataxia, tremor), dementia	Kayser-Fleischer rings on slit lamp. Serum copper elevated. Low serum ceruloplasmin < 0.2 g/L, penicillamine challenge test, gene mutation ATP7B

(continued on next page)

Table 1
(continued)

Condition	Characteristic	Distinction
Hereditary spastic paraparesis	Easily confused with primary progressive MS with progressive myelopathy	Peripheral nerve involvement MRI and CSF results are usually normal. Genetic testing not yet reliable
Porphyria	Progressive focal neurologic deficits usually including prominent ataxia	Psychiatric and behavior symptoms prominent. 24-h urine elevated ALA and PBG
Cerebral autosomal dominant arteriopathy with subcortical infarcts and leukoencephalopathy	Multifocal neurologic deficits, often associated with migraine and progressive dementia	Family history Genetic testing available; AD mutation in notch-3 gene
ONCOLOGY		
CNS lymphoma	Usually immunocompromised MRI lesions enhance and are highly sensitive to steroid treatment	CSF results positive cytology CSF results negative for IgG Brain biopsy may be necessary to differentiate
Paraneoplastic syndrome	Abrupt onset of ophthalmoplegia, ataxia. CSF oligoclonal band often present	MRI results usually normal Antibody serum positive Anti-Yo or Anti-Hu
STRUCTURAL		
Spondylosis	Easily mistaken for primary progressive MS, myelopathic	CSF and VEP results are normal. MRI shows spinal cord compression
Syringomyelia	Myelopathic symptoms, may involve lower cranial nerves	MRI imaging shows syrinx. Brain MRI and CSF normal
Spinal vascular malformation	Rare, but relapsing or progressive myelopathic symptoms with intrinsic cord abnormalities	MRI of brain, VEP, CSF results normal. Spinal angiogram may be necessary
ENVIRONMENTAL		
Toxin	Drug/exposure specific	CSF results normal. Usually monophasic with exposure

Abbreviations: NMO, neuromyelitis optica; PCR, polymerase chain reaction; PML, progressive multifocal leukoencephalopathy; VEP, visual evoked potential.

What are some of the key features of the presentation and findings on examination that would help confirm the diagnosis of optic neuritis?
Pain with ocular movement was present in 92% of patients in the Optic Neuritis Treatment Trial, distinguishing it from ischemic optic neuropathy, which is often painless. Patients may describe a dimming or bleaching of color (color desaturation). Visual acuity may or may not be affected. There may also be visual field loss. The optic disc often appears entirely normal, because inflammation is predominately retrobulbar, although a few patients may have optic disc swelling and edema (papillitis). An afferent pupillary defect is typically present on the swinging flashlight test. MRI of the orbits with T1, fat-suppressed sequences with gadolinium reveals optic nerve enhancement in most patients (**Fig. 1**).[23]

What is the appropriate treatment?
The Optic Neuritis Treatment Trial established the standard of care. Patients treated with high-dose intravenous (IV) glucocorticoid (methylprednisolone sodium succinate, 1 g, for 3 days) followed by an 11-day oral prednisone taper had a 50% improvement in time to next relapse, with significant delay in onset of clinically definite MS.[24] There was no difference in final visual acuity at 1 year comparing treated (high-dose versus low-dose steroid limbs) and untreated cases. Many neurologists currently use high-dose steroid regimens (either IV or oral) for the treatment of acute optic neuritis. The decision to use a taper, however, is a highly controversial and contentious area of MS therapeutics. In our center, we typically do not use steroid tapers, except in selected individuals who seem to not be improving to our satisfaction.

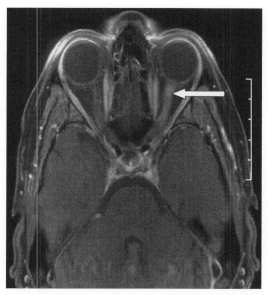

Fig. 1. Acute optic neuritis is associated with enhancement of the optic nerve in approximately two thirds of the patients. This axial T1-weighted, postgadolinium infusion MR image with fat-suppressed orbital view shows homogenous enhancement of the left optic nerve.

Are any diagnostic studies indicated in patients with a clinically isolated syndrome?
The most important investigation is MRI of the brain and spinal cord. It is recognized that up to 80% of patients with the first episode have evidence of pre-existing lesions.[25] The clinically isolated syndromes most likely to progress to clinically definite MS are partial spinal cord syndromes (50%), optic neuritis (25%), and brainstem syndromes (15%).[26]

What is the radiographic signature of multiple sclerosis?
Conventional MRI of the brain typically reveals lesions that are perpendicular to the ventricles and ovoid in shape, particularly when viewing sagittal T2-weighted (T2 and fluid-attenuated inversion recovery; FLAIR) sequences. Characteristically, such lesions often seem to emanate from the ependymal zone of the ventricles and extend upward into the white matter (so-called "Dawson's fingers") (**Fig. 2**). Lesions also occur in the corona radiata, corpus callosum, centrum semiovale, and juxtacortical areas and in gray matter (**Fig. 3**). The FLAIR MRI sequence is the most helpful in identifying lesions in the cerebral hemispheres, because there is greater contrast between dark CSF in the ventricles and white periventricular lesions (**Fig. 4**). In the spinal cord the lesions tend to be cigar-shaped, span one to two segments, and have a predilection for the cervical spinal cord. Brainstem lesions most commonly localize to the tegmentum, given the proximity to the fourth ventricle and cerebral aqueduct. We know that periventricular regions of the brain are areas for high lesion predilection, because most inflammatory trafficking occurs at postcapillary venules, and these microvessels are in greatest concentration in these ventricular zones. Gadolinium enhancement signifies a breach in the integrity of the blood-brain barrier endothelial tight junctions, which occurs in the acute inflammatory phase of the illness, and usually lasts only 2 to 4 weeks in any lesion, but sometimes up to a few months.

Would other studies be of benefit?
In cases of the clinically isolated syndrome, ancillary testing may be of benefit, especially if MRI results are normal or atypical. CSF analysis may be helpful, particularly if positive for oligoclonal bands and elevated IgG index. These findings are only

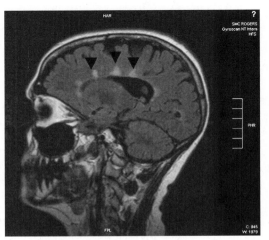

Fig. 2. A sagittal fluid-attenuated inversion recovery (FLAIR) MR image demonstrates subependymal hyperintensities radiating out into the deep white matter often referred to as "Dawson's Fingers".

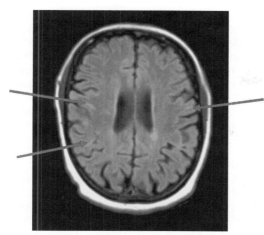

Fig. 3. An axial fluid-attenuated inversion recovery (FLAIR) MR image shows juxtacortical gray matter hyperintensities (*arrows*). Gray matter involvement is underrepresented by routine MR imaging and is involved early in the disease course.

characteristic of MS, however, and are not disease specific. Evoked potentials measure latency of neuronal responses to stimulation through visual, sensory, or auditory pathways; slowing of latencies suggests demyelination and identifies subclinical disease and helps confirm spatial dissemination in the CNS. Evoked potentials are nonspecific and can be normal in 40% to 50% of patients initially.[17]

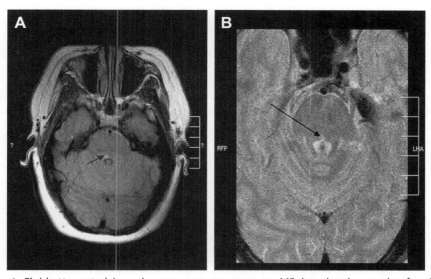

Fig. 4. Fluid-attenuated inversion recovery sequence on MR imaging is superior for the detection of MS plaques because the CSF appears black, which increases the contrast. On T2-weighted MRI, the MS plaques and CSF are white, which makes it more difficult to distinguish. (*A*) An axial FLAIR MR image demonstrates a periventricular MS plaque (*arrow*) with high contrast between black CSF and white MS plaque. (*B*) An axial T2-weighted MR image demonstrates low contrast between white CSF and white MS plaque (*arrow*).

Should a patient with clinically isolated syndrome be offered treatment with an immunomodulatory agent?

Several placebo-controlled phase III clinical trials (class I evidence) have studied patients with clinically isolated syndrome and evidence of silent lesions on MRI.[25] There was substantial reduction in new MRI lesions and risk of subsequent exacerbations in patients treated with interferon beta-1a (Avonex or Rebif), interferon beta-1b (Betaseron), and more recently with glatiramer acetate (Copaxone). [15,27] Patients initially treated with placebo and later transitioned to active treatment never achieved the magnitude of benefit seen in the patients who received early treatment with disease-modifying therapy.[15]

Was a disease-modifying agent started in this patient?

The patient was started on weekly intramuscular interferon beta-1a (Avonex). To avoid the postinjection flu-like syndrome commonly experienced with the use of all interferons, she was instructed to titrate the dose of interferon up slowly and premedicate with a nonsteroidal anti-inflammatory agent, such as controlled-release naproxen (Naprelan). Liver enzyme levels in blood, particularly transaminases, may be elevated in the first few months of treatment and are more common with higher dose, higher frequency, subcutaneous injection forms of interferon (Rebif and Betaseron). Mild leukopenia and lymphopenia are common but not usually clinically important, because the drugs modulate but do not suppress the immune system.[26,28] Another common side effect of interferon treatment is injection site reaction. To avoid the reaction, patients are instructed to allow the drug to come to room temperature, ice the skin over the planned injection site, apply diphenhydramine (Benadryl) cream, and rotate injections sites. Injection-site pain can be mitigated by using aerosolized ethyl chloride spray immediately before injection. Despite these precautions, skin necrosis and lipoatrophy have been reported with subcutaneously injected interferons and glatiramer acetate.[29,30] Rarely, intramuscular interferon can be associated with muscle abscess.[31]

2: Relapsing Remitting Multiple Sclerosis

A 38-year-old woman presented to her gynecologist after she noticed that warm water did not feel the same on the right breast as the left while showering. Over a few weeks, she also noted that a strange electrical sensation shooting down her back when she looked down and flexed her neck. In the past, she had double or blurred vision when hot or overfatigued. The first time she noticed this, she was driving cross-country without air conditioning after finishing college. It lasted only a few days, and she never sought medical attention. She denied any other symptoms, including loss of vision, muscle weakness, or bowel or bladder difficulties. She was referred to a neurologist for further evaluation.

Examination revealed bilateral hyperreflexia in the lower extremities, upgoing toes on plantar stimulation, diminished pain to pin prick below the nipple (T4 dermatome) on the right side, and left eye lag on adduction during horizontal saccades, without complaint of diplopia. There was no relative afferent pupil defect on swinging flashlight testing. MRI of the brain and cervical spine with and without gadolinium was obtained. The radiologist reported multiple periventricular lesions, an enhancing lesion of the mid-cervical cord without mass effect. The physical examination, clinical history, and MRI results were consistent with the diagnosis of relapsing remitting MS (ie, clinically definite MS) with dissemination in time and space.[12,13]

What is the Significance of Diplopia and Slow Adduction of the Left Eye?

Internuclear ophthalmoplegia Internuclear ophthalmoplegia results from a lesion of the medial longitudinal fasciculus located in the tegmentum of the midbrain and pons. It is the most common eye movement abnormality in patients who have MS. Patients may complain of double or blurred vision with left or right gaze. Examination may show slow adduction of the affected eye and horizontal nystagmus in the contralateral eye, which can be the only finding. The pyramidal tract (motor) and pontine micturition center (bladder function) are near the medial longitudinal fasciculus anatomically and may be affected, giving rise to symptoms of neurogenic bladder (urgency, frequency, urge incontinence, and bladder retention).

What is the significance of symptoms worsening in heat?

Uhthoff's phenomenon Exposure to heat, prolonged exercise, infection, perimenstrual and even psychologic stress may cause transient appearance or worsening of neurologic symptoms or dysfunction in chronically demyelinated pathways (Uhthoff's phenomenon) because of conduction slowing or block.[32–34] It is important to differentiate transient worsening (pseudoexacerbation) secondary to inciting factors (heat, fatigue, infection) from symptoms that represent a true acute relapse that may warrant therapy modification. Transient symptoms secondary to a pseudoexacerbation usually last less than 24 hours, fluctuate during the day, and resolve once the factor is removed. It is sometimes difficult to differentiate a pseudoexacerbation from a bona fide exacerbation, and clinical judgment must be exercised in deciding whether to pursue further investigation or modification of treatment.

What is the significance of the electrical sensation with neck flexion?

Lhermitte's phenomenon or sign The shock-like sensation with neck flexion (Lhermitte's phenomenon) suggests a cervical cord lesion precipitating ephaptic transmission ("cross talk" between demyelinated axons) with stretching or movement.[32–34] Although not specific to a demyelinating lesion, it is commonly associated with this pathologic condition and helps with localization of the lesion.

What treatments are available for relapsing remitting multiple sclerosis?

Six US Food and Drug Administration–approved drugs are currently available in the United States for the treatment of relapsing remitting MS. These drugs include three beta interferon formulations produced by commercial recombinant DNA techniques. Interferons are produced naturally in human lymphocytes and modulate the immune system by influencing the production of protein products. Avonex and Rebif are forms of interferon beta-1a, but the strength of the individual doses and the injection routes and differ. Avonex is prepackaged as a 30-μg dose that is given once a week intramuscularly. Rebif is provided in two dose strengths, 22 μg and 44 μg, and is injected subcutaneously three times a week, beginning therapy with the lower dose. Betaseron, interferon beta-1b, is given subcutaneously every other day. Beta interferons have been shown to be effective in multiple clinical and radiographic domains, including reduction of relapse rate, relapse severity, reduction of T2 and gadolinium-enhancing lesions on MRI, and prolonging time to progression to disability.[15,24–26,35,36] Glatiramer acetate (Copaxone) is a synthetic drug that interferes with antigen presentation.[37] It is given as a single, daily, 20-mg subcutaneous injection.

Natalizumab (Tysabri) is a recombinant monoclonal antibody directed against alpha 4-integrin, which inhibits the trafficking of immune cells into the CNS.[38] Naatalizumab has been shown to be a highly efficacious MS disease-modifying therapy across all studied clinical and radiographic domains. However, Tysabri was associated with development of progressive multifocal leukoencephalopathy (PML) when used in combination therapy regimens in MS (two cases when used in conjunction with Avonex) and in a single patient with Crohn's disease who was treated with various immunomodulators during clinical trials.[39,40] After the identification of these progressive multifocal leukoencephalopathy cases, the medication was voluntarily withdrawn from the market by the manufacturer on February 28, 2005 for further investigation. Tysabri was re-approved and re-released to market June 5, 2006. There have been no further reported cases of progressive multifocal leukoencephalopathy (monitored through the manufacturer's TOUCH program) with monotherapy as of the writing of this article. There have been two new cases of PML reported in Europe (August 2008). Europe is not using the TOUCH program, and the details of these cases are not entirely clear at this time. Tysabri is given once a month by IV infusion over 1 hour at approved infusion centers only.

Novantarone (mitoxantrone) is an anthrocenedione chemotherapeutic agent (similar to adriamycin) that has been approved for the treatment of relapsing remitting MS and secondary progressive MS. It is considered a second-line medication but can be effective when there is evidence of persistent disease activity.[41] Given the risk of cardiotoxicity, this agent can be used only for a finite period. Leukemia also has been confirmed as a serious sequela in a limited number of patients (most commonly acute promyelocytic leukemia).[42]

Multiple factors must be taken into account when formulating a treatment plan for MS. Each individual patient differs in evidence of disease activity (clinical and radiographic), level of disability, and social and psychologic capacity. All of these factors should be considered. It is beyond the scope of this article to cover this process in detail. It is important, however, to educate patients about the different treatment options, emphasizing that they are principally prevention and disease-mitigating strategies, not curative or restorative. Education regarding the rationale, potential side effects, and associated interventions available is crucial to optimize adherent drug-taking behavior and disease-modifying effects. To date, all approved, evidence-based therapies are available only in injectable forms. It is hoped that ongoing research will identify effective, well-tolerated treatments that are easier to administer. Other agents (without sufficient evidence-based studies to support their application in MS), such as periodic steroid pulses, IV immunoglobulin, plasma exchange, mycophenolate mofetil, azathioprine, and methotrexate, are not infrequently used by specialized clinics in selected patients.[43–45]

How was this patient treated?

The patient initially received methylprednisolone, 1 g IV, every day for 3 days, without oral glucocorticoid taper. Traditionally, a brief pulse (3–5 days) of high-dose glucocorticoid is given for acute exacerbations, which has been shown to decrease the duration of the symptomatic episode but does not necessarily reduce the severity of disease or alter long-term disability.[41] There is some evidence that high-dose pulse steroids given every 3 to 4 months for maintenance therapy may be effective in reducing disability and decreasing disease activity measured by MRI.[46] Multiple different steroid regimens are used in the United States (**Table 2**) without good evidence for superiority of any specific protocol.[47,48] Although pulse steroid therapy seems to reduce the risk of serious side effects when compared with long-term, lower, more frequent dosing, it is advisable to prescribe supplemental calcium and vitamin D. Serial bone density screening has been suggested,[49] and we believe it is a mandatory surveillance strategy (along with following vitamin D levels) to identify accelerated bone loss.

For maintenance immunomodulation therapy, a discussion between the treating physician and patient led to the decision to start treatment with glatiramer acetate (Copaxone). During the first week of treatment, she experienced shortness of breath and anxiety (idiosyncratic effects that occur in approximately 10% of patients treated with Copaxone).[50] The patient was given reassurance and the symptoms

Table 2 Steroid regimens		
Agent	**Adjunctive**	**Exacerbation**
Methylprednisolone	1-2 grams IV for 1-2 days monthly or every other month	1-2 grams IV daily for 3-5 days (with/without an oral taper)
Dexamethasone	*Monthly:* 80-160 mg for 2-4 days or 20-40 mg given weekly	*Primary Treatment:* 80 mg BID for three days *Taper:* 12 mg for 4 days, then 8 mg for 4 days, then 4 mg for 4 days, stop
Prednisone	Monthly 500 mg bid for 2-4 days	*Primary Treatment* 500 mg bid for three days

spontaneously resolved. A follow-up MRI was performed 4 months after the initial study and showed multiple new enhancing periventricular lesions despite clinical stability. This illustrates an important point that clinically apparent relapses under-represent the true burden of disease by up to ten times.[51–53] Newer MR techniques (spectroscopy, magnetic transfer, and diffusion tensor imaging) indicate that CNS inflammation in MS is actually a global phenomenon that affects gray and white matter and seems to occur constitutively.[54] In published trials, glatiramer acetate (Copaxone) exhibits a delayed effect in reducing new gadolinium-enhancing lesions. Consequently, the new MRI findings prompted the addition of IV methylpredniso-lone, 1 g, monthly for the next 6 months.

What are the options for treating breakthrough disease?

All of the disease-modifying agents available reduce—but do not eliminate—disease progression and relapses. There are no generally accepted guidelines for assessing when therapy should be augmented or changed. Ongoing relapses, recurrent MRI activity, or functional decline may indicate inadequate disease control. Adjunctive therapy may be initiated depending on the clinical circumstances (**Table 3**). There is little justification for switching between the interferons or glatiramer acetate, because efficacy is approximately equal.[27] We do recognize that some individual patients seem to do better with one therapy versus another disease-modifying therapy. As such, switching therapy should not be discouraged if, in the opinion of the treating neurologist, it seems warranted.

Patients on interferon treatment who exhibit disease progression should be checked for interferon neutralizing antibody activity. Some physicians routinely assess interferon antibody status regardless of the clinical and radiographic course to be certain that this resistance factor is not present, which may increase the risk of disease activity over time. The predilection for antibody formation is highest among patients using the subcutaneous injectable forms, Betaseron and Rebif (about 14%–33%), and is lowest with Avonex (approximately 5%).[27,55–57] The antibodies are cross-reactive among the interferons, and once they are detected (either at high titer or if they are persistent) the patient should be switched to an alternative form of therapy.[55] Neutralizing antibodies also may be found in patients treated with natalizumab (Tysabri); however, only approximately half of patients who are initially antibody positive remain positive. Patients who are antibody positive are also more likely to have infusion reactions.

Table 3
Adjunctive immunotherapy

Agent	Regimen	Laboratory	Adverse Event
Intravenous immunoglobulin	Induction 1 g/kg/d for 2 d Maintenance 0.2–1 g/kg/mo	Quantitative IgA, plasma viscosity, BUN, Cr, LFTs	Aseptic meningitis, anaphylaxis, viral hepatitis, hypercoaguable state
Azathioprine (Imuran)	Induction 50 mg/d × 1 wk Titration increase by 50 mg/wk until at target dose Target dose: 2–3 mg/kg or MCV > 100; lymphocyte count at 800–1000	Monitor WBC to goal WBC < 3000, lymphocyte 800–1000, MCV > 100 LFTs Test all patients for thiopurine methyltransferase effect before treatment to ensure they are not homozygous for the undermetabolic state	Allergic reaction 15% Lymphopenia Anemia Transaminitis Pancreatitis Alopecia Lymphoma (slight)
Methotrexate	Induction 0.2–1 g/kg/mo 2.5 mg/wk until at Maintenance 0.2–1 g/kg/mo 7.5–20 mg/wk Supplement folic acid 1 mg/d	Chest radiograph LFTs	Interstitial pneumonitis Transaminitis Cirrhosis Gastrointestinal upset Mucositis
Cyclophosphamide(CYP)	Preparation 1. Foley unless CIC 2. ABX suppression 3. Hydration Maintenance 1. IV Mesna at 20% CYP dose, 30 min before and 3 and 6 h after infusion 2. Antiemetic with each Mesna dose 3. IV CYP 0.5-1 g/m²	Check before and then 2 wk after each infusion: CBC with differential LFTs BUN, creatinine Electrolytes UA with micro PVR in all patients to ensure no urine retention If PVR is > 100 mL place Foley catheter during Rx	Nausea/vomiting Hepatorenal toxicity Hemorrhagic cystitis Myelosuppression Amenorrhea, risk of sterility and cancer

Mitoxantrone (Novantarone)	Preparation 1. EF > 50% 2. EKG Maintenance 5–12 mg/m² every 1–3 mo × 8–12 doses maximum	CBC with differential EF at 1 y, if decreases by 10%, stop therapy	Neutropenia, acute leukemia, cardiotoxicity, alopecia, nausea
Mycophenolate mofetil (Cellcept)	Induction Week 1: 250 mg twice daily Week 2: 500 mg twice daily Week 3: 750 mg twice daily Week 4: 1000 mg twice daily on empty stomach Maintenance 1000 mg twice daily	Mandatory surveillance laboratory (CBC, LFT, BUN, CRT, electrolytes) performed at baseline and then months 1,2,3, and then quarterly	*Diarrhea* *Transaminitis* *Recurrent urinary tract infections* *Hair loss* *Anemia* *Thrombocytopenia* *Shingles* *Beware of PML*

Abbreviations: ABX, antibiotics; BUN, blood urea nitrogen; CBC, complete blood count; CIC, clean intermittent catheterization; Cr, creatinine; EF, cardiac ejection fraction; EKG, electrocardiogram; LFTs, liver function tests; MCV, mean corpuscular volume; WBC, white blood cell count.

3: Relapsing Remitting Multiple Sclerosis Transitioning to Secondary Progressive

A 46-year-old man with a 15-year history of MS characterized by various relapses consisting of optic neuritis, diplopia, right hemiparesis, and trigeminal neuralgia presented with complaints of gradual worsening of gait, multiple falls, and urinary urgency. He denied any specific problems in his work as an architect but admitted it was taking him longer to complete tasks. His wife reported that he seemed more forgetful and irritable at home. He frequently had to go into the office on the weekends to finish work. He was maintained on glatiramer acetate (Copaxone) for 8 years and had not had any exacerbations for the past 5 years.

Many patients on disease-modifying agents eventually transition to the secondary progressive form of the disease despite years of apparent stability. Relapsing remitting MS is characterized histopathologically by perivenular inflammation, gliosis, and demyelination with episodic clinical worsening and radiographic activity (enhancing MRI lesions) In contrast, secondary progressive MS seems to be less inflammatory but there is prominent demyelination, gliosis, and axon loss. Although there is little or no clinical or radiographic disease activity (by conventional imaging techniques) in this stage, there is rapid acceleration of disability. Many of the therapies effective in modulation of the disease process early in MS have failed to show efficacy in the secondary progressive phase.[58]

Symptomatic therapy

Gait dysfunction Gait dysfunction may contribute to fatigue and increases the risk of injury from falling. Examination revealed bilateral lower extremity spasticity, heel cord tightness, and weakness of the ankle dorsiflexors. The patient was asked to participate in physical therapy, specifically for gait and balance training and muscle stretching. If bracing may be of assistance or a patient requires additional evaluation for assistive devices and therapy, there should be a low threshold for referral to a physician who specializes in physical rehabilitation medicine, preferably a practitioner who has some expertise in dealing with problems specific to this population of patients. Botulinum toxin injections of the posterior compartment calf muscles may be considered before intensive physical therapy to facilitate stretching and foot-ankle mobilization and dorsiflexion conditioning.[59,60]

In this case, 4-aminopyridine, a compounded medication that blocks potassium channels and prolongs axonal action potential duration, was added to help with strength and endurance.[61–63] The medication was prescribed orally and was titrated over several weeks. The patient was instructed to take it with meals to minimize peak dose side effects and risk of generalized seizure.

For muscle spasms and spasticity, muscle relaxant medications, including baclofen, tinazidine (Zanaflex), and benzodiazepines (clonazepam or diazepam), may be tried. These drugs should be titrated slowly, beginning at low doses, and the patient should be monitored for side effects, including oversedation, exacerbation of underlying weakness, and liver dysfunction. If spasticity is refractory or medication side effects are intolerable, placement of an intrathecal baclofen pump should be considered in selected patients. Falling is a major risk factor for significant injury in patients who have MS.[58,64] Normal balance is maintained through the synergistic action of systems, including vision, hearing, proprioception, vestibular mechanisms, motor coordination, and muscle tension. These systems are particularly compromised in MS.

Patients who have MS are at higher risk than the general population for bone loss (osteopenia/osteoporosis) from inactivity, steroid use, avoidance of the sun (usually related to heat sensitivity), and vitamin D deficiency.[64] Vitamin D levels should be checked and supplements prescribed if levels are low. Supplemental calcium, 1500 mg to 2000 mg/day, is also suggested, with the addition of bisphophate (Fosamax, Boniva, Actonel) and calcitonin (Miacalcin) if bone demineralization has already occurred. All patients capable of weight-bearing exercise should be strongly encouraged to pursue a regular exercise program. Patients who have severe bone loss or do not respond to antiresorptive agents should be referred to a bone and mineral metabolism specialist for further assessment and treatment.

What is the cause of fatigue in multiple sclerosis?

Fatigue is present in most patients who have MS. In fact, fatigue is the single most cited reason for disability and must be aggressively investigated and treated to minimize its adverse and compromising effects.[65] Fatigue is postulated to be mediated through inflammatory cytokines, although it is likely that a complex interplay of multiple factors influences the predilection for fatigue in this population. A careful history and investigation for other contributing factors should be made, including depression, sleep disruption (caused by obstructive apnea, restless legs syndrome, periodic limb movement disorder, nocturia, or muscle spasms, and spasticity), medication effects, poor sleep hygiene, substance use (caffeine, alcohol), nutritional deficiency, endrocrinopathies (hypothyroidism), anemia, deconditioning, and occult infection.

Several agents may aid in mitigating fatigue. For patients with exertional fatigue, 4-aminopyridine is particularly helpful. Amantadine (Symmetrel) increases dopamine levels and may be tried for mild fatigue. More potent activating medications include modafinil (Provigil), mixed salts of dextroamphetamine (Adderall), methylphenidate (Ritalin, Concerta), pemoloine (Cylert), Lisdexamfetamine dimesylate (Vyvanse), and Atomoxetine HCL (Straterra). Activating antidepressants such as venlafaxine (Effexor) and buproprion (Wellbutrin) also may be tried, depending on the particular needs of the patient. Studies also have demonstrated that an over-the-counter nutritional agent, acetyl-L-carnitine, can be helpful for fatigue in patients who have MS.[66]

Bladder, bowel, or sexual dysfunction

Approximately 90% of patients who have MS experience bowel, bladder, or sexual dysfunction at some time during the course of their disease. Patients may be reluctant to discuss these symptoms, particularly those related to sexual dysfunction, and these disease-related features must be actively sought by the practitioner.

Bladder Proper function of the bladder depends on the coordinated action of all levels of the nervous system. The function of the bladder is to store and then eliminate urine. Normally these actions are regulated by higher brain centers (cerebral cortex and pontine micturition center); in patients who have MS these pathways are frequently damaged. In the storage phase, somatic control through sacral segments (S2, 3, 4- Onuf's nucleus) contracts the rhabdosphincter, and sympathetic tone maintains contraction of the bladder neck and inhibits detrusor muscle contraction. In the voiding phase, stretching of the bladder wall with filling activates sensory afferents and the rhabdosphincter and bladder neck relax, followed by parasympathetic, cholinergic-mediated contraction of the detrusor muscle, emptying the bladder.

Detrusor hyperreflexia is similar to hyperactive muscle stretch reflexes, in which minimal stretch (bladder filling) results in vigorous muscle contraction. Patients report urgency, frequency, urge incontinence, and painful bladder spasm. If there is detrusor sphincter dysynergy there is contraction of the detrusor (bladder) without coordinated relaxation of the sphincter, which prevents emptying of the bladder. This can lead to urine retention, which results in chronic urinary tract infections and calculi and ultimately damage to the bladder wall sensory afferent nerves. If the detrusor loses the ability to sense filling, catheterization may be necessary to prevent further injury and involvement of the upper urinary tract and kidneys, resulting in hydronephrosis.

Treatment varies depending on the nature of the problem but may involve lifestyle modification, pharmacotherapy, and, if necessary, surgical intervention. Patients should be advised to avoid spicy foods (containing capsaicin) and caffeine, because they may irritate the bladder wall and precipitate spasm. Pelvic floor exercises may be helpful. Exercises should be continued for at least 3 months before determining efficacy. Instruct patients to do three sets of 8 to 12 slow, maximal contractions daily if possible at least four times a week. Bladder training with scheduled voiding also may be helpful in certain cases. Medications should be titrated slowly, and postvoid residual bladder volume should be monitored with medication changes (usually with bladder ultrasound).

Anticholinergic medications form the basis of pharmacotherapy for detrusor hyperactivity by reducing involuntary contractions. Oxybutynin (ditropan, ditropan XL), tolterodine (detrol, detrol LA), and imipramine (which most commonly prevents incontinence by increasing adrenergic tone at the bladder sphincter) are the most commonly used medications. Patients should be monitored for anticholinergic side effects (dry eyes, dry mouth, urine retention, blurred vision, flushed skin, and constipation). Anticholinergic medication may precipitate acute urine retention or confusion. Maneuvers that also may be helpful for more complete emptying are double voiding and localized application of vibration over the bladder (hypogastrium).

The following alpha-adrenergic medications are used for sphincter relaxation in detrusor-sphincter dysnergia: tamsulosin (Flomax), doxazosin (Cardura), and terazoxin (Hytrin). These medications may cause significant hypotension. Desmopressin (DDAVP) may be used (effectively) for persistent nocturia. Sodium levels should be monitored for development of hyponatremia (which is rare), and concurrent diuretics should be used with caution. DDAVP should not be used in patients with congestive heart failure or uncontrolled hypertension.

Patients with refractory dysnergia may ultimately need to do intermittent self-catheterization. Botulinum toxin A may be injected directly into the sphincter or detrusor by a urologist, gynourologist, or neurourologist with specialized expertise in these techniques.[67–69] Indwelling catheters should be avoided because of the risk of recurrent urinary tract infection, which may worsen MS symptoms and contribute to bladder cancer risk.[70] If urinary difficulties persist despite medical management, an evaluation by a neurourologist is recommended. Urodynamic studies of the storage and elimination phases of bladder function can aid in diagnosis and identify other problems, such as bladder outlet obstruction (tumor, prostatic hypertrophy), low volume bladder, and pelvic floor weakness. Renal ultrasound should be performed to evaluate for hydronephrosis with chronic urine retention. Surgical intervention may be considered as a last resort. Various surgical procedures, including urterointestinal cutaneous diversion, suprapubic catheter placement, stint prosthesis, and sphincter dilation, may be performed depending on the particular circumstances.

Bowel Bowel dysfunction in MS is multifactorial. Evidence indicates that normal neurogastrointestinal signaling, as in the gastrocolic reflex, is diminished in patients who have MS. Frank bowel incontinence is unusual but can occur and is usually secondary to a poor bowel program for chronic constipation. Diarrhea and urge incontinence can result from hyperexcitability of the bowel wall caused by decreased neuronal inhibition, but constipation is by far the most common problem. Multiple classes of medications commonly used for MS, including anticholinergics, antidepressants, supplements (calcium), and diuretics, may exacerbate poor neural reflexes.

Inadequate hydration, lack of exercise, pelvic floor weakness, or spasticity can further complicate the problem. Patients should be instructed on behaviors to alleviate constipation, including exercise, hydration, pelvic floor strengthening, and a high-fiber diet supplemented with a fiber-bulking agent such as psyllium (Metamucil, Fiberall). Laxatives also may be necessary, such as polyethylene glycol (MiraLax, GlycoLax), which has the advantage of minimal associated bloating. If the problem is poor rectal evacuation, glycerin, docusate, or mini-enemas (Theravac minidose enema) may be tried. Digital rectal stimulation is sometimes used by patients but should not be encouraged on a regular basis. The long-term use of laxatives, stool softeners, and stimulants should be avoided if possible.

Sexual dysfunction In women, diminished arousal, lubrication, and sensation and failure to orgasm are the most common complaints. Lubricants in combination with a high-frequency vibrator (outlet powered) may enhance sensation and allow for orgasm. Erectile dysfunction and diminished arousal are the primary complaints in men. Phosphodiesterase inhibitors such as sildenafil (Viagra, Revatio), tadalafil (Cialis), vardenafil (Levitra), alprostadil (penile suppository or injection), or hydraulic pumps, penile banding, and penile implants are effective options for erectile dysfunction. Decreased libido caused by testosterone deficiency can occur in men and women unrelated to MS (but it may occur in some who have hypothalamic-pituitary-gonadal defects). Blood levels should be checked and replacement prescribed if necessary. Multiple factors frequently associated with MS also may diminish libido, including sleep disruption, fatigue, depression, and dysfunctional relationship. These factors should be addressed individually. If medication is necessary to treat depression, try to use an agent with minimal sexual side effects, such as bupropion (Wellbutrin) or mirtazipine (Remeron). Referral to a counselor or psychotherapist may be helpful.

PAROXYSMAL NEUROLOGIC SYMPTOMS IN MULTIPLE SCLEROSIS

The sensory pathways are commonly affected, resulting in a wide variety of disturbing sensory symptoms. These symptoms may involve cranial nerve sensory afferents (trigeminal neuralgia, glossopharyngeal neuralgia) or consist of regional paresthesias, burning, or pruritis. On the motor side, episodic dystonia can be varied and disabling; patients may experience intermittent dysarthria, ataxia, hemifacial spasm, or task-specific dystonia (eg, writer's cramp). A careful history and examination usually are sufficient to distinguish from epileptic activity. In some cases, however, additional testing (electroencephalogram, MRI of the brain) may need to be performed. Membrane-stabilizing medications, such as anticonvulsant medications (gabapentin, pregabalin, topiramate, valproic acid, zonisamide, oxcarbazepine, carbazepine, lamotrigine, phenytoin, levetiracetum), can be efficacious. Medication should be chosen based on patient comorbidities and the practitioner's familiarity with the medication. Neuropathic pain syndromes may be exquisitely sensitive to therapy and may require only a small amount of medication, so start low and titrate slowly. Benzodiazepines (clonazepam, diazepam) may be helpful in some cases, particularly if symptoms disrupt sleep or the patient experiences painful spasms.

RESOURCES

Several national organizations are devoted to assisting not only patients and their families but also health care professionals who are interested in caring for individuals who have MS (**Table 4**). The National Multiple Sclerosis Society provides millions of dollars for MS research every year, and it hosts many successful fundraising events, such as

Table 4
Multiple sclerosis resource table

Resource	Education	Referrals	Research	Assistance, devices, evaluation
National Multiple Sclerosis Society Ph: 800-344-4867	■	■	■	■
www.nationalmssociety.org				
Multiple Sclerosis Society of America Ph: 800-532-7667	■	■		■
www.msassociation.org				
Multiple Sclerosis Foundation Ph: 888-673-6287	■	■		■
www.msfacts.org				
www.ms-cam.org Rocky Mountain MS Center Web site on complementary and alternative medicine for people with MS	■		■	
National Institute of Health Clinical Trial listing				
www.clinicaltrials.gov			■	
Assistive technology				
Abledata www.abledata.com				
Vehicle modification		■		■
National Highway Traffic Safety Administration www.nhtsa.dot.gov				
National Mobility Equipment Dealer's Association www.nmeda.org				
Comprehensive driving examination				
Association for Driver Rehabilitation Specialists www.driver-ed.org				
Caregivers				
National Family Caregiver's Association www.nfcacares.org	■			
National Caregiver's Library www.caregiverslibrary.org				

Disability

Social Security Ph: 800-772-1213 www.ssa.gov

www.disabilityinfo.gov Provided by the federal government

National Organization of Social Security Claimant's
Representatives Ph: 800-431-2804 www.nosscr.org

Advocacy

Equal Employment Opportunity Commission www.eeoc.gov

MS Workplace www.msworkplace.com

Job Accommodation Network (JAN) (Office of Disability
Employment Policy of the US Department of Labor)
Ph: 800-526-7234 www.jan.wvu.edu

Medication assistance programs for disease modifying agents

MS Active Source (Avonex and Tysabri) Ph: 800-456-2255

Shared Solutions (Copaxone) Ph: 800-887-8100

MS Lifelines (Rebif) Ph: 877-447-3243

Beta Plus (Betaseron) Ph: 800-788-1467

All other medications contact the manufacturing company or
go to:

www.Rxhope.com

www.rxasssist.org

www.needymeds.com

Partnership for Prescription Assistance Ph: 888-477-2669
www.pparx.org

The National Organization for Rare Disorders Ph: 800-999-6673
www.rarediseases.org

the 150-mile bike tour held each year in April. Local chapters can provide financial assistance and assist patients in locating other resources. They are also active in supporting and providing funding for fellowship programs to train physicians interested in specializing in the care of patients who have MS and, more recently, basic research. The Multiple Sclerosis Foundation also provides patients and health care professionals with not only educational grants but also home care programs, assistive technology, and telephone support. The Multiple Sclerosis Association of America has exceptional patient programs that include imaging (MRI), equipment, and lending library. These three organizations each have an educational magazine devoted to MS topics and facilitate local support groups. We also use local resources for our patients who have MS, including Meals on Wheels, United Way programs, the Salvation Army, legal aid, Easter Seals, local churches, the Veteran's Administration, mental health associations, fair housing, financial planners, YWCA, family counseling, benefits planning and outreach programs, and state work and rehabilitative programs.

FUTURE PROMISE AND DIRECTION

Research in MS is rapidly expanding our understanding of pathophysiology and our ability to accurately diagnose this disease in its various manifestations. Our ability to more effectively direct and monitor therapy is improving rapidly. Exciting new therapies are under development to not only better prevent progression but also repair existing damage. We already know that early identification and treatment of MS can translate into improved quality of life.[15,24,26,27,46,50,71,72] As new, effective therapies emerge, the importance of early recognition and treatment will only increase. Ophthalmologists, gynecologists, and primary care physicians will play an ever-increasing role in identifying patients with suspected inflammatory demyelinating syndromes. They are in a powerful position to favorably impact the natural history of MS. In collaboration, we can greatly enhance the quality of care and lives of our patients.

REFERENCES

1. Anderson DW, et al. Revised estimate of the prevalence of multiple sclerosis in the United States. Ann Neurol 1992;31(3):333–6.
2. Weinshenker BG, et al. The natural history of multiple sclerosis: a geographically based study. I. Clinical course and disability. Brain 1989;112(Pt 1):133–46.
3. Hayes CE, Donald Acheson E. A unifying multiple sclerosis etiology linking virus infection, sunlight, and vitamin D, through viral interleukin-10. Med Hypotheses 2008;71(1):85–90.
4. Kampman MT, Brustad M. Vitamin D: a candidate for the environmental effect in multiple sclerosis. Observations from Norway. Neuroepidemiology 2008;30(3):140–6.
5. Brex PA, et al. Assessing the risk of early multiple sclerosis in patients with clinically isolated syndromes: the role of a follow up MRI. J Neurol Neurosurg Psychiatry 2001;70(3):390–3.
6. Abramsky O, et al. Suppressive effect of pregnancy on MS and EAE. Prog Clin Biol Res 1984;146:399–406.
7. Devonshire V, et al. The immune system and hormones: review and relevance to pregnancy and contraception in women with MS. Int MS J 2003;10(2):44–50.
8. Starnawski M, et al [Pregnancy in women with multiple sclerosis (MS): a report of 2 cases]. Ginekol Pol 1998;69(12):1032–4.
9. Runmarker B, Andersen O. Prognostic factors in a multiple sclerosis incidence cohort with twenty-five years of follow-up. Brain 1993;116(Pt 1):117–34.

10. Kappos L, et al. Effect of early versus delayed interferon beta-1b treatment on disability after a first clinical event suggestive of multiple sclerosis: a 3-year follow-up analysis of the BENEFIT study. Lancet 2007;370(9585):389–97.

11. Lublin FD, Reingold SC. Defining the clinical course of multiple sclerosis: results of an international survey. National Multiple Sclerosis Society (USA) Advisory Committee on Clinical Trials of New Agents in Multiple Sclerosis. Neurology 1996;46(4):907–11.

12. McDonald WI, et al. Recommended diagnostic criteria for multiple sclerosis: guidelines from the international panel on the diagnosis of multiple sclerosis. Ann Neurol 2001;50(1):121–7.

13. Poser CM, et al. New diagnostic criteria for multiple sclerosis: guidelines for research protocols. Ann Neurol 1983;13(3):227–31.

14. Beck RW, et al. The effect of corticosteroids for acute optic neuritis on the subsequent development of multiple sclerosis: the Optic Neuritis Study Group. N Engl J Med 1993;329(24):1764–9.

15. Comi G, et al. Effect of early interferon treatment on conversion to definite multiple sclerosis: a randomised study. Lancet 2001;357(9268):1576–82.

16. Freedman MS, et al. Recommended standard of cerebrospinal fluid analysis in the diagnosis of multiple sclerosis: a consensus statement. Arch Neurol 2005; 62(6):865–70.

17. Martinelli V, et al. Paraclinical tests in acute-onset optic neuritis: basal data and results of a short follow-up. Acta Neurol Scand 1991;84(3):231–6.

18. Noseworthy JH, et al. Multiple sclerosis. N Engl J Med 2000;343(13):938–52.

19. Frohman EM, Racke MK, Raine CS. Multiple sclerosis: the plaque and its pathogenesis. N Engl J Med 2006;354(9):942–55.

20. Cannella B, Raine CS. The adhesion molecule and cytokine profile of multiple sclerosis lesions. Ann Neurol 1995;37(4):424–35.

21. Hauser SL, et al. B-cell depletion with rituximab in relapsing-remitting multiple sclerosis. N Engl J Med 2008;358(7):676–88.

22. Lucchinetti CF, et al. Distinct patterns of multiple sclerosis pathology indicates heterogeneity on pathogenesis. Brain Pathol 1996;6(3):259–74.

23. Guy J, et al. Enhancement and demyelination of the intraorbital optic nerve: fat suppression magnetic resonance imaging. Ophthalmology 1992;99(5):713–9.

24. Optic Neuritis Study Group. The 5-year risk of MS after optic neuritis: experience of the optic neuritis treatment trial. Neurology 1997;49(5):1404–13.

25. Jacobs L, Kinkel PR, Kinkel WR. Silent brain lesions in patients with isolated idiopathic optic neuritis: a clinical and nuclear magnetic resonance imaging study. Arch Neurol 1986;43(5):452–5.

26. PRISMS-4: long-term efficacy of interferon-beta-1a in relapsing MS. Neurology 2001;56(12):1628–36.

27. Jacobs LD, et al. Intramuscular interferon beta-1a therapy initiated during a first demyelinating event in multiple sclerosis. CHAMPS Study Group. N Engl J Med 2000;343(13):898–904.

28. Jacobs LD, et al. Intramuscular interferon beta-1a for disease progression in relapsing multiple sclerosis: the Multiple Sclerosis Collaborative Research Group (MSCRG). Ann Neurol 1996;39(3):285–94.

29. Beiske AG, Myhr KM. Lipoatrophy: a non-reversible complication of subcutaneous interferon-beta 1a treatment of multiple sclerosis. J Neurol 2006;253(3):377–8.

30. O'Sullivan SS, et al. Panniculitis and lipoatrophy after subcutaneous injection of interferon beta-1b in a patient with multiple sclerosis. J Neurol Neurosurg Psychiatry 2006;77(12):1382–3.

31. Frohman EM, et al. Disease modifying agent related skin reactions in multiple sclerosis: prevention, assessment, and management. Mult Scler 2004;10(3): 302–7.

32. Guthrie TC, Nelson DA. Influence of temperature changes on multiple sclerosis: critical review of mechanisms and research potential. J Neurol Sci 1995;129(1): 1–8.

33. Humm AM, et al. Quantification of Uhthoff's phenomenon in multiple sclerosis: a magnetic stimulation study. Clin Neurophysiol 2004;115(11): 2493–501.

34. Smith KJ, McDonald WI. The pathophysiology of multiple sclerosis: the mechanisms underlying the production of symptoms and the natural history of the disease. Philos Trans R Soc Lond B Biol Sci 1999;354(1390):1649–73.

35. The IFNB Multiple Sclerosis Study Group and The University of British Columbia MS/MRI Analysis Group. Interferon beta-1b in the treatment of multiple sclerosis: final outcome of the randomized controlled trial. Neurology 1995; 45(7):1277–85.

36. PRISMS (Prevention of Relapses and Disability by Interferon beta-1a Subcutaneously in Multiple Sclerosis) Study Group. Randomised double-blind placebo-controlled study of interferon beta-1a in relapsing/remitting multiple sclerosis. Lancet 1998;352(9139):1498–504.

37. Karandikar NJ, et al. Glatiramer acetate (Copaxone) therapy induces CD8(+) T cell responses in patients with multiple sclerosis. J Clin Invest 2002;109(5):641–9.

38. Calabresi PA, et al. The incidence and significance of anti-natalizumab antibodies: results from AFFIRM and SENTINEL. Neurology 2007;69(14):1391–403.

39. Kleinschmidt-DeMasters BK, Tyler KL. Progressive multifocal leukoencephalopathy complicating treatment with natalizumab and interferon beta-1a for multiple sclerosis. N Engl J Med 2005;353(4):369–74.

40. Stuve O, et al. Potential risk of progressive multifocal leukoencephalopathy with natalizumab therapy: possible interventions. Arch Neurol 2007;64(2): 169–76.

41. Goodin DS, et al. Disease modifying therapies in multiple sclerosis: report of the Therapeutics and Technology Assessment Subcommittee of the American Academy of Neurology and the MS Council for Clinical Practice Guidelines. Neurology 2002;58(2):169–78.

42. Ramkumar B, et al. Acute promyelocytic leukemia after mitoxantrone therapy for multiple sclerosis. Cancer Genet Cytogenet 2008;182(2):126–9.

43. Boster A, et al. Intense immunosuppression in patients with rapidly worsening multiple sclerosis: treatment guidelines for the clinician. Lancet Neurol 2008; 7(2):173–83.

44. Costello F, et al. Combination therapies for multiple sclerosis: scientific rationale, clinical trials, and clinical practice. Curr Opin Neurol 2007;20(3):281–5.

45. Frohman EM, et al. Therapeutic considerations for disease progression in multiple sclerosis: evidence, experience, and future expectations. Arch Neurol 2005;62(10):1519–30.

46. Zivadinov R, et al. Effects of IV methylprednisolone on brain atrophy in relapsing-remitting MS. Neurology 2001;57(7):1239–47.

47. Frohman EM, et al. Corticosteroids for multiple sclerosis: I. Application for treating exacerbations. Neurotherapeutics 2007;4(4):618–26.

48. Shah A, et al. Corticosteroids for multiple sclerosis: II. Application for disease-modifying effects. Neurotherapeutics 2007;4(4):627–32.
49. Chrousos GA, et al. Side effects of glucocorticoid treatment: experience of the Optic Neuritis Treatment Trial. JAMA 1993;269(16):2110–2.
50. Johnson KP, et al. Copolymer 1 reduces relapse rate and improves disability in relapsing-remitting multiple sclerosis: results of a phase III multicenter, double-blind placebo-controlled trial. The Copolymer 1 Multiple Sclerosis Study Group. Neurology 1995;45(7):1268–76.
51. Rudick RA, et al. Natalizumab plus interferon beta-1a for relapsing multiple sclerosis. N Engl J Med 2006;354(9):911–23.
52. Strasser-Fuchs S, et al. Clinically benign multiple sclerosis despite large T2 lesion load: can we explain this paradox? Mult Scler 2008;14(2):205–11.
53. Thompson AJ, et al. Patterns of disease activity in multiple sclerosis. BMJ 1990; 301(6742):44–5.
54. Miller DH, et al. The role of magnetic resonance techniques in understanding and managing multiple sclerosis. Brain 1998;121(Pt 1):3–24.
55. Khan OA, Dhib-Jalbut SS. Neutralizing antibodies to interferon beta-1a and interferon beta-1b in MS patients are cross-reactive. Neurology 1998;51(6):1698–702.
56. Rudick RA, et al. Incidence and significance of neutralizing antibodies to interferon beta-1a in multiple sclerosis. Multiple Sclerosis Collaborative Research Group (MSCRG). Neurology 1998;50(5):1266–72.
57. Runkel L, et al. Structural and functional differences between glycosylated and non-glycosylated forms of human interferon-beta (IFN-beta). Pharm Res 1998; 15(4):641–9.
58. European Study Group on interferon beta-1b in secondary progressive MS. Placebo-controlled multicentre randomised trial of interferon beta-1b in treatment of secondary progressive multiple sclerosis. Lancet 1998;352(9139):1491–7.
59. Giovannelli M, et al. Early physiotherapy after injection of botulinum toxin increases the beneficial effects on spasticity in patients with multiple sclerosis. Clin Rehabil 2007;21(4):331–7.
60. Ward AB. Spasticity treatment with botulinum toxins. J Neural Transm 2008; 115(4):607–16.
61. Goodman AD, et al. Fampridine-SR in multiple sclerosis: a randomized, double-blind, placebo-controlled, dose-ranging study. Mult Scler 2007;13(3):357–68.
62. Hayes KC. Fampridine-SR for multiple sclerosis and spinal cord injury. Expert Rev Neurother 2007;7(5):453–61.
63. Romani A, et al. Fatigue in multiple sclerosis: multidimensional assessment and response to symptomatic treatment. Mult Scler 2004;10(4):462–8.
64. Peterson EW, et al. Injurious falls among middle aged and older adults with multiple sclerosis. Arch Phys Med Rehabil 2008;89(6):1031–7.
65. Debouverie M, et al. Physical dimension of fatigue correlated with disability change over time in patients with multiple sclerosis. J Neurol 2008;255(5):633–6.
66. Lebrun C, et al. Levocarnitine administration in multiple sclerosis patients with immunosuppressive therapy-induced fatigue. Mult Scler 2006;12(3):321–4.
67. Justus N, et al [Treatment with botulinum toxin in neurologic pediatrics]. Kinderkrankenschwester 2007;26(7):274–6.
68. Smith CP, Somogyi GT, Boone TB. Botulinum toxin in urology: evaluation using an evidence-based medicine approach. Nat Clin Pract Urol 2004;1(1):31–7.

69. Thompson AJ, et al. Clinical management of spasticity. J Neurol Neurosurg Psychiatry 2005;76(4):459–63.

70. Litwiller SE, Frohman EM, Zimmern PE. Multiple sclerosis and the urologist. J Urol 1999;161(3):743–57.

71. Rudick RA, et al. Impact of interferon beta-1a on neurologic disability in relapsing multiple sclerosis: the Multiple Sclerosis Collaborative Research Group (MSCRG). Neurology 1997;49(2):358–63.

72. Tintore M. Rationale for early intervention with immunomodulatory treatments. J Neurol 2008;255(Suppl 1):37–43.

Low Back Pain

Michael Devereaux, MD, FACP

KEYWORDS

- Sciatica • Low back pain • Acute low back pain
- Chronic back pain • Spine • Pain

LOW BACK PAIN

General internists and family practitioners play an important role in the initial evaluation and treatment of acute low back pain and chronic low back pain. In the present managed care environment, it is doubtful that this role will decrease, and indeed it should not, because a large percentage of patients who have low back pain can be managed by the primary care physician without referral to a specialist. According to one study, the primary care physician is the initial provider of care for acute low back pain approximately 65% of the time and frequently is the sole provider of care.[1] Given the limited time in the present medical system the primary care physician often has available to evaluate a patient who has acute or chronic low back pain, it is imperative that the generalist have an understanding of the salient points in the history, the essentials of the physical/neurologic examination, the diagnostic testing options, and the effectiveness (or lack of effectiveness) of available treatments.

WHAT IS THE INCIDENCE AND PREVALENCE OF LOW BACK PAIN?

Epidemiologic studies of low back pain are an interpretive challenge because of the inconsistency and lack of standardization used to define back pain in different studies and the variability of criteria from one study to the next.[2] Both the prevalence and incidence of low back pain are high. Hart and colleagues[3] estimated the total number of annual adult visits for low back pain to a physician in the United States to be 15 million, making back pain the fifth most common reason for a physician office visit at the time of this study. The lifetime prevalence of an episode of significant low back pain is 60% to 90%.[2,4,5] Deyo and Tsui-Wu[6] reported a 13.8% lifetime prevalence of an episode of low back pain of 2 or more weeks' duration. About 1.6% of the same population (12% of the patients who had low back pain) reported sciatica.[6] An example of the interpretative challenge of the epidemiology literature is that the reported the annual incidence of developing an episode of low back pain ranges from 4% to 93%, depending on the study.[2] In one well-designed epidemiologic survey of adults age 20 to 69 years, 19% of 318 patients who did not have a history of back pain over a period of 6 months

Neurological Institute, University Hospitals, Case Medical Center, 11100 Euclid Avenue, Cleveland, OH 44106, USA
E-mail address: Michael.Devereauxi@UHhospitals.org

Med Clin N Am 93 (2009) 477–501
doi:10.1016/j.mcna.2008.09.013
0025-7125/08/$ – see front matter

medical.theclinics.com

before entry into the study developed an episode of low back pain (usually mild in intensity) over the 1-year study period.[7]

Low back pain has a major social impact in the industrialized world. In the United States, back pain is the second leading cause of work absenteeism. Spine symptoms are the reason for approximately 25% of all lost work days.[5] In 1988, approximately 175.8 million restricted activity days were caused by spine-related disorders.[4,8,9] At any one time an estimated 1% of adults in the United States are disabled temporarily, and 1% are disabled chronically as a result of low back pain. Approximately 400,000 compensated back injuries occur each year.[4,8,9]

WHAT ARE THE RISK FACTORS FOR LOW BACK PAIN?

Commonly accepted risk factors for acute low back pain (and often for chronic low back pain) include[5,10]

- Increasing age
- Heavy physical work (particularly involving long periods of static work postures, heavy lifting, twisting, and vibration)
- Psychosocial factors, including work dissatisfaction and monotonous work
- Depression
- Obesity (body mass index > 30%; possibly a more significant factor in women than in men)
- Smoking
- Severe (> 80%) scoliosis
- Drug abuse
- History of headache

Many other factors that commonly, but probably erroneously, are thought to increase the risk of low back pain include[5]

- Anthropometric status (height and body build)
- Posture, including kyphosis, lordosis, and modest scoliosis (< 80%)
- Leg-length differences
- State of physical fitness (Although physical fitness is not a predicator of acute low back pain, fit individuals have a lower incidence of chronic low back pain and tend to recover more quickly from episodes of acute low back pain than unfit individuals.)

WHAT ARE THE ANATOMIC ESSENTIALS THAT A PRIMARY CARE PHYSICIANS NEED TO KNOW HOW TO DIAGNOSIS AND TREAT THE CAUSES OF LOW BACK PAIN?

There are five lumbar vertebrae. Each is composed of a body, two pedicles, two laminae, four articular facets, and a spinous process. Between each pair of vertebrae are two openings, the foramina, through which pass a spinal nerve (the nerve "root"), radicular blood vessels, and the sinuvertebral nerves (**Fig. 1**). The spinal canal itself is formed posterolaterally by the laminae and ligamentum flavum, anterolaterally by the pedicles, and anteriorly by the posterior surface of the vertebral bodies and intervertebral disks. The midsagittal diameter of the lumbar canal averages about 18 mm. Narrowing as the result of spondylotic degeneration with superimposed additional narrowing secondary to extension of the trunk can compress the cauda equina. The conus medullaris, the tip of the spinal cord, is at the level of L1-L2.

The facets (the zygapophyseal joints) are true synovial joints. These joints, like all synovial joints, are subject to degenerative and inflammatory changes with resultant

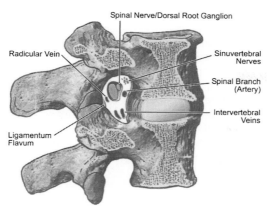

Fig. 1. The foramen. (*From* Levin KH, Covington EC, Devereaux MW, et al. Neck and back pain. Continuum: Lifelong Learning Neurol 2001;7:9; with permission.)

enlargement that, in association with thickening of the ligamentum flavum, can contribute to canal stenosis as a component of spondylosis. The exact role of the facet joint in the production of spine pain, particularly low back pain, remains somewhat controversial.[11,12]

The intervertebral disk has the dual role of providing the primary support for the column of vertebral bones while maintaining elasticity to permit the required mobility of the spine. Each disk is composed of a ring of elastic collagen, the annulus fibrosus, surrounding the gelatinous nucleus pulposus (**Fig. 2**). The aging or chronically injured disk contains increasing amounts of fibrous tissue that gradually replaces the highly elastic collagen fibers comprising the annulus fibrosis of the young disk. The older disk is less elastic, and its hydraulic recall mechanism is weakened. By age 50 years, the annulus becomes fissured, and ultimately the disk deteriorates into a desiccated, fragmented, and frayed annulus fibrosus surrounding a fibrotic nucleus pulposus. The intervertebral disk is avascular by age 20 years. The nucleus pulposus has no nerve

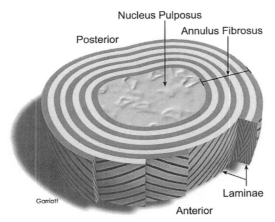

Fig. 2. The intervertebral disk. (*From* Levin KH, Covington EC, Devereaux MW, et al. Neck and back pain. Continuum: Lifelong Learning Neurol 2001;7:11; with permission.)

supply, but the outer lamellae of the annulus contains nerve endings derived from the sinuvertebral nerves (recurrent meningeal nerves).[5,13–18]

There is debate regarding the nociceptive nerve supply to the intervertebral disk and the role the disk plays as a generator of back pain. Korkala and colleagues[13] showed that the nerve endings entering the annulus fibrosus do not contain substance P and are not nociceptors. The authors noted that nociceptive nerve endings are located in the posterior ligament adjacent to the disk. Palmgren and colleagues,[19] in a study of normal human lumbar intervertebral disk tissue, demonstrated that nerve endings could be found at a depth of a few millimeters, whereas neuropeptide markers (eg, substance P) revealed nociceptive nerves only in the outermost layers of the annulus fibrous. This study supports the concept that the normal intervertebral disk is almost without nociceptive innervation.

This finding leads to the question of the mechanism of primary diskogenic pain, particularly in the lumbar spine. Damage to the intervertebral disk can produce pain, but no consensus exists on the mechanisms responsible. Radial tears and fissures in the annulus fibrosus occur as the disk ages. This change has been linked to the ingrowth of blood vessels and nerve fibers, leading to the concept that the ingrowth of these nerve endings may be the pathoanatomic basis for diskogenic pain.[16,20] If the ingrowth of nociceptive nerve fibers into the intervertebral disk is the neuroanatomic substrate for diskogenic pain, however, why are most degenerative disks not a source of pain? For example, diskography of degenerative disks does not uniformly induce pain.[20] Because disk degeneration alone is not the basis for diskogenic pain, contributing factors must be at play. Possibly a combination of focal damage to the annulus fibrosus, inflammation, neoinnervation, and nociceptor sensitization is necessary to induce diskogenic pain.[21]

Many ligaments lash the vertebrae together and, along with the paraspinous muscles, help control and limit spinal column motion. From a clinical perspective, some of the ligaments are more important than others. The posterior longitudinal ligament stretches from the axis (the tectorial membrane in the "high" cervical spine) to the sacrum and forms the anterior wall of the spinal canal. It is broad throughout the cervical and thoracic portions of the spine. At the L1 vertebral level, however, it begins to narrow, and at L5 it is one half its original width. It is attached firmly to each intervertebral disk and hyaline cartilage endplate, but only in the midline of the vertebral body by a septum to the periosteum. The open space between the posterior longitudinal ligament and the vertebral body is the anterior epidural space, which is important in the process of disk herniation. The narrowing of the ligament in the lumbar spine inadequately reinforces the lumbar disk, creating an inherent structural weakness. This narrowing, coupled with the great static and kinetic stress placed on the lumbar disks, contributes to their susceptibility to injury and herniation.

The ligamenta flava is composed of a series of strong, paired elastic ligaments that span the space between the laminae and are attached to the anterior inferior surface of the laminae above and the posterior superior margin of the laminae below. Each component stretches laterally, joining the facet joint capsule. The ligament stretches under tension, permitting flexion of the spine. It contains few, if any, nociceptive nerve fibers. It can be clinically important, because it can thicken with age and, along with other spondylotic degenerative changes, can contribute to canal stenosis that can produce myelopathy in the cervical spine and compression of the cauda equina in the lumbar spine.

With the exception of the atlas and axis, the range and type of movement in each segment of the spine is determined by the facet (zygapophyseal) joints, but spine stability and control of spine movement depends on muscles and ligaments. The movement itself, of course, is generated by muscle.

The spinal muscles are arranged in layers. The deeper layers comprise the intrinsic true back muscles, as defined by their position and innervation by the posterior rami of the spinal nerves. The more superficial extrinsic muscles insert on the bones of the upper limbs and are innervated by anterior rami of the spinal nerves.

The intrinsic muscles also are divided into superficial and deep groups. The superficial layer is comprised of the paraspinous erector spinae group, which spans the entire length of the spine from the occiput to the sacrum, and the splenius muscles of the upper back and neck. This superficial group functions collectively primarily to maintain erect posture. Deep to the erector spinae is the transversospinalis muscle group, which is composed of muscles made up of several smaller muscles that run obliquely and longitudinally. In essence, they form a system of guy ropes that provide lateral stability to the spine, contribute to maintenance of an erect posture, and rotate the spine. Deepest of all are the interspinal and intertransverse muscles, which are composed of numerous small muscles involved in the maintenance of posture.

The multiple subdivisions of muscle mass, numerous connective tissue planes, and multiple attachments of tendons over small areas of vertebral periosteum help explain the prevalence of neck and back pain and also the difficultly in localizing the source of that pain precisely. Given this difficulty in identifying muscle and tendon injury as the source of pain and the fact that there are other generators of low back pain besides muscles (eg, fascia, ligaments, facet joint, intervertebral disks), it is no wonder that, according to Deyo and colleagues,[9] the source of acute low back pain cannot be identified in 85% of patients. Also, when muscle is the source of pain, the pathophysiologic pain-generating process is unclear. In the clinic, muscle spasm often is the diagnosis offered. "Muscle spasm" generally is defined as a contraction of muscle that cannot be released voluntarily and is associated with electromyographic activity. Johnson[22] and Mense and Simons[23] have taken issue with increased muscle activity as a source of paraspinous pain, noting a lack of electromyographic evidence indicative of muscle spasm.

Localized spine pain is mediated through two peripheral nerve systems: the posterior rami of the spinal nerves and the sinuvertebral nerves. The sinuvertebral nerves supply structures within the spinal canal. These nerves arise from the rami communicantes and enter the spinal canal by way of the intervertebral foramina.[14] Branches ascend and descend one or more levels interconnecting with the sinuvertebral nerves from other levels and innervating the anterior and posterior longitudinal ligaments, the anterior and posterior portion of the dura mater, and blood vessels, among other structures (**Fig. 3**). This system also may supply nociceptive branches to degenerated intervertebral disks. Branches of the posterior rami of the spinal nerves provide nociceptive fibers to the fascia, ligaments, periosteum, and facet joints. The source of deep somatic neck and low back pain therefore can be the vertebral column itself, the surrounding muscle tendons, ligaments fascia, or a combination thereof.

Radicular pain, unlike spondylogenic pain, is mediated by the proximal spinal nerves rather than by the sinuvertebral nerves or the anterior or posterior rami of the spinal nerves.

WHAT TYPES OF PAIN ARE GENERATED BY LUMBAR SPINE DISORDER?

There are three major categories of pain related to the spine: localized, radiating, and referred.

Deyo and colleagues[9] noted that a definitive diagnosis of low back pain cannot be established in 85% of patients because of the weak association between the symptoms, pathologic changes, and imaging results. Nonetheless, it is widely assumed

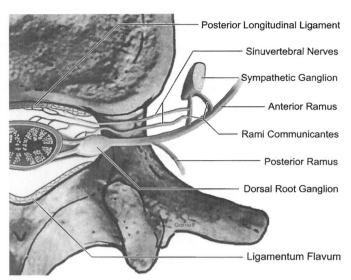

Posterior Longitudinal Ligament

Sinuvertebral Nerves

Sympathetic Ganglion

Anterior Ramus

Rami Communicantes

Posterior Ramus

Dorsal Root Ganglion

Ligamentum Flavum

Fig. 3. The sinuvertebral nerves. (*From* Levin KH, Covington EC, Devereaux MW, et al. Neck and back pain. Continuum: Lifelong Learning Neurol 2001;7:13; with permission.)

that much nonradiating low back pain is secondary to musculoligamentous injury, degenerative changes in the spine, or a combination of the two. As already noted. local spine pain is mediated primarily through the posterior rami of the spinal nerves and the sinuvertebral nerves.

The source of acute low back pain is most likely the result of increased tension of the paraspinous muscles related to physical activity, such as lifting, with resultant avulsion of tendinous attachments of the muscles to bony structures and/or rupture of the muscle fibers and/or tearing of muscle sheaths. Persistent overuse of a muscle group in the absence of muscle injury can result in pain and potential tonic contraction (spasm), probably reflecting increased metabolic activity and the production of chemical byproducts stimulating unmyelinated nerve fibers. This development is particularly likely with the persistent use of untrained, poorly conditioned muscles (as previously noted there is controversy regarding the existence of spasm).[22,23] The role of paraspinous muscles as a generator of chronic low back pain is uncertain but is likely to be much smaller than in acute low back pain.

As already stated, radiating or radicular pain is mediated not by the sinuvertebral nerves or the posterior rami of the spinal nerves but rather by the proximal spinal nerves. This radiating pain is the generator of "sciatica" (radicular pain into one or both lower extremities distal to the knee). At times, particularly in the case of high lumbar radiculopathies (L2 and L3), the radiating pain may be less well defined, with referral only into the thigh. Two major factors are involved in the generation of radicular-based radiating pain: compression and inflammation.

Compression of the nerve root produces local ischemia with a possible alteration in axoplasmic transport and resultant edema affecting the large mechanoreceptor fibers, resulting in loss of inhibition of pain and impulses carried by the unmyelinated fibers with resultant increased nociceptive input into the spinal cord (Gait theory).[5] Inflammation, which may be neurogenic or immunologic, develops at the site of compression, probably secondary to the previously isolated nuclear pulposous being herniated through the annulus fibrosus and exposed to the immune system for the first time, contributing to the generation of pain. The simultaneous involvement of the posterior ramus, the sinuvertebral nerves, and the compressed inflamed spinal nerve can result in the combination of low back pain and radiating pain into a lower extremity subserved by the anterior ramus.

Multiple processes affecting most organs in the abdomen as well as retroperitoneal structures (eg, dissecting aortic aneurysm, renal colic, tumors of many abdominal organs) can present with low back pain. Therefore, the examination of the abdomen is an important part of the initial assessment of a patient presenting with acute low pain.

WHAT ARE THE MOST COMMON CAUSES OF ACUTE NONRADIATING LOW BACK PAIN?

The exact generator of acute low back pain usually is not specifically diagnosable, as suggested by the lack of precision and specificity in the names given the syndromes: "back strain," "musculoskeletal pain syndrome," "back spasms," "myofascial pain syndrome," and, if pain is more widespread, "fibromyalgia." Tendon, ligament, muscle, and facet joints have all been implicated as sources of pain, but none can be readily documented in any given patient.

Muscle strain probably is the most common cause of neck and acute low back pain. Immediate or delayed-onset muscular strain often results from of some type of physical activity. This type of injury occurs when the muscles in question undergo forceful elongation, usually while being activated. Tearing of muscle fibers occurs primarily at the musculotendinous interface but can occur in the belly of the muscle as well.[12]

Ligamentous sprains are caused by stretching the ligament beyond its physiologic range. The pain of muscle strain and ligamentous sprain is described variously as aching, sharp, or dull and can be mild to severe. The key to the diagnosis in these patients is the absence of any significant radiating pain into either lower extremity and the absence of abnormalities on the neurologic and general examination.[24]

In this setting back pain generally is reduced significantly when the patient is recumbent. If such is the case, and there are no neurologic findings, an immediate diagnostic work-up usually is unnecessary. If pain does persist in recumbency, however, infections of the spinal column (osteomyelitis/epidural abscess) and metastatic cancer should be considered. An immediate diagnostic work-up in this setting usually is warranted.

HOW BIG A ROLE DOES DEGENERATIVE SPINE DISEASE PLAY IN THE GENERATION OF LOW BACK PAIN?

"Spondylosis" is the more correct term for degenerative changes that occur throughout the spine. These changes occur to the greatest degree in the lumbar and cervical portions of the spine, because these portions of the spine are more mobile (and hence subject to more "wear and tear") than the thoracic spine. "Spondylosis" is a more accurate term than "arthritis of the spine," because much of the degenerative change is not primarily inflammatory.[5] Spondylosis is a naturally occurring process in the aging spine, particularly the lumbar spine. By 79 years of age, nearly all individuals have some degree of spondylosis. By age 49 years, 60% of women and 80% of men have osteophytes and other changes indicative of early spondylosis. There is a poor correlation between the presence of spondylosis on radiographs of the lumbar spine and back pain. Some patients may have marked degenerative change with little or no pain. Disk herniation, a component of spondylosis, is a common finding in the absence of pain.[25,26] Other patients have significant low back pain in the absence of significant degenerative change. As with acute low back pain, it often is difficult to localize the source of nonradiating chronic low back pain, and lumbar spine surgery for nonradiating chronic low back pain often is unsuccessful. Progressive spondylosis with osteophyte formation, thickening of the ligaments (particularly the ligament of flavum), and bulging/transverse bar formation of aging lumbar intervertebral disks can lead to lumbar canal stenosis and ultimately to compression of individual nerve roots or of the cauda equina as a whole.

In summary, in dealing with patients who have low back pain and radiologic evidence of lumbar spondylosis, it is important to treat the patient and not the results of imaging procedures. Surgical treatment for chronic low back pain in patients who have a normal neurologic examination but with spondylosis (even severe spondylosis) on neuroimaging procedures often has a poor outcome.

WHAT IS THE DEFINITION OF SCIATICA AND WHAT CAUSES IT?

"Sciatica" refers to pain radiating into either lower extremity distal to the knee. It is associated most commonly with L5 and S1 radiculopathies, which together comprise more than 90% of all lumbosacral radiculopathies. L5 and S1 radiculopathies may result from a variety of pathophysiologic processes compromising the spinal nerve root/ roots, including acute disk herniation and spondylosis. Less common causes include compression by a benign or occasionally malignant tumor or epidural abscess. Although L5 and S1 radiculopathies combined are the most common cause of sciatica, there are other potential causes of radiating pain distal to the knee, including lesions involving the pelvic plexus or sciatic nerve (eg, the piriformis syndrome).

WHAT ARE THE ESSENTIALS IN THE HISTORY THAT HELP TO DEFINE THE NATURE OF LOW BACK PAIN?

The history of low back pain is of critical importance in assessing patients who have symptoms believed to be secondary to lumbar spine disorders, especially patients who have a nonfocal neurologic examination. The differential diagnosis frequently is based solely on the history in these patients. As with most pain syndromes, it is essential to establish a pain profile.[5,18]

Onset

In most instances, patients who present with acute-onset low back pain have a history of preceding pain, often for weeks, months, or longer. This is also true for patients who present with the acute onset of radicular pain. The onset of lumbosacral radicular pain in the absence of any prior history of low back pain is the exception rather than the rule. Radicular distribution pain into a lower extremity ("sciatica") often is the result of disk herniation. Slowly progressing pain is more typical of degenerative disorders of the spine and of slow-growing tumors.

Location

Musculoskeletal pain usually is localized to the paraspinal regions, spreading at time to the flanks and into the buttocks. In the case of lumbosacral radiculopathy, the pain usually radiates into a lower extremity. Occasionally, the distribution of the pain can point to the specific root involved (**Table 1**). For example, high lumbar (L2, L3) radiculopathic pain does not radiate distal to the knee, whereas the pain of an L4 radiculopathy can radiate distal to the knee to the medial leg. L5 and S1 radiculopathies tend to produce pain that radiates into the posterolateral thigh and posterolateral leg, often involving the foot. Pain may

Table 1
Symptoms and signs association with lumbar radiculopathy

Root	Pain Distribution	Dermatomal Sensory Distribution	Weakness	Affected Reflex
L1	Inguinal region	Inguinal region	Hip flexion	Cremasteric
L2	Inguinal region and anterior thigh	Anterior thigh	Hip flexion Hip adduction	Cremasteric thigh adductor
L3	Anterior thigh and knee	Distal anteromedial thigh including knee	Knee extension Hip flexion Hip adduction	Patellar thigh adductor
L4	Anterior thigh, medial aspect leg	Medial leg	Knee extension Hip flexion Hip adduction	Patellar
L5	Posterolateral thighLateral legMedial foot	Lateral leg, dorsal foot and great toe	Dorsiflexion foot/toes Knee flexionHip adduction	—
S1	Posterior thigh and leg, and lateral foot	Posterolateral leg and lateral aspect of foot	Plantar flexion foot/toesKnee flexionHip extension	Achilles

Data from Levin KH, Covington EC, Devereaux MW, et al. Neck and back pain. Continuum: Lifelong Learning Neurol 2001;7:16.

be maximum in the medial (L5 radiculopathy) or lateral (S1 radiculopathy) aspect of the foot.

Duration

Mechanical low back pain generally has a duration of days to weeks. Radicular pain often resolves more gradually over 6 to 8 weeks, if it resolves at all. A patient who presents with a history of chronic low back pain may not require a neurodiagnostic evaluation, but a careful history is required to rule out a new problem producing pain superimposed on chronic symptoms. These patients are a challenge even to the most experienced clinician, because such a patient, even with a history of chronic pain, may prove to be an exception and require an immediate neurodiagnostic evaluation.

Severity

As all clinicians recognize, the severity of pain often is difficult to interpret, because it can be colored by several factors, including the patient's personality. Nonradiating musculoskeletal pain may range from mild to incapacitating. Radicular pain secondary to a herniated disk often is severe but may not be. Severe low back pain not relieved when the patient is recumbent suggests metastatic cancer, pathologic vertebral fracture, or infection of a vertebra, disk, or in the epidural space.

Time of Day

In the absence of a history of trauma, new-onset of lumbar radiculopathy frequently is present upon awaking in the morning. Nonradiating pain that tends to be dull during the day often is the result of mechanical disorders (eg, muscle strain, degenerative disk disease/spondylosis). Tumors of the spine and spinal cord often produce pain that persists and occasionally increases in the supine position, sometimes increasing in bed at night.

Associated Symptoms

Paresthesia, weakness in one or both lower extremities, and bladder/bowel dysfunction may accompany low back pain, particularly radicular pain. Many patients who have radiating pain into a lower extremity complain of weakness. Distinguishing guarding secondary to pain from weakness caused by nerve root compromise can be challenging. Also, the patient should be questioned about abdominal pain and intestinal or genitourinary symptoms, because lesions in various abdominal organs may present with referred low back pain. Recognizing the presence of neurologic symptoms/signs is important and may lead to an expedited diagnostic work-up.

Triggers

Valsalva maneuvers (eg, coughing, sneezing, and bearing down at stool) often transiently aggravate lumbosacral radicular pain. Low back radicular pain generally is worse when the patient is seated or standing and often is relieved by lying in a supine position. If pain persists or increases in the supine position, the possibility of metastatic cancer or an infection must be considered. In the case of lumbar canal stenosis, the symptoms of neurogenic claudication often can be aggravated by standing erect (which tends to reduce the mid sagittal diameter of the lumbar canal) and by walking.

Motor Symptoms

In the face of pain, distinguishing between weakness and guarding by the history alone can be difficult. In the case of low back and lower extremity pain, however, weakness is suggested by the history of a foot slap when walking or falls secondary to a lower extremity "giving way." Although weakness usually is best appreciated on the neurologic examination, the history is a useful adjunct in helping distinguish weakness from guarding secondary to pain.

Sensory Disturbances

Patients who have radiculopathy often report numbness, tingling, and even coolness in the involved extremity. At times symptoms may suggest dysesthesia and allodynia. The distribution of a sensory disturbance by history, particularly numbness and tingling, sometimes may be more useful than the sensory examination itself in determining the presence and localization of radiculopathy.

Bladder and Bowel Disturbances

Sphincter disturbances in association with low back pain syndromes are uncommon, but a neurogenic bladder can be a component of a cauda equina syndrome. Disturbances of bowel and bladder control should serve as a warning of the need for an urgent neurodiagnostic work-up and, very probably, surgical intervention.

WHAT ARE THE ESSENTIALS OF THE PHYSICAL EXAMINATION?
General Examination

The necessity for a general physical assessment in a patient who complains of back pain cannot be overstated. The presence of low-grade fever, for example, may signal infection that involves the vertebral column, the epidural space, or the surrounding muscle (eg, psoas abscess). Inspection of the skin for lesions may yield diagnostic information (**Box 1**).

The rectal examination for sphincter tone, anal "wink," and the bulbocavernosus reflex may reflect changes in the spinal cord or cauda equina. An abnormal prostate examination may lead to a diagnosis of prostate cancer with spinal metastases. The abdominal examination is particularly important. In a patient who has low back pain. The presence of abdominal tenderness, organomegaly, or a pulsatile abdominal mass with a bruit signals the need for an urgent diagnostic evaluation that may lead to a potentially life-saving discovery, such as a leaking abdominal aneurysm. In patients who have low back pain and claudication, evaluation of the peripheral pulses in both lower extremities is essential to help distinguish neurogenic claudication from vascular claudication.

Neurologic Examination

The experienced clinician knows that the neurologic examination of a patient who has low back pain can be altered by the pain itself. For example, when testing strength, guarding must be taken into account. Tendon reflexes may be suppressed as a result of poor relaxation of the limb as a consequence of pain. Preparing the patient by explaining each step of the examination in advance may reduce anxiety and encourage relaxation, thereby reducing guarding and enhancing the reliability of the examination itself. The neurologic examination should include

Inspection of the low back: The presence of a tuft of hair over the lumbar spine suggests diastematomyelia/spina bifida occulta.

Posture: Splinting with a list away from the painful lower extremity is seen with a lateral lumbar disk herniation, whereas list toward the painful side can be seen with medial herniation. Tilting of the trunk to the side opposite the list by the examiner can cause additional nerve root compression with resultant accentuation of radicular distribution pain. Patients who have neurogenic claudication secondary to compression of the cauda equina may tend to stand and walk with the trunk flexed forward, a posture that reduces compression by widening the anterior-posterior dimension of the lumbar canal.

Percussion: Percussion over the lumbar spine may induce pain over a vertebral malignancy or infection.

Box 1
Skin lesions related to spine pain

Psoriasis—psoriatic arthritis

Erythema nodosum—inflammatory disease, cancer

Café-au-lait spots—neurofibromatosis

Hidradenitis suppurative—epidural abscess

Vesicles—herpes zoster

Needle marks (intravenous drug abuse)—vertebral column infections

Subcutaneous masses—neurofibroma, lymphadenopathy

Lumbar spine mobility: Lumbar spine mobility usually is reduced in patients who have low back pain, but a measurement of the degree of mobility usually is not useful because mobility varies so widely with conditioning and age.

Gait evaluation: An antalgic gait with splinting favors the side of a lumbar radiculopathy. Foot slap (ie, foot drop) secondary to weakness of dorsiflexors of the foot can be seen with an L5 radiculopathy. Heel and toe walking, toe tapping, and hopping on either foot may reveal additional evidence of weakness suggesting radiculopathy.

Motor testing: Individual muscle group testing around each joint in the lower extremity is important to elicit evidence of weakness within a specific myotome (**Table 1**).

Sensory testing: Sensory testing is usually done with a sharp object looking for evidence of sensory loss within a given dermatome (**Table 1**).

Reflexes: See **Table 1**.

Neuromechanical tests: Neuromechanical tests are an important adjunct to the traditional neurologic examination in patients who have low back pain radiating into a lower extremity.

Straight leg-raising test: With the patient in a supine position, the symptomatic lower extremity is elevated slowly off the examining table (**Fig. 4**). The spinal nerve and its dural sleeve, tethered by a herniated disk, are stretched when the lower extremity is elevated between 30° and 70°. The test is positive if radiating pain occurs within this range. Pain generated at less than 30° or more than 70° of elevation is nonspecific.

Lasegue test: A variation of straight leg-raising test. With the patient in a supine position, the symptomatic lower extremity is flexed to 90° at the hip and knee. The knee then is extended slowly, which produces radiating pain as a result of L5 and S1 nerve root compression.

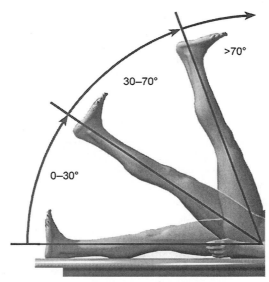

Fig. 4. The straight leg-raising test. (*From* Levin KH, Covington EC, Devereaux MW, et al. Neck and back pain. Continuum: Lifelong Learning Neurol 2001;7:20; with permission.)

Bragard's sign (test): If pain is generated by straight leg raising, the symptomatic extremity is lowered until the pain disappears (**Fig. 5**). At that point the foot is dorsiflexed. If this maneuver recreates radiating pain, the test is positive and supports the presence of a low lumbar radiculopathy.

Contralateral ("well") straight leg-raising test: Performed on the asymptomatic lower extremity, this test has specificity but low sensitivity for disk herniation.

Prone straight leg-raising test: With the patient in a prone position, the symptomatic lower extremity is slowly extended at the hip by the examiner (**Fig. 6**). Accentuation of pain in the anterior thigh suggests a high lumbar (L2, L3) radiculopathy.

Valsalva test: The Valsalva maneuver increases intrathecal pressure, which accentuates radicular pain in the presence of spinal nerve compression and inflammation.

Brudzinski test: With the patient supine, the examiner flexes the patient's head. In the presence of spinal compression, this flexion aggravates radicular pain.

Patrick (Faber) test: The lateral malleolus of the symptomatic lower extremity is placed on the patella of the opposite extremity, and the symptomatic extremity is slowly rotated externally (**Fig. 7**). Accentuation of the pain suggests that pain is caused by a lesion in the hip or sacroiliac joint rather than by radiculopathy.

Gaenslen test: With the patient supine and the symptomatic extremity and buttocks extending slightly over the edge of the examination table, the asymptomatic lower extremity is flexed at the hip and knee and brought to the chest (**Fig. 8**). The symptomatic lower extremity is extended at the hip to the floor. Increased nonradiating low back and buttocks pain indicates sacroiliac joint disease.

Waddell test: Excessive sensitivity to light pinching of the skin in the region of low back pain suggests a functional component.

WHAT ARE THE MOST COMMON LUMBOSACRAL RADICULOPATHIES?

L5 radiculopathy is the most common lumbosacral radiculopathy, with S1 radiculopathy a close second. The two combined account for about 90% to 95% of all lumbar radiculopathies. The next most common is L4 radiculopathy (< 5%). High lumbar radiculopathies constitute the remainder. The combination of clinical symptoms and

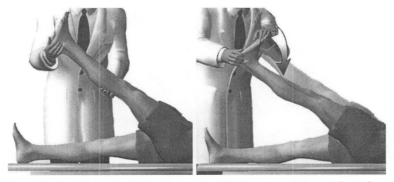

Fig. 5. Bragard's sign. (*From* Levin KH, Covington EC, Devereaux MW, et al. Neck and back pain. Continuum: Lifelong Learning Neurol 2001;7:20; with permission.)

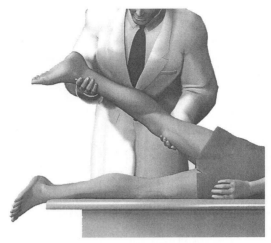

Fig. 6. Prone straight leg-raising test. (*From* Levin KH, Covington EC, Devereaux MW, et al. Neck and back pain. Continuum: Lifelong Learning Neurol 2001;7:21; with permission.)

signs (see **Table 1**) usually leads to the correct diagnosis. When appropriate, an MRI, and an electromyogram (EMG) with nerve conductions can give further support to the diagnosis.[5]

WHAT ARE THE MOST COMMON CAUSES OF LUMBAR RADICULOPATHY?

Although there are many potential causes of lumbar radiculopathy (**Box 2**), the most common are acute disk herniation and spondylosis or a combination of the two.[5,27,28] Most commonly, a herniated disk tethers the root exiting at the level below the disk herniation (L4-L5 disk herniation causing S1 radiculopathy).

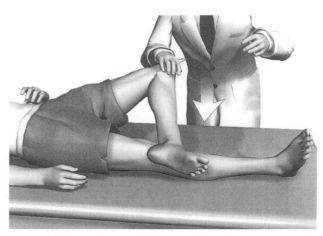

Fig. 7. Faber maneuver. (*From* Levin KH, Covington EC, Devereaux MW, et al. Neck and back pain. Continuum: Lifelong Learning Neurol 2001;7:22; with permission.)

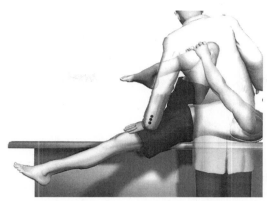

Fig. 8. Gaenslen test. (*From* Levin KH, Covington EC, Devereaux MW, et al. Neck and back pain. Continuum: Lifelong Learning Neurol 2001;7:22; with permission.)

In the case of disk herniation, the distribution of symptoms and signs depends on the level of herniation, the location of the herniation (midline, paramedian, lateral), and the size of the herniation. Disk herniation is common in asymptomatic patients.[25,26] Therefore in a symptomatic patient the presence of a herniated disk on MRI may be coincidental. It is imperative to link the symptoms with the identified herniated disk by a careful examination and additional tests (eg, EMG) where appropriate.

WHAT ARE THE CLINICAL MANIFESTATIONS OF LUMBAR CANAL STENOSIS?

Lumbar spinal stenosis can be caused by many conditions (**Box 3**).

Lumbar spinal stenosis is caused most commonly by spondylosis, at times superimposed over other causes of stenosis, particularly congenital. Spondylotic spinal stenosis often is asymptomatic. The presence and type of clinical manifestations reflect the degree of degenerative change and the location of the stenosis, affecting either the central canal of the spinal column or the lateral recesses of the canal. Symptomatic lateral canal stenosis typically presents as a radiculopathy. Although symptoms often are progressive at onset, they can appear suddenly as a result of an acute change, such as disk herniation superimposed over lateral stenosis.

Symptomatic central canal stenosis typically presents as neurogenic claudication/pseudoclaudication.[5,27] This condition is characterized by aching pain, often associated with paresthesia in the lower extremities precipitated by walking or standing erect. Sitting or flexing the trunk while standing often relieves the symptoms. As is the case with vascular claudication, the symptoms dissipate after a period of rest, and the patient can walk again before the symptoms recur.

Neurogenic claudication can be confused with vascular claudication of the lower extremities. Together, the presence of paresthesia (and occasionally motor weakness), reflex changes, relief of symptoms with trunk flexion, and preservation of the distal pulses can help distinguish neurogenic claudication from vascular claudication. Both types of claudication are seen most often in the elderly, and the two can occur together.

Treatment includes counseling and avoidance of activity that brings on symptoms. In severe cases surgical decompression may be necessary.

Box 2
Causes of lumbosacral radiculopathy
Degenerative
Disk herniation
Spondylosis
Neoplastic
Primary tumors
Metastatic tumors
Carcinomatous meningitis
Congenital/developmental
Arachnoid cyst
Synovial cyst
Spondylolisthesis
Infectious
Osteomyelitis
Epidural abscess
Tuberculosis
Herpes zoster
Lyme disease
HIV
Inflammatory
Sarcoidosis
Vasculitis
Endocrinologic/metabolic
Diabetic radiculopathy
Osteoporosis with vertebral fractures
Paget's disease
Acromegaly
Traumatic
Disk herniation
Vertebral fracture
Nerve root injury from spinal anesthesia
Arteriovenous malformation
Dural
Intradural

WHAT SHOULD BE THE APPROACH TO VERTEBRAL COMPRESSION FRACTURES?

Vertebral compression fracture is a common clinical problem in the elderly, usually secondary to osteoporosis and less frequently to osteolytic metastatic tumors and multiple myeloma.[5] There are approximately 700,000 vertebral compression fractures annually in the United States.[29] Vertebral compression fractures are most common in

---

Box 3
Lumbar spinal stenosis

Congenital

Acquired

Degenerative

Spondylosis

Spondylolisthesis

Adult scoliosis

Calcification of ligamentum flavum

Intraspinal synovial cysts

Spinal dysraphism

Metabolic/endocrinologic

Osteoporosis with fracture

Acromegaly

Renal osteodystrophy

Hypoparathyroidism

Epidural lipomatosis

Postoperative

Postlaminectomy

Postfusion

Postdiscectomy

Traumatic

Fracture

Spondylolisthesis

Miscellaneous

Paget's disease

Diffuse idiopathic skeletal hyperostosis

Amyloid

From Levin KH, Covington EC, Devereaux MW, et al. Neck and back pain. Continuum: Lifelong Learning Neurol 2001;7:34; with permission.

---

the thoracolumbar region (T12, L1), but they can occur throughout the thoracic and lumbar spine. A precipitating event, such as a fall or an automobile accident, occurs in perhaps 10% to 15% of patients who have osteoporosis. In most cases, however, there is no definable event or activity. The result of a fracture often is disabling pain. Although pain may be acute in onset and severe even in the absence of a precipitating event, the pain also may have a subacute onset, building gradually over days. The pain usually is localized over the fractured vertebra but occasionally can radiate in a radicular distribution. The severe pain generally lasts weeks but can last for months, often followed by low-grade discomfort that may persist for additional months. The pain usually is relieved by lying supine and often is aggravated by sitting, standing, or bodily motion. The diagnosis often is established by spine radiographs, although MRI and a technetium bone scan may be necessary to distinguish a pathologic fracture secondary to tumor from other causes.

Four treatment options for acute vertebral compression fractures are available:[30]

Medical management consists primarily of bed rest, pain management, and mobilization as soon as feasible to reduce muscle wasting.

Open surgery, often with placement of hardware to stabilize the spine, has a limited role.

Vertebroplasty is a percutaneous injection of a bone-filler material to stabilize the fractured vertebra. This treatment addresses the pain but not the vertebral deformity and resultant spinal deformity.

Balloon kyphoplasty is a promising, minimally invasive procedure in which an inflatable bone tamp (balloon) is inserted into the vertebra and inflated, reducing the compression fracture. The device is removed, and a bone filler is injected into the cavity created by the inflated balloon, stabilizing the vertebra. This treatment has the advantage of reducing the vertebral and spine deformity, pain, and length of hospital stay.

WHAT IS SPONDYLOLISTHESIS, AND WHAT IS ITS ROLE IN LOW BACK PAIN?

Spondylolisthesis, from the Greek "spondylous" (spine) and "olisthesis" (slip), is a condition in which a vertebra slips generally anteriorly with respect to the inferior vertebra. This slippage is termed an "anterolisthesis." When a vertebra slips posteriorly, the slippage is referred to as a "retrolisthesis."[12] The degree of slippage often is described as one of four grades:

Grade I: 0 to 25%
Grade II: 26% to 50%
Grade III: 51% to 75%
Grade IV: more than 75%

The lower lumbar vertebrae (L4-L5, L5-S1) are the usual sites of spondylolisthesis.

Spondylolysis is related to spondylolisthesis. It is a defect in the pars interarticularis without slippage. It is a common finding, present in more than 5% of individuals older than age 7 years.[31] It probably results from the combination of an inherited potential deficit in the pars and a stress fracture related to increased activity in later childhood. Spondylolysis is especially common in young athletes.[32]

Five types of spondylolisthesis have been described (**Box 4**).[5,33]

The most common type is isthmic spondylolisthesis, which is secondary to an acute fracture or deformity of the pars interarticularis. It has its greatest clinical impact in adults older than age 50 years. Other types of spondylolisthesis are caused by congenital disorders, degenerative changes, trauma, and pathologic fractures resulting from bone disease.

Although spondylolisthesis is a common cause of low back pain, it may remain asymptomatic for years. The onset of pain in a patient who has longstanding asymptomatic spondylolisthesis often is associated with an injury. Along with low back pain, spondylolisthesis may produce radiating pain into one or both lower extremities as a reflection of a build-up of a fibrocartilaginous mass at the site of the defect, with resultant nerve root compression at the level of the foramen.

Spondylolisthesis in the absence of neurologic compromise is treated much the same as nonspecific backaches from other causes. Acute low back pain secondary

> **Box 4**
> **Types of spondylolisthesis**
>
> Dysplastic: congenital defect of L5-S1 facets with resultant slippage
>
> Isthmic
>
>   Abnormality in pars interarticularis (most common variety)
>
>   Fatigue fracture of the pars interarticularis
>
>   Elongated pars interarticularis
>
>   Acute fracture of the pars interarticularis
>
> Degenerative: secondary to longstanding intersegmental instability
>
> Traumatic: secondary to acute fracture of "bony hook" (pedicle, lamina, facets)
>
> Pathologic: secondary to structural weakness of bones caused by localized or generalized disease
>
> *From* Levin KH, Covington EC, Devereaux MW, et al. Neck and back pain. Continuum: Lifelong Learning Neurol 2001;7:28; with permission.

to spondylolisthesis can be treated with rest and anti-inflammatory medications. Spondylolisthesis may be one condition in which brace therapy can be justified, although this treatment is debated. Surgical decompression with fusion may prove necessary in patients who develop chronic pain and in particular neurologic compromise (radiculopathy, cauda equina syndrome).

CAN A DAMAGED INTERVERTEBRAL DISK PRODUCE PAIN IN THE ABSENCE OF HERNIATION?

The condition referred to as "internal disk disruption" (IDD) is a controversial disorder. Many believe that degenerative disk disease may lead to IDD and resultant localized spine pain in the absence of deformity of the disk as seen with disk herniation/protrusion. With regard to this entity, two things must be kept in mind: healthy young disks may not contain nociceptive nerve endings, and patients who have severe degenerative disk disease by MRI scan may have no back pain at all. IDD most commonly affects the L4-L5 and L5-S1 intervertebral disks,[12,34] The pathophysiology underlying IDD is thought to be progressive annular deterioration and fissuring, ultimately involving the outer portions of the disk containing an ingrowth of nociceptive nerve endings.[12,19,35] There are no specific symptoms or findings on general and neurologic examinations to distinguish IDD from other causes of nonradiating low back pain.

The controversial diagnosis of IDD is established by the also controversial procedure, diskography. Diskography is a diagnostic test in which contrast material is injected under fluoroscopy into the disk thought to be the cause of low back pain. This evaluation often is followed by a CT scan. If the injection reproduces the low back pain and the disk architecture is disrupted by annular tears, the test is considered positive, and the diagnosis of IDD is established. As already stated, there is a significant amount of controversy surrounding provocative diskography and its value in predicting the outcome of spinal fusion to alleviate low back pain.[36,37]

WHEN IS DIAGNOSTIC TESTING INDICATED IN PATIENTS WHO HAVE LOW BACK PAIN, AND WHICH TESTS SHOULD BE PERFORMED?

Determining which diagnostic tests to perform and when to conduct them are among the more difficult decisions in the management of low back pain. As already stated, findings and diagnostic tests in a patient who has back pain may be misleading.[5,25,26]

A safe generalization is that initially patients who have "uncomplicated" low back pain with or without radiating pain into a lower extremity in the absence of physical findings on examination can be observed without diagnostic testing,[38] If pain persists for several weeks to a month, and particularly if the pain worsens, baseline diagnostic tests may be indicated even in the absence of physical findings.

Blood tests may be indicated, depending on the clinical setting, and can include a complete blood cell count, erythrocyte sedimentation rate, antinuclear antibody, prostate-specific antigen, and a metabolic panel. For patients who have persistent nonradiating low back pain, spine radiographs ultimately may be indicated, although generally the yield is low.[5,39] Nonetheless, spondylolisthesis, vertebral compression fractures, osteomyelitis/diskitis, and subtle evidence of metastatic cancer may be uncovered. In patients who have low back pain and neurologic findings, MRI has supplanted all other imaging techniques. In patients who have radiating pain, EMG and nerve conduction testing in skilled hands can prove useful, particularly when attempting to draw a correlation between symptoms, signs, and a specific abnormality on an MRI. Other diagnostic modalities, including bone scanning, CT scan/myelography, and possibly diskography (although this test remains controversial) may have a role; however, the primary care provider usually has called in a specialist before these tests prove necessary.

An immediate diagnostic work-up without delay usually is indicated when the presentation includes

Fever
Neuromuscular weakness
Significant trauma before the onset of back pain
Known malignancy
Pain when recumbent
Unexplained weight loss
History of drug and/or alcohol abuse

WHAT IS THE BEST APPROACH TO TREATMENT FOR THE PATIENT WHO HAS ACUTE, NONRADIATING LOW BACK PAIN AND A NORMAL EXAMINATION?

Acute low back pain is an enormously common problem. It usually is self limiting. If the history and physical examination do not reveal any reason to support an early diagnostic work-up, treatment aimed at pain management and early mobilization is the goal.[5,40] The natural history of acute low back pain favors conservative management.[5,10,38,41,42] Deyo and colleagues[9] noted that 50% of all patients resume normal activity in 4 to 6 weeks, and 95% return to normal activity in 6 months.

The literature supports the use of a short course of nonsteroidal antiinflammatory drugs (NSAIDs).[43] All NSAIDs seem to be equivalent for acute low back pain. In some patients acetaminophen may prove equally effective.[44] The analgesic and antiinflammatory benefits of NSAIDs must be balanced against the potential side effects. Long-term use should be avoided. For severe acute low back pain, the addition of a muscle relaxant may prove helpful but preferably for only a short time.[45,46] Non-benzodiazepine muscle relaxants such as cyclobenzaprine, methocarbamole, and carisoprodol are the best first choice.[46] Prolonged bed rest has not been shown to be of value, although bed rest for several days may be unavoidable for the patient who has severe back pain.[40,47,48] In this case, the patient should be advised to resume physical activity as soon as possible.[5,40]

Most treatment modalities for acute low back pain (eg, physical therapy,[38,40,49,50] traction,[51–53] hot or cold applications,[52,54] epidural steroid injections,[5,55]

transcutaneous electrical nerve stimulation[56,57] and acupuncture[58]) have not been proved conclusively to be effective. Some studies suggest a minor benefit from chiropractic manipulation, but it is controversial and is not cost effective.[49,59–63] The best and most cost-effective treatments are

Medications: acetaminophen, NSAIDs, a short-term opiate analgesic if necessary, and possibly, at some point, a muscle relaxant

Bed rest: only if necessary because of severe pain, followed as soon as possible by a gradual return to activities of daily living

Hot or cold packs (whichever the patient chooses): sometimes helpful, although not scientifically validated (One should avoid recommending electric heating pads because of the risk of burns.)

Follow-up examinations: As deemed necessary to include psychologic support and education

Physical therapy: May be of some value when the acute pain has dissipated

If pain persists, consider diagnostic testing and referral to a specialist when appropriate.

WHAT ARE THE AVAILABLE TREATMENT OPTIONS FOR CHRONIC LOW BACK PAIN?

A detailed description of treatment options is beyond the scope of this article. Management of chronic low back pain is difficult and demanding and generally is best shared by the primary care physician and one or more specialists. Patients who have chronic low back pain often have had one or more unsuccessful lumbar spine surgeries and often are categorized as having "failed back surgery syndrome" ("post lumbar laminectomy syndrome"). Often these patients are best treated in conjunction with a chronic pain management center.[5] In addition to failed back surgery, these patients frequently have failed courses of epidural blocks and sometimes failed spinal cord stimulation implants.

"Proceduralism" should be avoided or at least controlled as much as possible. Although procedures for chronic low back pain may be well intentioned, they all too often are unsuccessful, sometimes resulting in complications such as chronic arachnoiditis secondary to multiple surgeries, infection, and neurologic impairment. No single treatment approach for chronic low back pain is 100% successful. The best treatment approach includes education, exercise and physical reconditioning, psychotherapy and behavioral modification, and medications.

Medications useful in the management of chronic pain syndromes are serotonin reuptake inhibitors, certain anti-epileptic drugs, and sometimes NSAIDs. One must recognize the risk of potential significant side effects. Long-term administration of opiates, if determined to be necessary, should be done under strict supervision, preferably by a specialist in chronic pain management. Given the risk of addiction as well as analgesic rebound pain, the use of potentially addictive reactive medications should be avoided in the treatment of chronic pain.

Treatment also may include treatment for chemical dependence, if necessary; surgery, if clear-cut indications are uncovered; or the use of a spinal cord stimulator.

WHEN SHOULD A PATIENT WHO HAS LUMBAR RADICULOPATHY SECONDARY TO DISK HERNIATION BE REFERRED FOR SURGERY?

To some extent, social and occupational circumstances continue to play a role in determining whether a patient who has lumbar radiculopathy secondary to disk herniation requires surgery. A significant percentage of patients who have lumbosacral radiculopathy caused by a herniated disc can improve with medical/nonsurgical treatment.[5,10,38,64–66] A recent study[65] demonstrated greater improvement 3 months after surgery in patients who had surgically treated lumbar radiculopathy secondary to a herniated disk than in the medically treated control group. At 1 year, however, there was no difference between groups. The medical treatment for lumbar radiculopathy includes reduced activity with pain avoidance and the judicious use of nonaddictive medications for pain management, including NSAIDs and several different types of glucocorticoid injections. These injections include epidural glucocorticoid injections, facet joint injections, and medial branch blocks. Glucocorticoid injections, although generally safe, are expensive and of limited value. In a recent report, the Therapeutics and Technology Assessment Subcommittee of the American Academy of Neurology found that epidural steroid injections might result in some short-term improvement in radicular lumbosacral pain but did not recommend their routine use.[67] Studies supporting facet joint injections and medial branch blocks are small in number and inconclusive.[68,69]

In the absence of neurologic findings, a rush to surgical treatment for patients who have radiating pain and lumbar disk herniation should be avoided if at all possible to allow time for a potential satisfactory response to medical therapy.[5,10,38,64–66] Certainly a patient may become a surgical candidate in the following settings:

Low back pain radiating into a lower extremity not responding to conservative therapy

Neurologic deficits, particularly weakness in a radicular distribution (myotome) corresponding to the location/level of a herniated disk on a MRI scan

An EMG revealing active denervation in a radicular (myotome) distribution corresponding to the location/level of a herniated disk on a MRI scan even in the absence of neurologic deficits in a symptomatic patient

The presence of significant weakness in a specific myotome is perhaps the most important factor in the decision to perform a surgical procedure relatively early in the course of a patient who has sciatica. If the weakness is profound, delaying surgery increases the risk of permanent deficit, although all experienced neurologists, neurosurgeons, and orthopedic surgeons have seen occasional spectacular spontaneous recoveries of strength in patients who chose not to have surgery in this setting. Modest weakness often can resolve with conservative therapy. Unfortunately there are no foolproof criteria to guide the physician in the selection of patients for surgery.

To some degree modern neurosurgical techniques have made it easier to recommend surgery. A simple one-level lumbar laminectomy generally requires no more than a 24- to 36-hour hospitalization. This finding is not intended to suggest that surgery should be recommended only because of improvements in surgical technique. Studies suggest that spontaneous recovery without surgery occurs in 75% to 80% of all disk herniations.[64] Relief of nerve root impingement comes about in part from absorption and shrinkage of the displaced disk material, eliminating the need for surgery in many patients.[66]

REFERENCES

1. Praemer A, Furnes S, Rice D. Musculoskeletal conditions in the United States. Rosemont (IL): American Academy of Orthopedic Surgeons; 1992. p. 23–33.
2. Rubin DI. Epidemiology of risk factors for spine pain. Neurol Clin 2007;25:353–71.

3. Hart L, Deyo R, Churkin D. Physician office visits for low back pain. Spine 1995; 20:11–9.
4. Andersson GB. Epidemiology of low back pain. Acta Orthop Scand 1998; 281(Suppl):28–31.
5. Levin KH, Covington EC, Devereaux MW, et al. Neck and low back pain. Continuum (NY) 2001;7:1–205.
6. Deyo RA, Tsui-Wu Y-J. Descriptive epidemiology of low back pain and its related medical care in the United States. Spine 1987;12:264–8.
7. Cassidy JD, Cote P, Carroll LJ, et al. Incidence and course of low back pain episodes in the general population. Spine 2005;30:2817–23.
8. Frymoyer J, Cats-Baril W. An overview of the incidence and costs of low back pain. Orthop Clin North Am 1991;22:263–71.
9. Deyo RA, Cherkin D, Conrad D, et al. Cost, controversy, crisis: low back pain and the health of the public. Annu Rev Public Health 1992;12:141–55.
10. Devereaux MW. Approach to neck and low back disorders. In: Evans RW, editor. Saunders manual of neurologic practice. Philadelphia: Elsevier; 2003. p. 745–51.
11. Jackson R. The facet syndrome: myth or reality? Clin Orthop 1992;279:110–21.
12. Meleger AL, Krivickas LS. Neck and back pain: musculoskeletal disorders. Neurol Clin 2007;25:419–38.
13. Korkala O, Gronblad M, Liesi P, et al. Immunohistochemical demonstration of nociceptors in the ligamentous structures of the lumbar spine. Spine 1985;10:156–7.
14. Groen G, Baljet B, Drukker J. Nerves and nerve plexuses of the human vertebral column. Am J Anat 1990;188:282–96.
15. Roberts S, Evans H, Trivedi J, et al. History and pathology of the human intervertebral disc. J Bone Joint Surg Am 2006;88(Suppl 2):10–4.
16. Brisby H. Pathology and possible mechanisms of nervous system response to disc degeneration. J Bone Joint Surg Am 2006;88(Suppl 2):68–71.
17. Battie MC, Videman T. Lumbar disc degeneration: epidemiology and genetics. J Bone Joint Surg Am 2006;88(Suppl 2):3–9.
18. Devereaux MW. The anatomy and examination of the spine. Neurol Clin 2007;25: 419–38.
19. Palmgren T, Gronblad M, Virri J, et al. An immunohistochemical study of nerve structures in the annulus fibrosus of human normal lumbar intervertebral discs. Spine 1999;24:2075–9.
20. Coppes M, Marani E, Thomeer R, et al. Innervation of "painful" lumbar discs. Spine 1997;22:2342–9.
21. Lotz JC, Ulrich JA. Innervation inflammation and hypermobility may characterize pathologic disc degeneration: review of animal model data. J Bone Joint Surg Am 2006;88(Suppl 2):76–82.
22. Johnson E. The myth of skeletal muscle spasm. Am J Phys Med Rehabil 1989;68:1.
23. Mense S, Simons D. Muscle pain: understanding its nature, diagnoses and treatment. Baltimore (MD): Lippincott Williams & Wilkins; 2001. p. 117–8.
24. Scientific approach to the assessment and management of activity-related spinal disorders: a monograph for clinicians. Report of the Quebec Task Force on Spinal Disorders. Spine 1987;12:S1–59.
25. Boden SD, Davis DO, Dina TS, et al. Abnormal magnetic resonance scans of the lumbar spine in asymptomatic subjects: a prospective investigation. J Bone Joint Surg Am 1990;72:403–8.
26. Jensen M, Brant-Zawadzki M, Obuchowski N, et al. Magnetic resonance imaging of the lumbar spine in people without back pain. N Engl J Med 1994;331:69–73.

27. Dulaney E. Radiculopathy and cauda equina syndrome. In: Evans RW, editor. Saunders manual of neurologic practice. Philadelphia: Elsevier; 2003. p. 757–63.
28. Tarulii AW, Raynor EM. Lumbosacral radiculopathy. Neurol Clin 2007;25:387–405.
29. Riggs BL, Melton III IJ. The worldwide problem of osteoporosis: insights afforded by epidemiology. Bone 17:S505–11.
30. Ledlie JT, Renfro M. Balloon kyloplasty: one year outcomes in vertebral body height restoration, chronic pain, and activity levels. J Neurosurg (Spine 1) 2003;98:36–42.
31. Fredrickson BE, Baker D, McHolick WJ, et al. The natural history of spondylolysis and spondylolisthesis. J Bone Joint Surg Am 1984;66:699–707.
32. Rossi F. Spondylolysis, spondylolisthesis and sports. J Sports Med Phys Fitness 1978;18:317–40.
33. Matsunoga S, Sako T, Morizono Y, et al. Natural history degenerative spondylolisthesis: pathogenesis and natural course of the slippage. Spine 1990;15:1204–10.
34. Schwarzer AC, Aprill CN, Darby R, et al. The prevalence and clinical features of internal disc disruption in patients with chronic low back pain. Spine 1995;20:1878–88.
35. Bogduk N, Tynan W, Wilson AS, et al. The nerve supply of the lumbar intervertebral disc. J Anat 1981;132:39–56.
36. Carragee EJ. Volvo award winner in clinical studies: lumbar high-intensity zone and discography in subjects without low back problems. Spine 2000;25:2987–92.
37. Carragee EJ. Low-pressure positive asymptomatic of significant low back pain illness. Spine 2006;31:505–9.
38. Deyo RA, Weinstein JA. Low back pain. N Engl J Med 2001;344:363–70.
39. Surez-Almazor ME, Belseck E, Russell AS, et al. Use of lumbar radiographs for the early diagnosis of low back pain: proposed guidelines would increase utilization. JAMA 1997;277:1782–6.
40. Malmivarra A, Hakkinen U, Aro T, et al. The treatment of acute low back pain: bed rest, exercises, or ordinary activity? N Engl J Med 1995;332:351–5.
41. Levin KH. Nonsurgical interventions for spine pain. Neurol Clin 2007;25:495–505.
42. Venesy DA. Physical medicine and complementary approaches. Neurol Clin 2007;25:523–37.
43. van Tulder MW, Scholten RJ, Koes BW, et al. Nonsteroidal antiinflammatory drugs for low back pain. Cochrane Database Syst Rev 2000;2:CD000396.
44. Hancock MJ, Maher CG, Latimer J, et al. Assessment of diclofenac or spinal manipulative therapy, or both in addition to recommended first-line treatment for acute low back pain: a randomized control trial. Lancet 2007;370:1638–43.
45. van Tulder MW, Towroy T, Furian AD, et al. Muscle relaxants for nonspecific low back pain. Cochrane Database Syst Rev 2003;2:CD004252.
46. Beebe FA, Barkin RL, Barkin S. Clinical and pharmacologic review of skeletal muscle relaxants for musculoskeletal conditions. Am J Ther 2005;12:151–71.
47. Deyo RA, Diehl AK, Rosenthal M. How many days of acute bed rest for acute low back pain? A randomized clinical trial. N Engl J Med 1986;315:1064–70.
48. Hagen KB, Hilde G, Jamtvedt G, et al. Bed rest for acute low-back pain and sciatica. Cochrane Database Syst Rev 2004;4:CD001254.
49. Cherkin DC, Deyo RA, Battie M, et al. A comparison of physical therapy, chiropractic manipulation, and provision of an educational booklet for the treatment of patients with low back pain. N Engl J Med 1998;339:1021–9.
50. Beurskens AJ, de Vet HC, Koke AJ, et al. Efficacy of traction for non specific low back pain: 12-week and 6-month results of a randomized clinical trail. Spine 1997;22:2756–62.
51. Hayden JA, van Tulder MW, Malmivaara AV, et al. Meta-analysis: exercise therapy for non specific low back pain. Ann Intern Med 2005;142:765–75.

52. van Tulder MW, Waddell G. Conservative treatment of acute and subacute low back pain. In: Nachemson AL, Jonsson E, editors. Neck and back pain the scientific evidence of causes, diagnosis and treatment. Philadelphia: Lippincott Williams & Wilkins; 2000. p. 241–69.

53. Clarke JA, van Tulder MW, Blomberg SE, et al. Traction for low-back pain with or without sciatica. Cochrane Database Syst Rev 2005;4:CD003010.

54. French SD, Cameron M, Walker BF, et al. Superficial heat or cold for low back pain. Cochrane Database Syst Rev 2006;1:CD004750.

55. Carette S, Leclaire R, Marcoux S, et al. Epidural corticosteroid injections for sciatica due to herniated nucleus pulposus. N Engl J Med 1997;336:1634–40.

56. Deyo RA, Walsh NE, Martin DC, et al. A controlled trial of transcutaneous electrical nerve stimulators (TENS) and exercise for chronic low back pain. N Engl J Med 1990;322:1627–34.

57. Khadilkar A, Milne S, Brosseau L, et al. Transcutaneous electrical nerve stimulation (TENS) for chronic low-back pain. Cochrane Database Syst Rev 2005;3:CD003008.

58. Rabinstein AA, Shulman LM. Acupuncture in clinical neurology. Neurologist 2003; 9:137–48.

59. Shekelle PG, Adams AH, Chassin MR, et al. Spinal manipulation for low-back pain. Ann Intern Med 1992;117:590–8.

60. Assendleft WJJ, Morton SC, Yu EL, et al. Spinal manipulative therapy for low back pain: a meta-analysis of effectiveness relative to other therapies. Ann Intern Med 2003;138:871–81.

61. Cherkin DC, Sherman KJ, Deyo RA, et al. A review of the evidence for the effectiveness, safety, and cost of acupuncture, massage therapy, and spinal manipulation for back pain. Ann Intern Med 2003;138:898–906.

62. Ernst E, Canter PH. A systematic review of systematic reviews of spinal manipulation. J R Soc Med 2006;99:192–6.

63. Assendleft WJJ, Morton SC, Yu EL, et al. Spinal manipulative therapy for low-back pain. Cochrane Database Syst Rev 2008;3:CD000447.

64. Fager CA. Observations on spontaneous recovery from intervertebral disc herniation. Surg Neurol 1994;42:282–6.

65. Peul WC, van Houwelingen HC, van den Hout WB, et al. Surgery versus prolonged conservative treatment for sciatica. N Engl J Med 2007;356:2245–56.

66. Deyo RA. Back surgery—who needs it? N Engl J Med 2007;356:2239–43.

67. Armon C, Argoff CE, Samuels J, et al. Assessment: use of epidural steroid injections to treat radicular lumbosacral pain. Report of the therapeutics and technology sassessment subcommittee of the American Academy of Neurology. Neurology 2007;68:723–9.

68. Nelemans PJ, Bie De, De Vert HC, et al. Injection therapy for subacute and chronic benign low back pain. Spine 2001;26:501–15.

69. Casette S, Marcoux S, Truchon R, et al. A controlled trial of corticosteroid injections into facet joints for chronic low back pain. N Engl J Med 1991;325:1002–7.

Index

Note: Page numbers of article titles are in **boldface** type.

A

Acetaminophen, for migraine, 254
Acetazolamide, for dizziness, 269
Actigraphy, in sleep disorders, 418
Acupuncture, for neck pain, 282
Acyclovir, for dizziness, 269
Adjustment insomnia, 412
Adson's test, in neck pain, 276
Akathisia, drug-induced, 381–382
Akinesia, in Parkinson disease, 371
Almotriptan, for migraine, 254–255
Alprazolam, for dizziness, 268
Alzheimer's disease
    clinical features of, 396
    definition of, 395
    detection of, 392
    diagnosis of, 392–397
    pathology of, 396
    prevention of, 398
    treatment of, 397–398
    vascular dementia with, 398
Amantadine, for Parkinson disease, 373–374
4-Aminopyridine, for multiple sclerosis, 466–467
Amitriptyline
    for migraine prevention, 258–259
    for neuropathic pain, 329
    for sensory neuropathy, 328
Ammonium tetrathiomolybdate, for Wilson disease, 383
Aneurysm, brain, subarachnoid hemorrhage in, 357
Ankle
    peroneal neuropathy at, 299–300
    tarsal tunnel syndrome in, 303–306
Anticholinergics
    for bladder dysfunction, 468
    for Parkinson disease, 373–374
Antidepressants
    for Alzheimer's disease, 397
    for insomnia, 413
    for multiple sclerosis, 467
    for narcolepsy, 416–417
    for parasomnias, 419

Med Clin N Am 93 (2009) 503–525
doi:10.1016/S0025-7125(09)00011-X
0025-7125/09/$ – see front matter © 2009 Elsevier Inc. All rights reserved.

medical.theclinics.com